ANXIETY DISORDERS

Anxiety Disorders: A Guide for Integrating Psychopharmacology and Psychotherapy is a comprehensive reference for the psychology and psychiatry student, intern or resident, early-career psychologist or psychiatrist, and the busy clinician. It distills the most important information regarding combined treatments for anxiety and presents the material in an easily accessible, understandable, and readable format. Each chapter addresses a specific type of disorder: posttraumatic stress, panic, generalized anxiety, obsessive-compulsive, and others, and is authored by prominent clinicians with years of experience in providing integrated, individualized treatments. With its thorough exploration of psychopharmacological treatments, psychosocial treatments, and, crucially, the integration of the two, *Anxiety Disorders* is a text no 21st-century clinician or student can afford to be without.

Stephen M. Stahl, MD, is the author of over 450 articles and chapters and more than 1,300 scientific presentations and abstracts. He is an internationally recognized clinician, researcher, and teacher in psychiatry with subspecialty expertise in psychopharmacology. He has edited eight books and written more than 30 others, including the best-selling and award-winning textbook *Stahl's Essential Psychopharmacology*, the clinical manual *The Prescriber's Guide*, now in its fourth edition, and the series of clinical cases *Case Studies: Stahl's Essential Psychopharmacology*. Dr. Stahl is adjunct professor of psychiatry at the University of California San Diego and honorary visiting senior fellow at the University of Cambridge.

Bret A. Moore, PsyD, is board-certified in clinical psychology by the American Board of Professional Psychology, and adjunct associate professor in psychiatry at the University of Texas Health Science Center at San Antonio. He is the author or editor of nine books, including *Pharmacotherapy for Psychologists: Prescribing and Collaborative Roles*, *Handbook of Clinical Psychopharmacology for Psychologists*, and *Treating PTSD in Military Personnel: A Clinical Handbook*. His views and opinions on clinical psychology have been quoted in *USA Today*, the *New York Times*, the *Boston Globe*, and on NPR, the BBC, CNN, Fox News, and the CBC.

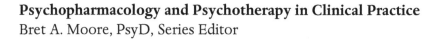

Psychopharmacology and Psychotherapy in Clinical Practice
Bret A. Moore, PsyD, Series Editor

Anxiety Disorders: A Guide for Integrating Psychopharmacology and Psychotherapy, by Stephen M. Stahl and Bret A. Moore

ANXIETY DISORDERS

A Guide for Integrating Psychopharmacology
and Psychotherapy

Edited by
Stephen M. Stahl and Bret A. Moore

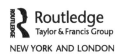

NEW YORK AND LONDON

First published 2013
by Routledge
605 Third Avenue, New York, NY 10017
4 Park Square, Milton Park, Abingdon, Oxon OX14 4RN

Library of Congress Cataloging in Publication Data
Stahl, S. M., author.
Anxiety disorders : a guide for integrating psychopharmacology and
psychotherapy / author, Stephen M. Stahl and Bret A. Moore.
   pages ; cm. – (Psychopharmacology and psychotherapy in clinical
   practice)
   Includes bibliographical references and index.
   1. Anxiety–Chemotherapy. 2. Cognitive therapy. I. Moore, Bret A.,
   author. II. Title.
   RC531.S682 2013
   616.852206–dc23   2012032019

ISBN: 978-0-415-50982-4 (hbk)
ISBN: 978-0-415-50983-1 (pbk)
ISBN: 978-0-203-12459-8 (ebk)

Typeset in Dante
by Wearset Ltd, Boldon, Tyne and Wear

Dedication

To my wife Cindy and my daughters Jennifer and Victoria

S.M.S.

To my wife Lori and my daughter Kaitlyn

B.A.M.

Contents

PART II
TREATMENT   95

Contributors

Jonathan S. Abramowitz, PhD, professor and associate chair of psychology, University of North Carolina at Chapel Hill.

Claire Advokat, PhD, professor emerita, department of psychology, Louisiana State University, Baton Rouge, Louisiana.

Christopher R. Bailey, Johns Hopkins University School of Medicine, Baltimore, Maryland.

Christopher S. Brown, PsyD, captain, United States Army, clinical psychology resident, department of behavioral health, Madigan Army Medical Center, Tacoma, Washington.

Richard A. Bryant, PhD, University of New South Wales, Sydney, Australia.

Eric Bui, MD, PhD, research fellow in psychiatry, Massachusetts General Hospital and Harvard Medical School.

Meredith E. Charney, PhD, assistant in psychology, Massachusetts General Hospital and an instructor in psychiatry at Harvard Medical School.

Joseph E. Comaty, PhD, MP, director, division of quality management, Louisiana State Department of Health and Hospitals, Baton Rouge, Louisiana.

Tara E. Galovski, PhD, department of psychology, Center for Trauma Recovery, University of Missouri–St. Louis.

Clare Gaskins, PhD, Metropolitan Center for Cognitive Behavioral Therapy and New York Presbyterian Hospital–Columbia University Medical Center, New York, New York.

Allison M. Greene, New York University.

S. Cory Harmon, PhD, clinical research psychologist, department of behavioral health, Madigan Army Medical Center, Tacoma, Washington.

Ryan J. Jacoby, University of North Carolina at Chapel Hill.

Robert M. Julien, MD, PhD, Lake Oswego, Oregon.

George M. Kapalka, PhD, ABPP, professor and chair, department of psychological counseling, Monmouth University, West Long Branch, New Jersey; director, Center for Behavior Modification, Brick, New Jersey.

Catherine M. Kariuki, MBChB, FCPsych (SA), senior registrar, Eastern Health Adult Mental Health Services at Melbourne, Australia.

M. Alexandra Kredlow, research assistant, Massachusetts General Hospital.

Jessica Levitt, PhD, Metropolitan Center for Cognitive Behavioral Therapy, New York, NY.

Christina Lipinski, MA, Metropolitan Center for Cognitive Behavioral Therapy and St. John's University, New York, NY.

Bret A. Moore, Psy.D., ABPP, adjunct associate professor of psychiatry, University of Texas Health Science Center at San Antonio.

Mark D. Muse, EdD, ABPP, Muse Psychological Associates, Rockville, Maryland.

Alexander Neumeister, MD, professor of psychiatry and radiology and director, NYU Molecular Imaging Program, New York University School of Medicine.

Angela Nickerson, PhD, University of New South Wales, Sydney, Australia.

Callandra Peters, department of psychological counseling, Monmouth University, West Long Branch, New Jersey.

Greer Richardson, MD, assistant clinical professor, department of psychiatry, Yale University.

David S. Shearer, PhD, director of behavioral sciences, family medicine residency, department of family medicine, Madigan Army Medical Center, Tacoma, Washington.

Naomi M. Simon, MD, MSc, director, Center for Anxiety and Traumatic Stress Disorders, Massachusetts General Hospital and associate professor of psychiatry, Harvard Medical School.

Stephen M. Stahl, MD, PhD, adjunct professor of psychiatry, University of California San Diego and honorary visiting senior fellow, University of Cambridge.

Dan J. Stein, MD, PhD, professor and chair, department of psychiatry and mental health, University of Cape Town, Cape Town, South Africa.

Michael Sweeney, PhD, Metropolitan Center for Cognitive Behavioral Therapy, New York, New York.

Robert Westerholm, PhD, Metropolitan Center for Cognitive Behavioral Therapy and New York Presbyterian Hospital–Columbia University Medical Center, New York, New York.

Amy M. Williams, PhD, independent practice, Flower Mound, Texas.

Robert D. Younger, PhD, MP, ABPP, captain, United States Navy; chief of staff, behavioral health directorate; chief, Behavioral Health Consultation and Liaison Service, Fort Belvoir Community Hospital, Fort Belvoir, Virginia.

Series Editor's Foreword

Psychopharmacology and Psychotherapy in Clinical Practice, an innovative and timely series of handbooks for both the student and the practitioner, is published by Routledge, one of the world leaders in mental health texts. The focus of Psychopharmacology and Psychotherapy in Clinical Practice is expansive. Broadly, the series encompasses topics relevant to clinical practice as well as clinical and translational research in psychopharmacology and psychotherapy. More specifically, a major aim of the series is to advance the area of integrating pharmacological and psychosocial interventions. A growing, albeit slow, body of literature on the integration of the traditionally separate modalities is appearing in both the psychiatric and the psychological literature. This series will help bridge the gap between the two disciplines and provide practitioners from diverse backgrounds with the most up-to-date information to inform best clinical practices.

Anxiety Disorders: A Guide for Integrating Psychopharmacology and Psychotherapy is the first in the series. Stephen M. Stahl, MD, PhD, one of the most prominent psychiatrists and psychopharmacologists today, takes the lead in this impressive volume. Calling on top experts in psychology, psychiatry, and psychopharmacology, *Anxiety Disorders* covers the intricacies of combined treatments for all major anxiety disorders. With my support, Dr. Stahl draws on his years of clinical, teaching, and research experience to formulate arguably the most comprehensive and useful text of its kind. It is unique in its scope as well as thorough in its coverage of the most salient research on individual and combined treatments in this area. The clinical vignettes used throughout the text illuminating successes and failures when individual treatments are applied, as well as the effects of combined treatments, are priceless.

In summary, *Anxiety Disorders* is an excellent inaugural volume for what will be a robust, acclaimed, and, most importantly, clinically useful series. You can rely on the promise that Psychopharmacology and Psychotherapy in Clinical Practice will solicit and include only top-tier experts in their respective fields. This will ensure that you have access to the latest and most accurate information in the fields of psychology, psychiatry, and psychopharmacology. As you begin to utilize this volume, we hope you will share our enthusiasm for this important series.

Bret A. Moore, PsyD, ABPP
Series Editor
Psychopharmacology and Psychotherapy in Clinical Practice

Foreword

Treatment of the anxiety disorders over the past century has reflected an implicit Cartesian dualism. Early conceptualizations of psychopathology dominated by psychoanalytic theory posited the primacy of a variety of unconscious impulses and conflicts, necessitating a psychodynamic approach to treatment that at times seemed to belie the patients' presentation and experience. In the last quarter of the 20th century, as emergent technology and analytic techniques resulted in an explosion of interest in the underlying neurobiological correlates of anxiety, the pendulum swung to an often reductionistic focus on dysregulation of neurotransmitters and a search for pharmacologic interventions that would eradicate disorders. Emergent psychological interventions, including cognitive and behavioral interventions drawn from conditioning theories, demonstrated efficacy but were often presented as antithetical to psychodynamic or pharmacotherapeutic approaches and suffered from a lack of dissemination for a variety of reasons, including the lack of providers adequately trained in the myriad of disorder-specific interventions.

Over the past couple of decades, however, scientific advances in our understanding of the underpinning of the anxiety disorders have evolved into a recognition of pathologic anxiety as the product of dysregulated fear circuitry in the brain. This dysfunction represents the confluence of an underlying neurobiologic diathesis likely reflecting familial and/or genetically transmitted predispositions that interact with an array of developmental, conditioning, and other life experiences and, through epigenetic and additional pathways, promote either the activation of pathologic anxiety or apparent resilience to the noxious impact of stress.

The recognition that both pharmacologic and psychological interventions impact the same brain circuitry and perhaps genetic factors relevant to anxiety disorders, supports a more nuanced rather than dualistic view of the pathogenesis of these conditions and speaks to the possibility of additive and synergistic effects of combined treatment approaches to optimize outcomes. Further, though pharmacotherapy and psychological interventions are each effective for the treatment of anxiety disorders, many patients receiving either class of interventions respond to them only partially or not at all. Therefore, we need to evaluate the relative benefits and limitations of combined treatment relative to monotherapy, and consider that combined interventions often show incremental rather than additive benefits. Novel combination strategies such as the addition of the partial glutamatergic NMDA receptor agonist to exposure-based cognitive-behavioral therapies for anxiety disorders raise the possible of innovative combination strategies in which pharmacologic therapies work by enhancing learning-based therapies rather than through the addition of two effective but distinct interventions. Thus, the confluence of emerging scientific insights and continued unmet clinical need makes this book, examining the integration of psychopharmacology and psychotherapy for the treatment of anxiety disorders, and edited by experts in these areas, timely and critical to our evolving understanding of the treatment of the anxiety disorders and the goal of optimizing the well-being of our affected patients.

Mark H. Pollack, MD
Grainger Professor and Chairman
Department of Psychiatry
Rush University Medical Center

Preface

The motivation for this book was frustration. The fields of psychology and psychiatry have traditionally functioned independently of each other for reasons that go beyond the scope of this preface. The unfortunate consequence of this separation, however, is that patients in need of comprehensive mental health care have often been relegated to either medication management or psychosocial therapies.

Combined treatment, or what is also referred to as integrated treatment, is the practice of utilizing both pharmacological and psychological interventions in the treatment of psychiatric disorders. Instead of relying on a sole treatment approach, practitioners utilize best practices from the fields of psychology and psychiatry. Sometimes this is done by a single practitioner, but in most cases it involves two professionals: one provides psychotherapy while the other prescribes medication. Although combined treatment is acknowledged by most mental health providers as an effective way to treat myriad psychiatric conditions—particularly those most resistant to treatment—there is relatively little research and guidance on the practice. This book fills the gap for the latter with regard to anxiety disorders.

In Chapter 1, Muse, Moore, and Stahl highlight the benefits as well as the challenges of combined treatments for anxiety disorders. The two tables comparing and contrasting monotherapy versus combined treatments for the major psychiatric disorders and the integrative model for anxiety disorders are alone worth the cost of the book.

Chapter 2, by Greene, Bailey, and Neumeister, covers in brilliant detail the biological, psychological, and social correlates of anxiety and its disorders. Although most concepts will be familiar to the student and practitioner, the authors' review will remind the reader of the complex nature of anxiety.

Robert M. Julien brings his vast knowledge of pharmacology to Chapter 3 and outlines the history of pharmacological treatment of anxiety as well as pharmacological interventions spanning from *in utero* to late life. Consistent with the author's conversational writing style, this chapter is a gem.

Chapter 4, "Psychosocial Treatment of Anxiety Disorders across the Lifespan," authored by Sweeney, Levitt, Westerholm, Gaskins, and Lipinski, has a similar goal to Chapter 3. However, instead of outlining pharmacological treatments across the lifespan, these experts use vignettes to showcase psychosocial therapies from childhood to adulthood, with developmental "nuggets" dispersed throughout.

Comaty and Advokat provide the first of eight treatment-focused chapters. Covering sole and combined treatments for generalized anxiety disorder, Chapter 5 is filled with useful clinical vignettes showcasing successful and less than successful examples of solitary treatments as well as positive effects of combined treatment. Chapters 6–12 follow suit, covering the remaining major anxiety disorders: obsessive-compulsive disorder (Abramowitz and Jacoby); acute stress disorder (Nickerson and Bryant); posttraumatic stress disorder (Williams, Richardson, and Galovski); panic disorder (Charney, Kredlow, Bui, and Simon); social anxiety disorder (Kariuki and Stein); specific phobia (Shearer, Harmon, Younger, and Brown); and separation anxiety disorder (Kapalka and Peters).

Anxiety Disorders: A Guide to Integrating Psychopharmacology and Psychotherapy is the first volume in a new series dedicated to the clinical practice of psychopharmacology and psychotherapy. We are grateful that the first book is focused on such an important and timely topic. However, there are many emerging trends in the treatment of psychiatric disorders that warrant attention. One prime example is the notion that psychotherapy can be viewed as an epigenetic "drug" (Stahl, 2012). Not unlike medications, research is beginning to illuminate the potential for cognitive and behavioral therapies to alter brain circuits. This is more reason for the mental health practitioner to be well versed in all treatment modalities.

REFERENCE

Stahl, S. M. (2012). Psychotherapy as an epigenetic "drug": Psychiatric therapeutics target symptoms linked to malfunctioning brain circuits with psychotherapy as well as with drugs. *Journal of Clinical Pharmacy and Therapeutics, 37,* 249–253.

Acknowledgments

Without the support of many people, this book would not have been possible. First, we would like to thank Anna Moore, Sam Rosenthal, and the rest of the staff from Routledge for providing us with the opportunity to develop this book. Second, we are grateful to the authors of this volume for their patience, hard work, and excellent chapters. An edited book is only as good as its authors. Last, we would like to thank our families for their unwavering and unconditional support. An editor is only as good as his or her loved ones behind the scenes.

Part I

The Nature of Anxiety

CHAPTER 1

Benefits and Challenges of Integrated Treatment

Mark D. Muse, Bret A. Moore, and Stephen M. Stahl

The interest in integrating biological interventions with psychosocial therapies in the area of mental health is a rather recent phenomenon. In contrast, the effort to integrate different psychotherapeutic approaches has a longer history which began in the late 1970s, when a proliferation of discrete psychotherapy schools became divisive to a professional consensus on best practices, creating the impression that therapists had to pick sides and choose to become a specialist in a particular school of psychotherapy. There was a tendency for practitioners to adhere clarkto a particular school's theory of psychopathology, and to study little or nothing of other, "competing" schools. Yet, as the multitude of psychotherapies became increasingly unwieldy, and the factionism of practitioners along party lines engendered intransigence, a subset of clinicians, usually referred to as "eclecticists," studied the gamut of psychotherapies and found that the different therapies had many common tenets and approaches, although their jargons were often different (Marks, 2010; Marks et al., undated).

To try to make sense of the smorgasbord of techniques and approaches, the International Academy of Eclectic Psychotherapists (IAEP) was formed in 1981 "to bring more practitioners towards rapprochement in an effort to break the 'only truth' barrier" (IAEP, 1991). Subsequently, the Society for the Exploration of Psychotherapy Integration (SEPI) was formed in 1983 (Stricker, 2010) "to promote the development and evaluation of approaches to psychotherapy that are not limited by a single orientation." These two organizations promoted communication across schools, and recognized that many therapies were, in fact, observing the same phenomena and responding to them with similar approaches, though such similarities were hard to appreciate among "adherents" to a particular approach.

Apart from these schools' theoretical differences, data started to become available in the 1970s (Luborsky, Singer, & Luborsky 1975; Smith & Glass, 1977), and were substantiated throughout the 1980s and 1990s (Asay & Lambert, 1999), on the comparative effectiveness of the different schools of psychotherapy (Wampold et al., 1997). Unsettling data emerged from meta-analyses of controlled studies comparing seemingly different treatments with similar results (Humble, Duncan, & Miller, 1999). This lack of major difference in therapeutic outcome among various psychotherapies lent support to the idea that the various schools of psychotherapy might be more similar than previously suspected, and this in turn gave rise to a search for commonalities among the therapies. A common factors theory (Messer & Wampold, 2002) was postulated which proposed that different approaches to psychotherapy have common components that account for outcome better than components that are unique or specific to each approach (Imel & Wampold, 2008). While several common factors have been identified, including empathy and relationship components, as well as the effect of placebo (Stefano, Fricchione, Slingsby, & Benson, 2001), patient variables are believed to exert the single greatest effect on therapy outcome (Tallman & Bohart, 1999).

The discovery of similar equivalent effectiveness among various medications within the same class of psychotropics has highlighted a parallel lack of specificity among pharmacotherapies, and led to the speculation that there may also be a "central" or common factor operating in the pharmacologic treatment of psychiatric conditions (Moncrieff & Cohen, 2009). Such a factor, or factors, has yet to be adequately identified in the case of pharmacotherapy, but some of the same factors affecting psychotherapeutic outcome, such as empathy (Riess, 2010) and placebo, have been speculated to have an effect on medical procedure outcomes. Moreover, in many cases different psychosocial treatments appear to be as effective as pharmacotherapy for the same condition, and this lack of difference begs the question of whether pharmacotherapy and psychotherapy are not both obtaining results by and large through shared common factors, rather than through specific mechanisms unique to the interventions. The Wampold hypothesis (Wampold, 2001) that the true difference among treatments is zero provides an alternative to the medical model, which assumes that there is a specific underlying neurological mechanism for each psychiatric condition and that drugs are effective because their respective mechanism of actions differentially address specific imbalances inherent to the disorder under treatment (Muse & Moore, 2012). In contrast to the strict biological model, the alternative view suggests that whether norepinephrine or serotonin is targeted, or whether cognitive-behavioral or psychodynamic therapies are implemented in the treatment of depression (Swartz, Frank, & Cheng, 2012), or whether placebo is employed as an active treatment (Baskin, Tierney, Minami, & Wampold, 2003), the interpersonal relationship with a provider and the ensuing patient's expectation for positive change are what largely drive condition improvement. This is aided somewhat by a nonspecific psychobiosocial change inherent in all treatment approaches, as well as by spontaneous recuperation in which the organism's innate ability to heal itself, divorced from any therapeutic intervention, tends to return the person to premorbid functioning (Posternak et al., 2006).

In general, it might be assumed that no matter which treatment is selected and applied, outcome will generally be positive for a certain number of patients receiving attention for a given condition. While there is ample evidence to suggest that this may be true to an extent, we are far from recommending picking an intervention strategy at random. In fact, the push to discover specificity of treatment outcome is very much alive, and although results have not been singularly encouraging, certain discoveries are worth reviewing for those clinicians who value making evidence-based decisions regarding the selection of treatments.

Muse (2010) reviewed efforts at integrating pharmacotherapy with psychotherapy and offered an impression of evidence-based indications for when one modality might be chosen over the other, or combined for synergic effect. Table 1.1 summarizes these tentative findings.

INTEGRATING PSYCHOBIOSOCIAL TREATMENTS OF ANXIETY DISORDERS

With reference to anxiety, the indications and cautions derived from Table 1.1 can be summarized as follows: (1) Psychosocial approaches are to be favored over pharmacotherapy for the majority of anxiety disorders. (2) When used, pharmacological interventions are mainly adjunctive and supportive of psychotherapy, the exception being with severe obsessive-compulsive disorder (OCD) or posttraumatic stress disorder (PTSD). (3) There are several specific instances where pharmacotherapy of anxiety may be contraindicated, owing to its tendency to cause interference with the therapeutic goal of patient-generated management of response to anxiety symptoms. (4) While cognitive-behavioral approaches to psychosocial treatments are overrepresented in controlled clinical studies, they are, nonetheless, a well-validated treatment modality, especially in the treatment of anxiety disorders. (5) Monotherapy is generally to be preferred to combination therapy because of multiple factors including cost, exposure to side effects, and limited data supporting the superiority of a combined approach over judiciously assigned monotherapy. Table 1.2 summarizes several points in the selection of monotherapy versus combined therapy in integrated psychobiosocial intervention with anxiety disorders.

A basic assumption in the management of anxiety is the need for the patient to tolerate and accept the experience of anxiety, without catastrophizing about improbable dire outcomes, and without using avoidance as an escape strategy. With social anxiety, the patient is encouraged to challenge fantasies of irreparable damage to reputation or career because of anxiety in public speaking engagements, just as the patient experiencing panic is encouraged to challenge assumptions about disastrous physical/medical outcomes from exposure to

TABLE 1.1

Monotherapy vs. Combined Therapy in Integrated Psychobiosocial Intervention

Research:

A) Medication's efficiency is hard to calculate since the greater part of its effect is placebo, which also accounts for the greater part of psychotherapy's effect, and which appears to be culturally bound and, as such, fluctuates over time as a function of cultural beliefs.

B) Research designs have been inadequate in identifying and separating the effects of medication and psychotherapy on various disorders.

C) Side effects of medication, which are demonstrably greater than with psychotherapy, are not adequately weighed as (negative) outcomes in research that compares this modality to psychotherapy.

Treatment:

A) Medication is important in:

1) Treating positive signs of schizophrenia
2) Treating mania in bipolar disorder
3) Treating depression with psychotic features
4) Treatment of ADHD, especially hyperactive type

B) edication is of comparable importance to psychotherapy in:

1) Treatment of major depression
2) Treating depressive end of bipolar disorder
3) Panic disorder
4) Tourette's

C) Medication is of secondary importance to psychotherapy in:

1) Treating negative signs of schizophrenia
2) Treating depressions other than major depression (adjustment disorder, depression NOS)
3) Treating obsessive-compulsive disorder
4) Treating eating disorders

D) Medication is generally not indicated in:

1) Treating simple phobias
2) Treating dysthymia
3) Treating chronic insomnia

E) Combining both medication and psychosocial therapy might be indicated for:

1) Schizophrenia, in which neuroleptics are augmented with systemic, family, or milieu therapy for overcoming the poor social integration involved in negative symptoms, and for reducing discontinuation of therapy
2) Bipolar disorder I, in which mood stabilizers are augmented by cognitive-educational approaches, intended to help the patient gain insight into the advantage of medication compliance
3) Major depression, in an effort to increase engagement and activity level
4) ADHD, in which analeptic medication is paired with cognitive-behavioral approaches aimed at time management, impulse control, and executive functions
5) Panic disorder, in which cognitive-behavioral approaches emphasize tolerance of anxiety while SSRI medications raise the threshold for manifest panic
6) Obsessive-compulsive disorder with a strong obsessive component, in which obsessive symptoms may be adjunctively treated with serotonin-specific reuptake inhibitors (SSRIs) or tricyclic medication while compulsive components are simultaneously treated with behavioral approaches

continued

TABLE 1.1 continued

Limitations:

A) Current research is dominated by attempts to match diagnosis with treatment modality, paying little attention to subject variables and life event interplay.

B) Little research has been done to optimize the behavioral administration of medications in an effort to integrate medication into behavioral approaches.

C) Cognitive-behavioral therapy is over-represented in controlled studies, leading to the question of how effective are psychosocial interventions in general when only a limited sampling of such interventions is compared to placebo and medication.

D) The medical model has emphasized symptom reduction, reducing the value of emotional distress as a motivator for therapeutic change.

Conclusions:

A) Medication is overused in the primary care setting, given its limited efficacy, its deleterious effects, and the availability of alternative psychosocial treatments of proven value with significantly less-marked side-effect profiles.

B) Much more research is needed on the differential effects of medication and psychotherapy on various diagnoses, patient populations, and presenting/underlying life issues before specific, empirically based, authoritative statements can be made with any degree of confidence as to which treatment or combination of treatments might be preferentially recommended.

Source: Adapted from Muse (2010); Muse and Moore (2012).

anxiety. Cognitive-behavioral treatment of anxiety emphasizes controlled exposure to anxiety-producing situations and/or cognitions in such a way that eventually leads to a weakened conditioned response. This can only be achieved through exposure to real situations and to real anxiety, and through the prevention of avoidance responses such as ritualistic compulsions and phobic fugue. The use of drugs which attenuate, mitigate, or eliminate anxiety should occur in a way that furthers the therapeutic goals, rather than derailing psychosocial treatment by encouraging artificial avoidance of anxiety and dependency on an outside agent.

Research on integrated psychobiosocial treatment of anxiety disorders is not as extensive as one might wish. Conclusions, therefore, are quite tentative, and aim at identifying which interventions are effective enough to be considered first-line, and which of these might best be employed alone or in combination with other therapies.

Posttraumatic Stress Disorder (PTSD)

Perhaps with no other of the anxiety disorders has the controversy over common factors versus specificity in treatments been waged more than with PTSD. Meta-analyses of different trauma-focused treatments for PTSD have consistently found no difference among the efficacy of these treatments (Bisson & Andrew, 2009), yet the American Psychiatric Association (2004) and the Institute of Medicine of the National Academies (2008) currently recommend trauma-focused psychological therapies as first-line treatment. Nonetheless, Benish, Imel, & Wampold (2008) have presented a meta-analysis which concluded that "psychotherapies produce equivalent benefits for patients with PTSD" regardless of whether they are trauma-focused. The Benish et al. study has been challenged by some (Ehlers et al., 2010) and defended by others (Wampold et al., 2010).

Williams, Richardson, & Galovski (this book, Chapter 8) provide a good review of anxiety intervention approaches for treating PTSD. They point out that, while pharmacotherapy can be beneficial, it rarely provides complete remission of PTSD. Indeed, a variety of medications have shown adjunctive benefit in reducing PTSD symptoms, but the consensus is that at this time there is no clear drug treatment for PTSD (Maxmen & Ward, 2002). On the other hand, there is an array of psychosocial approaches, most notably cognitive-behavioral approaches, which have proved to be effective in treating PTSD in individual and group psychotherapy. While these approaches frequently reduce the severity of symptoms, they often do not provide complete remission; nevertheless, psychosocial treatments of PTSD may be considered first-line, and may be initially chosen over pharmacotherapy because they do not have the accompanying side-effect profile of medication, and because

TABLE 1.2

Integrative Psychobiosocial Intervention with Anxiety Disorders

Research:

A) There is long-standing confirmation of the effectiveness of behavioral approaches in the treatment of all of the anxiety disorders. More research on other psychosocial approaches is needed.

   1) Such research would ideally compare different psychosocial and pharmacologic treatments, rather than simply show superiority over placebo.

B) Much more research is needed with the child and adolescent population to show benefits and adverse reactions to pharmacotherapy in anxiety disorders.

C) Greater research on the reinforcing aspects of medications is needed, with particular focus on dispensing contingencies that may lead to reliance on medication and undermine self-reliance in recovery from anxiety disorder.

D) Medical marijuana needs evidence-based research to establish its comparative therapeutic value in the treatment of anxiety disorders.

Treatments:

A) Anxiety conditions best treated without drugs:

   1) OCD, mild to moderate severity

   2) GAD, panic with/without agoraphobia

   3) Phobias, and situations in which drugs may interfere with performance (e.g., test anxiety, fear of driving)

B) Anxiety conditions in which drugs may speed recovery:

   1) Severe social anxiety, in conjunction with cognitive behavioral social skills training

   2) Severe psychosexual dysfunction, in conjunction with sex therapy

C) Anxiety conditions in which drugs could be first-line:

   1) Chronic, intractable OCD

   2) Persistent, pervasive PTSD

   3) One-time (fear of flying, visit to the dentist) or transient, situational anxieties (e.g., awaiting trial, dealing with the tax authorities)

D) Monotherapy is generally indicated over combination therapy, except in the case of unresponsiveness to monotherapy. Nonetheless, monotherapy with pharmacotherapy alone, without any psychosocial component, is rarely, if ever, optimum practice.

Conclusions:

A) Psychosocial therapy is the treatment of choice for the great majority of anxiety disorders, and may be augmented with medication for a combined treatment regimen in the case of limited, specific diagnoses (severe obsessive-complusive disorder, posttraumatic stress disorder), or when the anxiety condition is unresponsive to psychosocial approaches alone.

psychotherapy provides greater maintenance of therapeutic gain without necessarily requiring continual treatment, as is the case with medication. One possible drawback to psychotherapies using exposure techniques among PTSD patients, however, is the high dropout rate (Rothbaum et al., 2006).

Combining medication with psychotherapy for the treatment of PTSD is probably the norm in most clinical settings. Yet, there is little evidence that this is superior to monotherapy with psychosocial approaches, and in our opinion it is best reserved for PTSD patients who prove to be non-responsive to psychotherapy.

Panic Disorder and Agoraphobia

Although psychiatry texts present serotonin-specific reuptake inhibitors (SSRIs) as first-line treatment for panic disorder (Hales, Yudofsky, & Gabbard, 2011), the use of medication in general in the treatment of panic disorder, with or without agoraphobia, is questionable as first-line therapy since good success without medication side effects and potential for drug dependency is attained with psychological treatments. When evidence of the plausibility of antidepressants for the treatment of panic disorder is presented, the studies used do not usually compare such compounds to effective psychosocial therapy outcomes, but merely against placebo controls (Serretti et al., 2011). In general, cognitive-behavioral treatment of panic disorder and agoraphobia is well documented, with remission rates around 80% with follow-up at one year (D. M. Clark & Ehlers, 1993; Margraf, Barlow, Clark, & Telch, 1993). Marks et al. (1993), for example, found exposure therapy to be twice as effective as alprazolam. One NIMH-sponsored, extensive multisite study on panic disorder with mild to moderate agoraphobia concluded that patients did better *without* concurrent use of antidepressant medication while in psychotherapy (Woods et al., 1998). The possibility of a deleterious effect of benzodiazepines when combined with exposure therapy in the treatment of panic disorder has been noted (Schmidt, Koselka, & Woolaway-Bickel, 2001), and unwanted, but often-encountered.

There may be some validity in the argument that pharmacotherapy is more convenient for the patient looking for a quick therapeutic intervention with little patient investment of effort or tolerance of distress (Charney, Kredlow, Bui, & Simon, this book, Chapter 9). For such patients, usually seen in medical settings, the allure of a rapid-acting agent may enlist greater compliance and be, at least in the short run, more effective than trying to sell the patient a psychological treatment. Nonetheless, a fast-acting benzodiazepine—the fastest of all FDA-approved psychotropic medications for the treatment of panic—is no faster-acting than implosion exposure therapy. The deconditioning effects of exposure are rapid when the exposure is intensive, and substantial decrease in anxiety from single-trial exposure is the norm. Systematic desensitization, on the other hand, may require longer to provide significant results, but latency to recovery can be greatly decreased by increasing the frequency of visits. Considering that antidepressants require upwards of a month of dose adjustment to attain therapeutic effects, and usually require ill-defined maintenance dosing for indefinite periods to prevent relapse (Batalaan, Van Balkom, & Stein, 2012), it is not clear that a patient on the fast track to recovery from panic disorder would arrive at efficacious, sustainable symptom abatement any more quickly with pharmacotherapy than with behavioral treatment. Once again, the question is more one of fitting the treatment to the patient, for there will certainly be those patients who would rather try a medication before psychotherapy; and the sensitive clinician never minimizes patient variables, one of the most important being patient preference, in considering treatment of choice.

Generalized Anxiety Disorder (GAD)

Comaty and Advokat (this book, Chapter 12) note that the treatment of generalized anxiety disorder with pharmacotherapy alone is replete with difficulties, including mixed clinical results, higher rates of dropout (Mitte, 2005), difficulty in maintaining gains, and potential for abuse and discontinuation syndrome. Because psychotherapy has proved to be as effective as pharmacotherapy, to work as fast or faster, and to have improved remission rates with fewer side effects, it must be considered the treatment of choice with this form of anxiety disorder. For example, a meta-analysis of 35 studies shows cognitive-behavioral therapy (CBT) to be more effective in the treatment of GAD in the long term than pharmacologic treatment, and while both treatments reduce anxiety, CBT is more effective in reducing depression associated with GAD (Gould, Otto, Pollack, & Yap, 1997). Relaxation training appears to be especially well adapted for the treatment of diffuse anxieties and its collateral symptoms, such as insomnia (Borkovec & Weerts, 1976). Not only can relaxation be used in desensitization work either with cognitive or behavioral goals (Goldfried, 1971), but it is a bona fide anxiolytic treatment in itself (Öst, 1987), which has been shown for decades to achieve many of the same benefits as benzodiazepines but without the side-effect profile of medication. In fact, relaxation has been instrumental in aiding in the reduction of benzodiazepine use. Lick and Heffler (1977), for example, found progressive muscle relaxation to be more effective than placebo in the treatment of severe insomnia, and to be effective also in reducing the use of anxiolytic sleep aids.

As with other conditions, the range of psychotherapies submitted to controlled studies with GAD is extremely truncated, with CBT receiving the vast majority of attention. As of yet, there is little indication that one psychotherapy is more effective than another with GAD. There is some evidence, however, that cognitive approaches that attempt a mere suppression of worrisome thinking may actually enhance worrying through rebound (Wegner, 1994; Wang & Clark, 2008). While the effectiveness of cognitive therapy with GAD is well established (D. A. Clark & Beck, 2010), this kind of cognitive approach may need to be tailored to GAD: techniques that prolong exposure to worrisome thoughts while embracing and accepting the anxiety accompanying the cognition (Hayes & Wilson, 1994) may be indicated over techniques aimed at distraction or thought stopping.

Obsessive-Compulsive Disorder (OCD)

One of the first systematic applications of response prevention in the treatment of OCD has been attributed to the British psychologist Victor Meyer, who established a hospital-based program for treating OCD with behavioral approaches in 1966 (Hyman & Pedrick, 2010). Meta-analytic evaluation of the effectiveness of cognitive-behavioral therapy in the treatment of OCD established this approach as effective and efficacious nearly 15 years ago (Abramowitz, 1998) and, indeed, cognitive-behavioral therapy has been considered first-line for the treatment of OCD for quite some time. In general, data do not support the use of combination treatments over monotherapy treatment of OCD (Antony & Swinson, 2001). Simpson and Liebowitz (2011) argue in a review of six studies comparing psychotherapy to medication that CBT can be more effective than SSRIs when employed by skilled clinicians, but that SSRIs have also proven to be effective treatments. The data, however, do not support using combination therapy as a general first-line treatment for OCD; yet, expert consensus treatment guidelines for OCD (March, Frances, Kahn, & Carpenter, 1997), while recommending response prevention CBT monotherapy as first-line treatment for adults and adolescents with mild OCD, suggest that an exception be made in providing combined treatment of SSRI plus CBT in severe OCD for adults and adolescents. For prepubescent children, CBT is the first-line recommendation for all severities of OCD.

Abramowitz and Jacoby (this book, Chapter 6) correctly point out that avoidance is the motivator for compulsive responses in the OCD syndrome. The avoidance is rather straightforward in a compulsion that allows the patient to reduce anxiety by, for example, washing his or her hands. However, avoidance is also a primary component of obsessions; the obsession is meant to mitigate anxiety, just as the compulsion does. In a way, the patient who obsesses can be conceptualized as entertaining "cognitive compulsions." Although the obsessions might be experienced as egodystonic, the patient is nearly always actively involved in keeping them going.

At least one study suggests that cognitive therapy which targets misinterpretations associated with beliefs, without a behavioral exposure-response prevention (ERP) component, is effective in reducing OCD symptoms (Wilhelm et al., 2009). The authors of the Wilhelm study suggest that cognitive therapy may be an alternative to CBT and/or SSRI therapy when the patient develops side effects to medication or finds exposure therapy too invasive. Other psychosocial therapies that have proved to be effective in treating OCD include group therapy and family treatment interventions (Van Noppen & Steketee, 2004).

Phobias

John B. Watson demonstrated classical conditioning acquisition and extinction of phobic anxiety in 1920 (Watson & Rayner, 1920). With phobias, behavioral approaches have been singularly effective and efficacious, and it is hard to imagine why any other approach would be considered first-line. Certainly, many other therapies are adjunctive to behavioral therapy in the treatment of phobias, especially in the case of agoraphobia, where issues of personal autonomy might be addressed through self-concept-building approaches, independence may be fostered through treatment of family misalignments and co-dependencies, and social skills may be improved through assertiveness training and social skills groups.

Despite arguments positing pharmacotherapy as first-line treatment (Blanco, Bragdon, Schneier, & Liebowitz, 2012), with cognitive-behavioral therapy proposed only as an adjunct to pharmacotherapy in medication-resistant patients, medication might best play an adjunctive role to psychotherapy in phobia reconditioning; but even this is the exception rather than the rule. For example, with a patient who is too anxious to perform minimally well in public speaking or social/sexual relating, a short-acting benzodiazepine may be a first step in systematic desensitization. The idea here is to lower the level of Subjective Units of Distress (SUDs) on those hierarchical items that cannot be approached through previous half-steps leading to full exposure to the phobic situation. By temporarily reducing the anxiety associated with an item, the patient may be partially exposed to the situation, later to be followed with a greater degree of exposure by reducing the anxiolytic. In all cases, the dosing of the benzodiazepine should be such that the patient is dealing with as much anxiety as can be functionally tolerated (Sartory, 1983). If the patient is drugged to the extent that he or she is impervious to the situation, there will be no new learning and, what is more, the benzodiazepine is likely to impede memory and recall of the experience, and could contribute to "state-dependent learning" (Reus, Weingartner, & Post, 1979), a situation in which learning occurs under a specific internal environment and level of consciousness, and implies that the same state of consciousness must be recreated to access or recall the new state-specific learned response. Learning while under the influence of a drug may give reason to question generalizability of therapeutic gains when not taking the drug (Goodwin, Powell, Bremer, Hoine, & Stern, 1969; Overton, 1969; Muse, 1984; Colpaert & Koek, 1995).

BEHAVIORALLY MANAGED MEDICATION

The dichotomous debate over medication versus psychotherapy in the treatment of anxiety or, indeed, in the treatment of psychiatric conditions in general is obviated by the reflection that, while there might be psychotherapy without medication, there can be no prescribing of medication without psychotherapy occurring. Whether intentional or not, the way in which psychotropics are prescribed—the psychology of prescribing, if you will—affects the outcome that any particular chemical agent will have on the patient. Beyond the issues of placebo (Leuchter, Cook, Hunter, & Korb, 2009; Leuchter, Cook, Witte, Morgan, & Abrams, 2002) and therapeutic alliance as strong intervening "common" variables in the practice of pharmacotherapy, perhaps the most overlooked, yet potent, psychosocial component to medication dispensing is its reinforcing qualities. The way in which a drug is taken can reinforce therapeutic goals, or undermine them (Muse, 2008; Muse & McFarland, 1998).

Behavioral scientists have long studied the reinforcing qualities of temporal pairings in classical conditioning and in reward/punishment contingencies in operant conditioning paradigms. These are not theoretical postulates, but verified laws of behavior. The temporal assignment and reinforcing circumstances in which medication is used inevitably become significant components in the outcome of such interventions. The agoraphobic patient who carries around a bottle of benzodiazepines in her purse "just in case" she feels panic coming on is an example of poor outcome to a treatment in which the use of medication reinforced a sense of vulnerability and the need to avoid anxiety or panic, as is the example of a patient with GAD who has been on an SSRI for more than 10 years because he is apprehensive of an increase in anxiety if the medication were to be discontinued. Neither of these patients is anxiety-free, yet both are fearful of anxiety and rely on medication not as a temporary coping strategy that at one point facilitated recovery but, rather, as a defense mechanism which engenders dependency—psychological and, in some cases, physical.

There are numerous examples of how medication can be used behaviorally toward therapeutic gains (Muse, 2010; Muse & Moore, 2012), but none more convincing than their powerful reinforcing effect in the treatment of chronic pain. Fordyce (1976) outlined the operant contingencies of therapeutic interventions in general for patients suffering from benign pain syndromes, giving examples of how PRN medications, improperly prescribed, can lead to an increase in pain behavior (Berni & Fordyce, 1977). The question of whether malprescribed medications actually increase phenomenological perception of pain—so hard to measure—does not need to be answered in order to appreciate an increase in pain behavior such as moaning, rocking, pacing, complaining, and movement restriction associated with poor practices in prescribing. If the patient "needs to be in pain" in order to justify dispensing a reinforcing narcotic agent, then, quite predictably, for the behaviorist anyway, pain will reappear at the instrumental time. On the other hand, providing "dispensed" relief by administering a short-acting muscle relaxant such as diazepam *after* completing prescribed exercises is an example of using a pharmacologic agent to support therapeutic direction. In one instance, narcotic agents extend dependency and other dysfunctional pain behaviors, acting as a detour to recovery, whereas in the second example the judicious administration of a short-acting agent reinforces and rewards more functional behavior, and promotes progress toward the therapeutic goal of greater mobility and greater independence.

While not much research has been done on the deleterious effects of improperly prescribed anxiolytics in the maintenance of anxiety syndromes, it is apparent that such potential exists. The agoraphobic patient who is given a benzodiazepine long enough to become physically dependent on the drug may find phobia perpetuated as an instrumental behavior for obtaining the drug. On the other hand, the housebound patient who follows a behavioral program to manage agoraphobia, and who is prescribed a benzodiazepine to use *after* returning to the home, is likely to make greater progress as a result of the reinforcing nature of this contingency.

BENEFITS AND CHALLENGES OF INTEGRATIVE CARE

An oftentimes overlooked argument for the cautious use of psychotropic medications (Bhalerao et al., 2012), especially for the use of antidepressants in the treatment of anxiety disorders, is their propensity to cause side effects such as an increase in anxiety or the appearance of sexual dysfunction, as well as adverse events such as prolonged Q-T interval, as recently identified for citalopram (FDA, 2012). Such occurrences in treatment are iatrogenic setbacks, and may lead to abandonment of treatment or, at the least, compromise the therapeutic relationship. Evidence suggests that those patients who experience an adverse effect from SSRIs are even more likely to experience the same kind of adverse reaction if the antidepressant is switched to another one (Katz et al., 2012), which would tend to argue for desisting from multiple trials of such drugs with anxiety patients. When weighing the evidence for choosing monotherapy over combined therapy, the risks of side effects associated with medication should be considered, and the decision to combine pharmacotherapy with psychotherapy should, therefore, not be an automatic one based on the assumption that more is better.

As an aside, marijuana, as a treatment for anxiety, should be considered along with other pharmacotherapies (Tambaro & Bortolato, 2012); for, although still a Schedule I drug with the Drug Enforcement Administration in the United States, it would appear from anecdotal sources that it is being increasingly prescribed within jurisdictions with local medical marijuana laws. Until recently, studies on marijuana have nearly always focused on its pernicious effects (side effects, if you will) and on the recovery from marijuana abuse (discontinuation syndrome). If cannabis and derivatives are to become increasingly available for medical treatment, then it behooves the clinical psychopharmacologist to know of these substances' potential therapeutic uses, as well as their potential for adverse effects (Leung, 2011). The few studies examining marijuana's medical use tend to focus on physical maladies, most notably Gilles de la Tourette syndrome, and conditions involving spasticity and/or pain. Of evident absence are studies exploring its well-known anxiolytic characteristics. While at least one study substantiates marijuana as a powerful anxiolytic (Fabre & McLendon, 1981), and a separate preliminary study (Ganon-Elazar & Akirav, 2009) hints at the cannabinoid receptor's role in mitigating acquisition of, and facilitating recovery from, PTSD, the integration of this substance within the balanced treatment of anxiety would tend to argue, as with all pharmacology in the realm of anxiety disorder, for an adjunctive role to complement first-line behavioral therapy.

CONCLUSION

Our survey of integrated care in the treatment of anxiety leaves one with the feeling that the preferred mode of therapy is not combined, but rather monotherapy involving psychosocial interventions; this is largely the impression because the evidence to date points us in that direction. The discerning use of medication has a role in managing certain anxiety disorders, but clearly it is a secondary role in most cases. On the other hand, the evidence is quite different with other nosologic categories such as psychosis and bipolar disorder, where medication many times plays the lead role; or in depression, where a combined treatment approach is often the preferred approach. These conclusions are not ideological posturing over a contrived psychotherapy versus medication controversy; rather, the scientist-practitioner must go where the evidence leads, and in the case of anxiety disorders the data suggest that integrative care should incorporate psychosocial interventions as first-line in the treatment of most cases of anxiety while combining pharmacotherapy with psychosocial approaches only in those cases that warrant the exception.

Clinical Points to Remember

1. The integration of biopsychosocial aspects in the treatment of mental health conditions requires the practitioner to have the flexibility of mind to embrace the entire individual, and to become knowledgeable in all three areas (biological, psychological, and social) of the person's functioning.

2. Integrative treatment is not the same as multidiscipline treatment, but implies that a single mental health professional is proficient enough in the biological, psychological, and sociological aspects of mental and emotional well-being to recognize maladies in all of the spheres that impact on mental health.

3. Evidence to date has rarely established specific treatments for particular conditions. Indeed, most evidence points to "common factors" in treatments which yield similar results. Pharmacotherapy, like psychotherapy, appears to exert its therapeutic effect largely from non-specific variables.

4. The fact that there are common factors to all treatment approaches does not rule out the possibility of specific "active ingredients" for individual therapies. Although the specific effects of different therapies are generally small, some studies have been able to indicate that certain therapies are more effective than others for certain conditions.

5. Cognitive-behavioral approaches have been shown to be effective in the treatment of all anxiety disorders. Pharmacotherapy has also been shown to be effective in the reduction of anxiety and accompanying symptoms. Nonetheless, concerns over side effects, dependency, and long-term recovery associated with pharmacotherapy of anxiety tip the scale in favor of psychotherapy in the treatment of anxiety disorders.

6. Exceptions to the above rule include persistent, chronic, intractable OCD and persistent, pervasive PTSD, as well as other conditions that have not responded to psychotherapy.

REFERENCES

Abramowitz, J. S. (1998). Does cognitive-behavioral therapy cure obsessive-compulsive disorder? A meta-analytic evaluation of clinical significance. *Behavior Therapy, 29*, 339–355.

American Psychiatric Association. (2004). Treatment of patients with acute stress disorder and posttraumatic stress disorder. Retrieved from www.psychiatryonline.com/pracGuide

Antony, M. M., & Swinson, R. P. (2001). Comparative and combined treatments for obsessive-compulsive disorder. In M. M. Sammons & N. B. Schmidt (Eds.), *Combined Treatments for Mental Disorders: A Guide to Psychological and Pharmacological Interventions.* Washington, DC: American Psychological Association.

Asay, T. P., & Lambert, M. J. (1999). The empirical case for the common factors in therapy: Quantitative findings. In M. A. Humble, B. L. Duncan, & S. D. Miller (Eds.), *The heart and soul of change: What works in therapy.* Washington, DC: American Psychological Association.

Baskin, T. W., Tierney, S. C., Minami, T., & Wampold, B. E. (2003). Establishing specificity in psychotherapy: A meta-analysis of structural equivalence of placebo controls. *Journal of Consulting and Clinical Psychology, 71,* 973–979.

Batelaan, N. M., Van Balkom, A. J. L. M., & Stein, D. J. (2012). Evidence-based pharmacotherapy of panic disorder: An update. *International Journal of Neuropsychopharmacology, 15,* 403–415.

Benish, S. G., Imel, Z. E., & Wampold, B. E. (2008). The relative efficacy of bona fide psychotherapies for treating post-traumatic stress disorder: A meta-analysis of direct comparisons. *Clinical Psychology Review, 28,* 1281.

Berni, R., & Fordyce, W. E. (1977). *Behavior Modification and the Nursing Process.* St. Louis, MO: C. V. Mosby.

Bhalerao, S., Seyfried, L. S., Kim, H. M., Chiang, C., Kavanagh, J., & Kales, H. C. (2012). Mortality risk with the use of atypical antipsychotics in later-life bipolar disorder. *Journal of Geriatric Psychiatry and Neurology, 25,* 29–36.

Bisson, J., & Andrew, M. (2009). *Psychological treatments of post-traumatic stress disorder (PTSD).* The Cochrane Library.

Blanco, C., Bragdon, L. B., Schneier, F. R., & Liebowitz, M. R. (2012). The evidence-based pharmacotherapy of social anxiety disorder. *International Journal of Neuropsychopharmacology, 15,* 1–15.

Borkovec, T. D., & Weerts, T. C. (1976). Effects of progressive relaxation on sleep disturbance: An electroencephalographic evaluation. *Psychosomatic Medicine, 38,* 173–180.

Clark, D. A., & Beck, A. T. (2010). *Cognitive therapy of anxiety disorders: Science and practice.* New York: Guilford Press.

Clark, D. M., & Ehlers, A. (1993). An overview of the cognitive theory and treatment of panic disorder. *Applied and Preventive Psychology, 2,* 131–139.

Colpaert, F. C., & Koek, W. (1995). Empirical evidence that the state dependence and drug discrimination paradigms can generate different outcomes. *Psychopharmacology, 120,* 272–279.

Ehlers, A., Bisson, J., Clark, D. M., Creamer, M., Pilling, S., Richards, D., et al. (2010). Do all psychological treatments really work the same in posttraumatic stress disorder? *Clinical Psychology Review, 30,* 269–276.

Fabre, L. F., & McLendon, D. (1981). The efficacy and safety of nabilone (a synthetic cannabinoid) in the treatment of anxiety. *Journal of Clinical Pharmacology, 21,* 377S–382S.

FDA (2012). Celexa (citalopram hydrobromide): Drug Safety Communication: Revised recommendations, potential risk of abnormal heart rhythms. Washington, DC: *Medwatch: The FDA Safety Information and Adverse Event Reporting Program.*

Fordyce, W. E. (1976). *Behavioral methods for chronic pain and illness.* St. Louis: C. V. Mosby.

Ganon-Elazar, E., & Akirav, I. (2009). Cannabinoid receptor activation in the basolateral amygdala blocks the effects of stress on the conditioning and extinction of inhibitory avoidance. *Journal of Neuroscience, 29*, 11078–11088.

Goldfried, M. R. (1971). Systematic desensitization as training in self-control. *Journal of Consulting and Clinical Psychology, 37*, 228–234.

Goodwin, D. W., Powell, B., Bremer, D., Hoine, H., & Stern, J. (1969). Alcohol and recall: State-dependent effects in man. *Science, 163*, 1358–1360.

Gould, R. A., Otto, M. W., Pollack, M. H., & Yap, L. (1997). Cognitive behavioral and pharmacological treatment of generalized anxiety disorder: A preliminary meta-analysis. *Behavior Therapy, 28*, 285–281.

Hales, R. E., Yudofsky, S. C., & Gabbard, G. O. (2011). *Essentials of Psychiatry* (3rd ed.). Arlington, VA: American Psychiatric Publishing.

Hayes, S. C., & Wilson, K. G. (1994). Acceptance and commitment therapy: Altering the verbal support for experiential avoidance. *Behavior Analyst, 17*, 289–303.

Hubble, M. A., Duncan, B. L., & Miller, S. D. (1999). *The heart and soul of change: What works in therapy.* Washington, DC: American Psychological Association.

Hyman, B. M., & Pedrick, C. (2010). *The OCD workbook: Your guide to breaking free from obsessive-compulsive disorder* (2nd ed.). Oakland, CA: New Harbinger Publications.

IAEP (1991) Society statement. *Journal of Integrative and Eclectic Psychotherapy, 10*, 264.

Imel, Z. E., & Wampold, B. E. (2008). The importance of treatment and the science of common factors in psychotherapy. In S. D. Brown & R. W. Lent (Eds.), *Handbook of counseling psychology* (4th ed., pp. 249–266). Hoboken, NJ: John Wiley.

Institute of Medicine of the National Academies (2008). *Committee on Treatment of Posttraumatic Stress Disorder.* Washington, DC: National Academies Press.

Katz, A. J., Dusetzina, S. B., Farley, J. F., Ellis, A. R., Gaynes, B. N., Castillo, W. C., et al. (2012). Distressing adverse events after antidepressant switch in the Sequenced Treatment Alternatives to Relieve Depression (STAR*D) trial: Influence of adverse events during initial treatment with citalopram on development of subsequent adverse events with an alternative antidepressant. *Pharmacotherapy, 32*, 234–243.

Leuchter, A. F., Cook, I. A., Hunter, A. M., & Korb, A. S. (2009). A new paradigm for the prediction of antidepressant treatment response. *Dialogues in Clinical Neuroscience, 11*, 435–446.

Leuchter, A. F., Cook, I. A., Witte, E. A., Morgan, M., & Abrams, M. (2002). Changes in brain function of depressed subjects during treatment with placebo. *American Journal of Psychiatry, 159*, 122–129.

Leung, L. (2011). Cannabis and its derivatives: Review of medical use. *Journal of the American Board of Family Medicine, 24*, 452–462.

Lick, J. R., & Heffler, D. (1977). Relaxation training and attention placebo in the treatment of severe insomnia. *Journal of Consulting and Clinical Psychology, 48*, 153–161.

Luborsky, L., Singer, B., & Luborsky, L. (1975) Comparative studies of psychotherapies: Is it true that "everybody has won and all must have prizes"? *Archives of General Psychiatry, 32*, 995–1008.

March, J. S., Frances, A., Kahn, D. A., & Carpenter, D. (Eds.). (1997). The expert consensus guidelines: Treatment of obsessive-compulsive disorder. *Journal of Clinical Psychiatry, 58* (Supplement 4).

Margraf, J., Barlow, D. H., Clark, D. M., & Telch, M. J. (1993). Psychological treatment of panic: Work in progress on outcome, active ingredients, and follow-up. *Behaviour Research and Therapy, 31*, 1–8.

Marks, I. (2010). *Common language for psychotherapy procedures: The first 80.* Rome: Centro per la Ricerca in Psicoterapia.

Marks, I. M., Swinson, R. P., Başoğlu, M., Kuch, K., Noshirvani, H., O'Sullivan, G., et al. (1993). Alprazolam and exposure alone and combined in panic disorder with agoraphobia: A controlled study in London and Toronto. *British Journal of Psychiatry, 162*, 776–787.

Marks, I. M., Tortella-Feliu, M., Fernández de la Cruz, L., Fullana, M.-A., Sungar, M., & de Wit, L. (undated). Classifying what psychotherapists do: A first step. Common language for psychotherapy. Unpublished manuscript. Retrieved from www.commonlanguagepsychotherapy.org

Maxmen, J. S., & Ward, N. G. (2002). *Psychotropic drugs: Fast facts* (3rd ed.). New York: W. W. Norton.

Messer, S. B., & Wampold, B. E. (2002). Let's face facts: Common factors are more potent than specific therapy ingredients. *Clinical Psychology: Science and Practice, 9*, 21–25.

Mitte, K. (2005). Meta-analysis of cognitive-behavioral treatments for generalized anxiety disorder: A comparison with pharmacotherapy. *Psychological Bulletin, 131*, 785–795.

Moncrieff, J., & Cohen, D. (2009). How do psychiatric drugs work? *British Medical Journal, 338*, 1535–1537.

Muse, M. (1984). Narcosynthesis in the treatment of posttraumatic chronic pain. *Rehabilitation Psychology, 29*, 113–118.

Muse, M. (2008). Convergencia de psicoterapia y psicofarmacología: El uso de regímenes conductistas en el manejo de medicamentos psicoactivos. *Revista de Psicoterapia, 69*, 5–10.

Muse, M. (2010). Combining therapies in medical psychology: When to medicate and when not. *Archives of Medical Psychology, 1*, 19–27.

Muse, M., Brown, S., & Cothran-Ross, T. (2012). Psychology, psychopharmacology, and pediatrics: When to treat and when to refer. In G. M. Kapalka (Ed.), *Pediatricians and pharmacologically trained psychologists: Practitioner's guide to collaborative treatment.* New York: Springer.

Muse, M., & McFarland, D. (1994, June 22–26). The convergence of psychology and psychiatry: The use of behaviorally prescribed medications. Paper presented at the Second International Congress of Eclectic Psychotherapy, Lyon, France.

Muse, M., & Moore, B. A. (2012). Integrating clinical psychopharmacology within the practice of medical psychology. In M. Muse & B. A. Moore (Eds.), *Handbook of clinical psychopharmacology for psychologists* (pp. 17–44). Hoboken, NJ: John Wiley.

Öst, L.-G. (1987). Applied relaxation: Description of a coping technique and review of controlled studies. *Behaviour Research and Therapy, 25*, 397–409.

Overton, D. A. (1968). Dissociated learning in drug states (state-dependent learning). In D. H. Efron et al. (Eds.), *Psychopharmacology: A review of progress 1957–1967.* Washington, DC: U.S. Government Printing Office.

Posternak, M. A., Solomon, D. A., Leon, A. C., Mueller, T. I., Shea, M. T., & Keller, M. B. (2006). The naturalistic course of unipolar major depression in the absence of somatic therapy. *Journal of Nervous and Mental Disease, 194*, 324–329.

Reus, V. I., Weingartner, H., & Post, R. M. (1979). Clinical implications of state-dependent learning. *American Journal of Psychiatry, 136,* 927–931.

Riess, H. (2010). Empathy in medicine: a neurobiological perspective. *JAMA: Journal of the American Medical Association, 304,* 1604–1605.

Rothbaum, B. O., Cahill, S. P., Foa, E. B., Davidson, J. R. T., Compton, J., Connor, K. M., et al. (2006). Augmentation of sertraline with prolonged exposure in the treatment of posttraumatic stress disorder. *Journal of Traumatic Stress, 1,* 625–638.

Sartory, G. (1983). Benzodiazepines and behavioural treatment of phobic anxiety. *Behavioural Psychotherapy, 11,* 204–217.

Schmidt, N. B., Koselka, M., & Woolaway-Bickel, K. (2001). Combined treatments for phobic anxiety disorders. In M. T. Sammons and N. B. Schmidt (Eds.), *Combined treatments for mental disorders: A guide to psychological and pharmacological interventions* (pp. 81–110). Washington, DC: American Psychological Association.

Serretti, A., Chiesa, A., Calati, R., G. Perna, L. Bellodi, & DeRonchi, D. (2011). Novel antidepressants and panic disorder: Evidence beyond current guidelines. *Neuropsychobiology, 63,* 1–7.

Simpson, H. B., & Liebowitz, M. R. (2011). Combining pharmacotherapy and cognitive-behavioral therapy in the treatment of OCD. In J. S. Abramowitz & A. C. Houts (Eds.), *Concepts and controversies in obsessive-compulsive disorder* (pp. 359–376). New York: Springer.

Smith, M. L., & Glass, G. V. (1977). Meta-analysis of psychotherapy outcome studies. *American Psychologist, 32,* 752–760.

Stefano, G. B., Fricchione, G. L., Slingsby, B. T., & Benson, H. (2001). The placebo effect and relaxation response: Neural processes and their coupling to constitutive nitric oxide. *Brain Research Reviews, 35,* 1–19.

Stricker, G. (2010). A second look at psychotherapy integration. *Journal of Psychotherapy Integration, 20,* 397–405.

Swartz, H. A., Frank, E., & Cheng, Y. (2012). A randomized pilot study of psychotherapy and quetiapine for the acute treatment of bipolar II depression. *Bipolar Disorders, 14,* 211–216.

Tallman, K., & Bohart, A. C. (1999) The client as a common factor: Clients as self-healers. In M. A. Hubble, B. L. Duncan, & S. D. Miller (Eds.), *The heart and soul of change: What works in therapy* (pp. 91–131). Washington, DC: American Psychological Association.

Tambaro, S., & Bortolato, M. (2012). Cannabinoid-related agents in the treatment of anxiety disorders: Current knowledge and future perspectives. *Recent Patents on CNS Drug Discovery, 7,* 25–40.

Van Noppen, B. L., & Steketee, G. (2004). Individual, group, and multifamily cognitive-behavioral treatments. In M. Tortora Pato & J. Zohar (Eds.), *Current treatments of obsessive-compulsive disorder* (2nd ed., pp. 133–172). Washington, DC: American Psychiatric Publishing.

Wampold, B. E. (2001). *The great psychotherapy debate: Models, methods, and findings.* Mahwah, NJ: Lawrence Erlbaum.

Wampold, B. E., Imel, Z. E., Laska, K. M., Benish, S., Miller, S. D., Flückiger, C., et al. (2010). Determining what works in the treatment of PTSD. *Clinical Psychology Review, 30,* 923–933.

Wampold, B. E., Mondin, G. W., Moody, M., Stich, F., Benson, K., & Ahn, H. (1997). A meta-analysis of outcome studies comparing bona fide psychotherapies: Empirically, "all must have prizes". *Psychological Bulletin, 122*, 203–215.

Wang, A., & Clark, D. A. (2008). The suppression of worry and its triggers in a nonclinical sample: Rebound and other negative effects. Unpublished manuscript. Department of Psychology, University of New Brunswick.

Watson, J. B., & Rayner, R. (1920). Conditioned emotional reactions. *Journal of Experimental Psychology, 3*(1), 1–14.

Wegner, D. M. (1994). *White bears and other unwanted thoughts: Suppression, obsession, and the psychology of mental control.* New York: Guilford Press.

Wilhelm, S., Steketee, G., Fama, J. M., Buhlmann, U., Teachman, B. A., & Golan, E. (2009). Modular cognitive therapy of obsessive-compulsive disorder: A wait-list controlled trial. *Journal of Cognitive Psychotherapy, 23*, 294–305.

Woods, S. W., Barlow, D. H., Gorman, J. M., & Shear, M. K. (1998). Follow-up results six months after discontinuation of all treatment. In D. H. Barlow (Ed.), *Results from the multi-center clinical trial on the treatment of panic disorder: Cognitive behavior treatment versus imipramine versus their combination.* Washington, DC: Symposium presented at the 32nd Annual Convention of the Association for Advancement of Behavior Therapy.

CHAPTER 2

A Biopsychosocial Approach to Anxiety

**Allison M. Greene, Christopher R. Bailey, and
Alexander Neumeister**

PSYCHOLOGICAL PERSPECTIVE

Foundations of Learned Fear

Classical conditioning

As humans, our adaptive functioning depends largely on our ability to form emotional responses to environmental stimuli based on our knowledge of the events that those stimuli predict. Such responses can facilitate interpersonal communication, assist in memory formation, and promote decision making and subsequent action (Hartley & Phelps, 2010). More broadly and perhaps more importantly, the ability to learn associations between aversive events and the environmental cues that predict them is crucial for our survival. The concept of learned associations provides a useful framework for understanding the nature of emotional responsiveness in humans.

In the first half of the 20th century, Russian physiologist Ivan Pavlov first introduced the concept of learned associations in his well-known experiments on classical conditioning. While studying digestive reflexes in dogs, Pavlov (1927) recognized that the animals responded predictably to salient cues in their environment, such as salivating at the sight of food. He also observed that the natural salivation response to food could be elicited by random stimuli that attained significance through repeated pairings with the food. Pavlov trained his research subjects to associate the sound of a bell with the presentation of food by presenting the two stimuli simultaneously or within close temporal proximity. Further, the dogs learned to associate the presentation of food with the environments in which they were experimentally trained, salivating at the mere sight of Pavlov's laboratory even in the absence of food.

In Pavlovian, or classical, conditioning, the salient environmental cue is called the unconditioned stimulus (US) and the involuntary, natural response it produces is the unconditioned response (UR). The neutral stimulus that attains significance through repeated parings with the US is the conditioned stimulus

(CS), and the response elicited by the CS is the conditioned responses (CR). In the case of Pavlov's experiments, the UR and the CR are physiologically similar insofar as both involve salivation and are both automatic. However, while the UR is an innate response to the sight of food, the CR is a learned response elicited by stimuli other than the food itself.

Our cognitive faculties are more sophisticated than those of Pavlov's research subjects, but the processes that govern the way we acquire information about our environments and use it to construct emotional responses are similar in an important way: we use the associations we learn between environmental stimuli and events to guide our emotional behavior. Indeed, the conditioning paradigm Pavlov used to train his dogs almost a century ago has had a ubiquitous influence on contemporary research on anxiety in both animals and humans.

Fear conditioning

Of considerable interest to psychologists and neuroscientists is fear conditioning, a particular form of classical conditioning whereby organisms learn to form relationships between stimuli and aversive or threatening events. Fear conditioning was first studied empirically almost a century ago by researchers John Watson and Rosalie Rayner at Johns Hopkins University. Their experiment represents one of the earliest studies involving experimental manipulations of emotion and a striking demonstration of how quickly and effectively fear can be established using Pavlovian mechanisms. By simultaneously showing an 11-month-old child, Little Albert, a white rat (CS) and hitting a steel bar with a hammer (US) out of the boy's sight loudly enough to startle him (UR), Watson and Rayner effectively trained Albert to fear the rat (1920). The effect of the fear conditioning was so pronounced that Albert transferred the emotional response to a fur coat, crying in its presence and "withdrawing his body as far as possible, pushing ... with his feet." Importantly, the experiment on Little Albert would not be acceptable under current ethical or legal standards. The scientists' purpose was to demonstrate that fear is primal in nature, and to offer a novel explanation for psychopathologic phobias. In fact, the idea that pathological anxiety is an extension of the normal fear response continues to be studied extensively.

In contemporary fear-conditioning studies, a consenting individual is conditioned to fear a neutral stimulus after several conjugate presentations of the stimulus with an aversive or threatening event. After fear is established, the neutral stimulus elicits an automatic emotional response that would normally only occur in the presence of danger or threat (LeDoux, 2003). For instance, a stimulus such as a tone (CS) might be paired repeatedly with a light foot shock (US), which automatically elicits a range of responses such as increased heart rate or freezing (UR) (Hartley & Phelps, 2010). After several pairings of the shock with the tone, the tone elicits the fear response in the absence of the shock (CR). Effectively, the fear-conditioning paradigm makes it possible for neutral stimuli to acquire the capacity to elicit evolutionarily tuned responses to danger (LeDoux, 2003).

Fear conditioning is one of the most widely used and successful paradigms in experimental research on anxiety. Its utility is underscored by its versatility. For example, neuroscientists have used fear conditioning in conjunction with positron emission tomography (PET) (Linnman et al., 2012) and functional magnetic resonance imaging (fMRI) (Bonne et al., 2008) to explore the neuro-circuitry of fear. Other lines of research employ fear-conditioning paradigms in symptom provocation studies to investigate physiological responses to fear (Acheson, Forsyth, & Moses, 2012). In its most fundamental use, many researchers use fear conditioning to study the nature of fear acquisition and maintenance. Indeed, much of the knowledge available on fear and anxiety is the result of research that has employed fear conditioning in one form or another (Beckers, Krypotos, Boddez, Effting, & Kindt, in press).

Fear and Memory

Consolidation

For an organism to interact successfully with its environment, it must use its knowledge of event–outcome associations to approach or avoid various types of situations. This process depends on an ability to acquire and store memories of stimuli and the outcomes they predict. Consolidation refers to the conversion of conscious experience to memory (Amiel, Mathew, Garakani, Neumeister, & Charney, 2009).

Memory retention can be short-term, in which case cognitive representation of a conscious experience is transient. In the mid 20th century the human capacity for short-term memory was quantified experimentally as approximately seven pieces of information at a given time (Miller, 1956), though more recent studies suggest that it might be even smaller (Cowan, 2001). Consolidation, by contrast, refers to conversion of conscious experience to long-term memory storage, which has a much larger capacity than short-term storage and results in memories that are more permanent.

On the molecular level, short-term memory is associated with small changes in the glutamatergic neurotransmission pathway (Amiel et al., 2009). Specifically, short-term memory acquisition involves enhancement of glutamatergic transmission resulting in increased sensitivity of the α-amino-3-hydroxy-5-methylisoxazole-4-propionic acid (AMPA) receptor. Long-term memory consolidation, on the other hand, is associated with lasting changes in synaptic potentiation. Glutamatergic stimulation of sufficient quantity and appropriate quality results in postsynaptic changes in the N-methyl-D-aspartate (NMDA) receptor that initiate a signaling cascade ending gene transcription and protein synthesis (Amiel et al., 2009; Malenka & Bear, 2004). This process is known as long-term potentiation (LTP).

The amygdala and hippocampus are key areas in which LTP occurs, and therefore play critical roles in memory acquisition and storage (Hartley & Phelps, 2010). The function of the hippocampus in memory consolidation was illustrated in the well-known 1957 case study of patient H.M., who, following a bilateral medial temporal lobe resection to treat epilepsy, suffered from severe memory deficits (Scoville & Milner, 1957). Additionally, damage to the hippocampus has been shown to disrupt the acquisition of declarative information about the relationships between stimuli and outcomes (Bechara et al., 1995). Similar results implicating the hippocampus in memory consolidation have been replicated in animal studies (Whitlock, Heynen, Shuler, & Bear, 2006).

The role of the amygdala in memory consolidation has been explored extensively and has also been indicated as a crucial area for encoding and storing fearful memories. Case studies have indicated that damage to the amygdala can result in a failure to acquire conditioned autonomic responses to fearful stimuli (Bechara et al., 1995). Interestingly, damage to both the amygdala and the hippocampus results in failure to acquire both declarative information about stimuli and autonomic responses to them. Studies using fMRI to investigate neural responses in conditioning paradigms have demonstrated increased activity in the amygdala during associative learning (Büchel, Dolan, Armony, & Friston, 1999), further implicating its importance in learning and memory.

Extinction

Cognitive flexibility enables an individual to adjust to a dynamic environment. For instance, it is beneficial for an individual to unlearn the association between a stimulus and an aversive event if cause–effect relationships change. Extinction refers to the gradual depression of a conditioned fear response that occurs when the CS is presented repeatedly without reinforcement by the aversive US (Hartley & Phelps, 2010). When this process occurs, the CS that previously predicted danger no longer does, and it no longer produces a fear response when presented to the conditioned individual.

Importantly, extinction does not erase the initially formed memory of the CS and the aversive event, but instead facilitates the formation of a novel stimulus–outcome association. The persistence of the CS–US memory is evidenced by the capacity for the CR to reemerge in various experimental phenomena such as renewal, the reemergence of the CR in novel contexts; spontaneous recovery, the reemergence of the CR after a passage of time; and reinstatement, the reemergence of the CR following an unsignaled presentation of the CS (Hartley & Phelps, 2010).

Like consolidation, extinction involves increased sensitivity of glutamatergic NMDA receptors in the amygdala (Amiel et al., 2009). The process of extinction can be blocked by an NMDA receptor antagonist such as AP5 or γ-aminobutyric acid (GABA) (Falls, Miserendino, & Davis, 1992; Akirav, 2007), or enhanced by agonists of the same receptors, such as D-cycloserine (Langton & Richardson, 2008). In fact, several lines of research propose targeting the NMDA receptor in conjunction with exposure therapy for the treatment of anxiety disorders including phobias, social anxiety, and obsessive-compulsive disorder (Amaral & Roesler, 2008).

Reconsolidation

Classic theories of memory suggested that when a memory is first learned, it is fragile and labile until it has gone through a consolidation period, after which it becomes permanent (Hartley & Phelps, 2010). During consolidation, a memory can be disrupted, but once it is consolidated it cannot be eliminated. Forty years ago, however, researchers at the University of California challenged the idea that consolidated memories are invincible and discovered that by delivering electroconvulsive shocks to rats just after reinstating memory cues, they could disrupt well-established memories (Lewis, Bregman, & Mahan, 1972). The discovery that consolidated memories are not permanent suggested that a memory trace returns to a transient state each time it is retrieved, and if it is to become stable again, it requires an additional period of consolidation. This phenomenon, originally called "cue-dependent amnesia," is now known as reconsolidation.

Historically, studies on reconsolidation were limited to animals because their invasive techniques such as the administration of electroconvulsive shocks or protein synthesis inhibitors were not ethical or safe for use in humans (Schiller et al., 2010). More recently, researchers have discovered that propranalol, a β-adrenergic antagonist that has been shown to block reconsolidation in rats (Debiec & LeDoux, 2004), is safe for use in humans. In 2009, Kindt, Soeter, and Vervliet discovered that oral administration of propranolol before memory reactivation in humans erased the behavioral expression of fear in response to a CS presented 24 hours later. Non-medical techniques have also been used to explore reconsolidation in humans. For example, updating a fearful memory with non-fearful information during reconsolidation has been shown to prevent the return of fear (Schiller et al., 2010).

Normal Fear and Models of Abnormal Anxiety

The normal fear response

It is necessary to experience fear in the face of threat because fear motivates individuals to escape dangerous situations. For instance, when an animal encounters a threatening stimulus such as a predator, an adaptive fear response triggers the animal to act in order to remove the negative emotion and consequently free itself from an unfortunate fate (Rosen & Schulkin, 1998). Despite its key role in survival, normal fear is not always adaptive. Public speaking is not a dangerous situation, yet it elicits anxiety or apprehension from many individuals. Importantly, normal anxiety subsides during or shortly after a public presentation. A similar example is test anxiety.

Though the perception of fearful stimuli is moderated by voluntary action and the emotion of fear manifests as a conscious experience, the brain mechanisms that appraise environmental cues and regulate the fear response are automatic and unconscious (LeDoux, 2003). Indeed, the cognitive experience of fear is just one component of an intricate network of biological processes that mediate this complex emotion.

When a threatening stimulus is encountered, the information obtained by an individual's perceptual faculties is transmitted to the thalamus, a forebrain structure responsible for relay and integration of sensory information. Once it is there, the signal is simultaneously transmitted to brain stem nuclei for initiation of automatic reflexes, and to the amygdala for both rapid and higher-order processing. This system is maintained via a reciprocal neural circuit between the amygdala and hippocampus and the primary sensory cortex through which continued processing and learning take place (Amiel et al., 2009).

Afferent pathways transmit information from sensory organs to the brain, and efferent pathways deliver information from the brain to other systems in the body once the information has been processed by the amygdala. Specifically, if a stimulus is deemed threatening by the amygdala, a fear response is expressed through efferent pathways targeting the motor and neuroendocrine systems (Amiel et al., 2009).

Circuits involving the hypothalamus, a forebrain structure near the thalamus implicated in neuroendocrine functioning and autonomic arousal, and the pituitary gland, a structure extending from the hypothalamus whose secretions influence hormone activity in other glands of the body, stimulate autonomic activation of the central nervous system. Physiological responses to this process include, for example, increased heart rate and blood pressure, pupil dilation, and opening of respiratory passages.

The fear response also includes projections to motor pathways. In fact, the physiological manifestations of autonomic activation function to mobilize an individual for action. Eighty years ago, physiologist Walter Cannon (1929) coined the term "fight or flight response" to describe the two biological tools an organism can use to avoid danger. Autonomic activation of the central nervous system prepares an organism to employ either, depending on which is more feasible in a given situation.

In a normally functioning individual, this network of perceptual, chemical, and motivational processes offers protection from danger (Amiel et al., 2009; Rosen & Schulkin, 1998). Importantly, the repertoire of physical and physiological changes associated with the normal fear response as well as the cognitive sensations of fear such as hypervigilance subside once the threatening stimulus has been removed. Dysregulation of the fear regulation process can result in pathological anxiety.

Dysregulation of fear processing

Fear is associated with cognitions such as hyperarousal and vigilance, as well panic, escape, and avoidance behaviors. While anxiety involves analogous cognitive constructs, it does not involve defensive action (Rosen & Schulkin, 1998). As such, fear is understood as an alarm response to current danger, while anxiety is an emotional state associated with preparation for future aversive events (Rauch, Shin, & Phelps, 2009). One perspective on the etiology of anxiety disorders suggests that pathological anxiety extends directly from the normal fear response (Rosen & Schulkin, 1998). Importantly, this perspective indicates that the psychological constructs of fear and not the defensive behaviors associated with it are associated with pathological anxiety.

Normal anxiety is transient, and it is generally manageable by self-coping strategies such as reappraisal, selective attention, and suppression (Hartley & Phelps, 2010). However, during and following intense or prolonged psychological stress, neural fear circuits may be overactivated and hyperresponsive. The hyperreponsive fear circuit is more easily triggered until ultimately fear activation becomes independent from any external stimuli (Rosen & Schulkin, 1998).

For example, posttraumatic stress disorder (PTSD) occurs in some people following acute or prolonged exposure to a traumatic event (APA, 2000). Substantial evidence suggests that PTSD is associated with overactivation of the amygdala—a central structure of the neural fear circuit that evaluates sensory information for appropriate emotional responsiveness (Rauch et al., 2006). Furthermore, fMRI studies of patients with PTSD have indicated underactivation of areas of the prefrontal cortex that inhibit fear responsiveness by moderating fear signals from the amygdala with higher levels of reasoning (Kent & Rauch, 2003).

The diathesis–stress model

Although significant evidence indicates a relationship between dysregulation in neural fear-processing circuits and pathological anxiety, modern etiological models of anxiety emphasize both internal risk factors and external stressors in the development of anxiety disorders. The diathesis–stress model conceptualizes pathological anxiety as the product of dispositional vulnerabilities that increase one's likelihood of developing particular disorders and negative external circumstances or internal stressors to which individuals can be exposed (Mineka & Oehlberg, 2008).

Several lines of research suggest that certain personality traits represent significant diatheses for clinical anxiety (Mineka & Oehlberg, 2008). For example, decreased assertiveness has been linked to anxiety severity in several populations (Chambless, Hunter, & Jackson, 1982; Reiter, Otto, Pollack, & Rosenbaum, 1991), as it might represent a communicative challenge for individuals or cause distress in the face of interpersonal issues (Calkins et al., 2009). Additionally, several longitudinal studies have revealed that high levels of neuroticism are correlated with subsequent anxiety (Weinstock & Whisman, 2006). Characteristics of perfectionism, such as concerns about one's mistakes and doubts about one's decisions, have also been shown to predict anxiety in both adults (e.g., Enns & Cox, 2002) and children (Moser, Slane, Alexandra, & Klump, 2012; O'Connor, Rasmussen, & Hawton, 2009). Interestingly, correlational studies of twins have revealed that both anxiety and perfectionism are moderately heritable (Moser et al., 2012).

Genetic variables are also recognized as potential diathesis for the development of anxiety disorders. For example, a recent study on genetic risk profiles for psychiatric disorders found that small effects contributed by several genetic loci influence both anxiety and depression in elderly and middle-aged populations (Demirkan et al., 2011). Concerning PTSD in particular, the fact that only a subset of individuals who are exposed to traumatic life events acquire PTSD suggests that stress alone does not determine the development of this anxiety disorder. Rather, it is likely that genetic variants contribute to individual differences in responsiveness to trauma that make some individuals more susceptible to PTSD than others following trauma exposure (Yehuda & Seckl, 2011).

THE BIOLOGY OF ANXIETY

Neuroanatomy

Several brain regions are involved in the detection, processing, integration, and response to stressful or fearful stimuli. Visual, auditory, gustatory, and somatosensory receptors detect sensory information, which is then relayed to the thalamus for distribution. The thalamus transmits signals to the brain stem to respond to stimuli through automatic reflexes and to the amygdala and regions of the prefrontal cortex, hippocampus, and insula (LeDoux, 2003). The latter regions represent the brain's fear-processing neurocircuitry. This circuit is responsible for higher-order fear processing and mediating an appropriate response to fearful or stressful stimuli.

Theories about the pathophysiology of anxiety have focused on dysfunction within the aforementioned fear-processing neurocircuitry. The amygdalocentric anxiety model, a theory of pathological fear processing, stresses the amygdala's role in producing an appropriate response to fearful stimuli through its connections with other brain areas associated with fear processing, such as the prefrontal cortex (PFC) and the hippocampus (Rauch et al., 2006). This model hypothesizes that the amygdala is hyperresponsive in an anxious individual when they are presented with threatening or fearful stimuli, resulting in symptoms of hyperarousal, including being easily startled, feeling tense, and having trouble sleeping (National Institute of Mental Health [NIMH], 2008). The amygdalocentric model also posits decreased control over the amygdala by ventral/medial PFC (vmPFC), including the anterior cingulate cortex, subcallosal cortex and orbitofrontal cortex, and hippocampus (Rauch et al., 2006). In a healthy individual, fear-related amygdala activation is reduced by the vmPFC and hippocampus to prevent a prolonged and disadvantageous fear response. In contrast to psychiatrically healthy people, anxious patients may be unable to activate the vmPFC and hippocampus, leading to inappropriate fear responses characterized by an inability to suppress attention to fearful stimuli and an overgeneralization of fear to non-threatening stimuli (Figure 2.1).

Multiple clinical, psychophysiological, and neuroimaging studies support the amygdalocentric model of anxiety. To investigate abnormal fear processing in anxiety, investigators have used different paradigms designed to activate brain areas related to fear, including exposing PTSD patients to aversive and trauma-specific stimuli. Classical fear-conditioning paradigms have also been used to investigate fear processing in anxiety. In general, these studies demonstrate hyperactivation within the amygdala and attenuated activation in PFC and hippocampus in individuals with anxiety disorders compared to healthy controls.

Neurochemistry

Multiple lines of evidence implicate several neurochemical systems in the pathophysiology of anxiety disorders. These systems respond to stressful stimuli by releasing a variety of neurochemicals that mediate various intricate interactions between anxiety-processing neurocircuitry. Some of the chief neurochemical systems implicated in anxiety will now be briefly outlined.

Corticotropin-releasing hormone

Corticotropin-releasing hormone (CRH) is a polypeptide hormone secreted by the hypothalamus that is traditionally implicated as a cardinal neurochemical in an individual's physiological and behavioral responses to stress. CRH mediates stress activation of the hypothalamic–pituitary–adrenal (HPA) axis, a neuroendocrine system involved in stress, by stimulating the synthesis of adrenocorticotropic hormone (ACTH) in the pituitary gland, which ultimately leads to corticotropin and glucocorticoid release (Bonfiglio et al., 2011). CRH neurons are distributed throughout the brain; however, with regard to stress, a particular CRH circuit has been theorized. This circuit originates in the lateral hypothalamus, dorsal raphe, and the central nucleus of the amygdala (CeA) (Lee & Davis, 1997), which then projects to the bed nucleus of stria terminalis (BNST), which then in turn signals the paraventricular nucleus of the hypothalamus (PVN), activating the HPA axis. In response to stressful stimuli, CRH levels increase and exert their effect by activating CRH_1 and CRH_2, G-coupled protein receptors throughout the brain, to mediate an adaptive physiological and behavioral response (Bonfiglio et al., 2011).

Multiple lines of evidence from animal models indicate that there are functional differences between CRH_1 and CRH_2 activation. Injections of CRH into rodent brains or mice reveal over-expression of CRH, the animals displaying anxiety-like behavior such as psychomotor agitation, decreased appetite, sleep disturbances, decreased sexual interest, etc. (Heinrichs & Koob, 2004). CRH_1

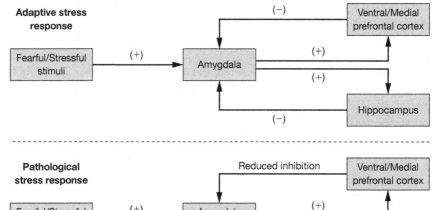

FIG. 2.1 The Amygdalocentric Model of Stress.

(Top) Fearful or stressful stimuli cause activation of the amygdala, whose activation leads to higher processing of the stimuli in the hippocampus and ventral/medial prefrontal cortex (vmPFC), which in turn act directly on the amygdala to reduce its activation and mediate an adaptive response to threat.

(Bottom) The amygdala is hyperresponsive to the fearful or stressful stimuli and the hippocampus and vmPFC are unable to reduce or inhibit its activation, leading to anxious symptoms.

receptor knockout mice displayed decreased anxiety-like behaviors and attenuated stress responses, indicating the CRH_1 receptor's role in controlling anxiety behaviors and its potential as a novel anxiolytic drug target for pharmacological antagonism (Holsboer & Ising, 2008). Conversely, CRH_2 receptor knockout mice display increased anxiety-like behaviors; however, the role of these receptors in stress and anxiety is not currently clear (Bale et al., 2000).

In humans, CRH elevation occurs in response to stress; however, early life exposure can produce chronically elevated CRH levels and increased sensitivity to stressful stimuli (DeSantis et al., 2011). The individual response, however, is variable and depends on socioeconomic factors and trauma history, meaning that those with early life stress may be at higher risk for psychiatric illness but do not necessarily end up in a pathological state (De Young, Kenardy, & Cobham, 2011). Several clinical studies indicate that CRH is elevated in depression and anxiety disorders. For instance, increased CRH in CSF- and CRH-producing neurons in the hypothalamus have been found in patients with major depression (Merali et al., 2004). Similar elevations in CSF CRH levels have been observed in PTSD patients compared to healthy controls. CRH_1 receptors remain a target of interest for the treatment of depression and anxiety disorders; however, data from CRH-modulating drug studies are limited; thus, further experimentation will be needed before efficacious and effective treatments are developed (Ising & Holsboer, 2007).

Cortisol

Cortisol is a glucocorticoid, a class of steroid hormone, released from the zona fasciculata of the adrenal gland in response to stressful stimuli (Radley et al., 2011). The release of cortisol is controlled by the HPA axis. As already described, CRH secretion by the hypothalamus triggers the release of ACTH from the pituitary gland, which subsequently travels through the blood to the adrenal gland, resulting in glucocorticoid secretion. Cortisol has a multitude of functions in the body, including suppression of the immune response, increasing blood glucose levels, and aiding metabolism. Of greater interest in recent years is cortisol's role in an adaptive response to stress. Cortisol is secreted during the body's "fight or flight" response to danger or threat (Korte, Koolhaas, Wingfield, & McEwen, 2005). The transient release of cortisol during a response to stressful or fearful stimuli results in several advantageous changes to aid in survival, substantiated by several lines of clinical evidence, such as increased energy, resourceful emotional memory encoding, hypervigilance, and heightened attention (Munck, Guyre, & Holbrook, 1984). While the release of cortisol to mediate an adaptive response to danger is beneficial in the short term, high levels of cortisol in the long term can have harmful physical and psychological effects.

During an adaptive, non-pathological response to threat, cortisol release is inhibited through a negative feedback loop in which cortisol binds to receptors on the hypothalamus to inactivate the HPA axis and the consequent release of cortisol (Munck et al., 1984). When negative feedback fails and cortisol secretion persists, several pathologies can result, such as compromised immune function, hypertension, obesity, lipid imbalance, cardiovascular diseases, and osteoporosis (Karlamangla, Singer, McEwen, Rowe, & Seeman 2002). Prolonged cortisol exposure also alters neuronal survival and morphology, with particular neurotoxicity in the hippocampus (Tang, Kenyon, Seckl, & Nyirenda, 2011). For example, magnetic resonance imaging (MRI) has revealed that patients with Cushing's disease, which involves excessive prolonged cortisol release, have reductions in hippocampal volume and display declarative memory impairment (Starkman, Gebarski, Berent, & Schteingart, 1992). Cortisol levels in anxiety disorders are incompletely understood. Some studies have reported normal or decreased serum and urine cortisol levels in PTSD patients and HPA axis hyperreactivity in panic disorder patients following stress-related stimuli (reviewed by Yehuda & Seckl, 2011). These decreased cortisol levels are hypothesized to represent a predisposition toward developing PTSD (Yehuda & Seckl, 2011). The link between cortisol levels and the pathophysiology of PTSD and other anxiety disorders is complicated by some rare findings of elevated cortisol levels in PTSD (Radley et al., 2011). Cortisol remains an intriguing target toward understanding the complex pathophysiology of anxiety disorders and could represent a novel therapeutic target for anxiety disorders.

Dopamine

Dopamine (DA) is a catecholamine that serves as a neurotransmitter in the brain. DA is involved in several emotional processes, such as mood, memory, and attention, and plays a major role in the brain's reward system. Dopaminergic neurons originate in the substantia nigra, ventral tegmental area (VTA), and hypothalamus, and divide into four pathways: the mesocortical, mesolimbic, nigrostriatal, and tuberoinfundibular pathways. In response to stressful stimuli, DA metabolism is increased in the prefrontal cortex and decreased in the nucleus accumbens. Animal models of depression have shown that stressed mice that display depressive symptoms have high prefrontal DA metabolism and low metabolism in the nucleus accumbens (Ventura, Cabib, & Puglisi-Allegra, 2002); however, lesioning studies have shown that low DA metabolism in the prefrontal cortex inhibits fear extinction (Morrow, Elsworth, Rasmusson, & Roth, 1999). From this evidence, it appears that dopamine must remain within a narrow range; high DA leads to depressive behaviors, and low DA inhibits extinction (Amiel et al., 2009). DA is hypothesized to be necessary to preserve reward function in the nucleus accumbens while allowing aversive memories to be extinguished (Fricks-Gleason, Khalaj, & Marshall, 2012).

Human studies have not provided much insight into DA dysfunction in anxiety; however, genetic association studies have identified genetic polymorphisms in an enzyme involved in DA metabolism which are associated with high incidences of certain anxious phenotypes (McGrath et al., 2004; Rothe et al., 2006).

γ-Aminobutyric acid

γ-Aminobutyric acid (GABA) is the chief inhibitory neurotransmitter of the central nervous system. GABA exerts its inhibitory effect by binding to specific pre- and postsynaptic receptors, causing ion channels to open up and to let negatively charged chloride ions enter the cell and positively charged potassium ions to flow out of the cell. This combination of chloride influx and potassium efflux leads to the hyperpolarization of the cell or inhibition (Watanabe, Maemura, Kanbara, Tamayama, & Hayasaki, 2002). The $GABA_A$ and $GABA_C$ receptors are ligand-activated chloride channels, and $GABA_B$ receptors are G-coupled protein receptors that can open or close these channels (Schwartz, 1988). GABA's inhibitory effect largely counteracts the excitatory effect of glutamate, another neurotransmitter released in excess in response to stress, indicating its role in anxiety disorders (Nemeroff, 2003a).

Benzodiazepines, a type of anxiolytic drug, have been shown to enhance the inhibitory effect of GABA through binding to $GABA_A$ receptors, resulting in prolonged opening of chloride channels and thereby reducing neuronal excitability (Nemeroff, 2003b). Furthermore, GABA's anxiolytic effect has been supported by PET data showing decreased $GABA_A$ receptor binding in patients with panic disorder (Malizia et al., 1998). In addition, lower plasma GABA plasma and CSF levels have been also reported in certain patients with major depression, leading some to hypothesize that low GABA may represent a vulnerability to developing mood and anxiety disorders.

Glutamate

In contrast to GABA, glutamate serves as the major excitatory neurotransmitter of the central nervous system. Glutamate is involved in mechanisms of synaptic plasticity such as long-term potentiation and depression (Stanton, 1996). Because of its involvement in plasticity, glutamate is also involved in learning and memory. Glutamatergic pyramidal cells innervate brain regions involved in mediating responses to anxiety in fear such as the amygdala, hippocampus, and anterior cingulate cortex (McDonald, 1996). In pathological anxiety states, glutamate is released in concert with increased glucocorticoid levels. This excess release of glutamate exerts a neurotoxic effect on the brain by increasing intracellular calcium levels, particularly in the hippocampus (Sapolsky, 2003). The neurotoxic effects of glutamate often lead to neuronal atropy in the hippocampus. For example, animal studies have shown that repeated stress leads to decreased dendritic branching and neural regeneration in the hippocampus. Furthermore, multiple clinical studies have shown decreased hippocampal density in patients with PTSD (Bremner et al., 2003). Drugs that act on glutamate have also provided support for its role in anxiety. Specifically, psychoactive drugs that are believed to modulate glutamate have been shown to be anxiolytic in a variety of anxiety disorders (Bremner et al., 2004; Coric et al., 2005). The mechanism of these compounds is not yet understood; however, there is ongoing research into new glutamate-modulating drugs and applications, and the mechanisms of gluamatergic dysfunction in the pathophysiology of anxiety disorders.

Noradrenaline/norepinephrine

Noradrenaline or norepinephrine (NE) is a catecholamine that functions as a hormone and a neurotransmitter. As a neurotransmitter, NE is released in response to stressful stimuli and affects a variety of body systems throughout the central nervous system and cardiovascular system. Specifically, it directly causes increased heart rate, along with increasing energy utilization, during the "fight or flight" response (Guyton & Hall, 2006). In the brain, NE is synthesized in the adrenal medulla, post-ganglionic neurons of the sympathetic nervous system, and the locus coeruleus, a region of the brain stem and the origin of norepinephrine pathways in the central nervous system. Pathways from the locus coeruleus act on adrenergic receptors in regions of the limbic system and cerebral cortex (O'Donnell, Hegadoren, & Coupland, 2004). In response to threat, the locus coeruleus is activated by the amygdala and hypothalamus. NE is then released and stimulates several limbic and cortical regions to mediate an appropriate adaptive response to threatening stimuli. Clinical studies demonstrate that an exaggerated release of NE in response to threat results in anxiety symptoms such as panic attacks, hyperarousal, exaggerated startle, and insomnia (reviewed by Southwick et al., 1999).

The development of pathological anxiety with respect to the noradrenergic system is hypothesized to occur through sensitization of the locus coeruleus. Sensitization is a process that occurs when a receptor, in this case adrenergic receptor, is more apt to respond to particular stimuli after repeated stimulation of the receptor. The locus coeruleus is sensitized by repeated exposure to fearful or threatening stimuli, resulting in increased NE release when presented with a subsequent negative stimulus (Simson & Weiss, 1988). Patients with PTSD often have psychiatric histories filled with multiple traumatic events. Multiple trauma exposures are regarded as a risk factor for the development of PTSD, which is largely in line with the aforementioned hypothesis of sensitization within the locus coeruleus (O'Donnell et al., 2004). Other risk factors related to the noradrenergic system in developing anxiety are related to a genetic polymorphism in a gene encoding in a particular adrenergic receptor.

In short, individuals who possess this genetic deletion have higher levels of NE release and anxiety when the system is pharmacologically activated, and a distinct pattern of neural activation in the limbic system, amygdala, and its related regions (Neumeister et al., 2005, 2006). These findings suggest that perhaps this polymorphism may be a crucial predictor of the development of depression and anxiety disorders after exposure to repeated stress.

Neuropeptide Y

Neuropeptide Y (NPY) is a polypeptide with several functions in the central nervous system such as inflammatory response, tissue growth, energy, sleep regulation, and the stress response. The role of NPY in the pathophysiology of anxiety disorders has been of increasing interest in recent years. In response to stress, NPY is released and believed to mediate an appropriate adaptive reaction to fear through inhibition of the stress response (reviewed by Wu et al., 2011). Intracerebroventricular (ICV) administration of NPY into the central nervous system of rats provided the most compelling evidence of the anxiolytic effect of NPY. For example, in several animal models of anxiety, rats receiving ICV NPY have shown decreased fear-potentiated startle, and more exploratory behaviors in light–dark compartment paradigms, which are behaviors that are indicative of decreased anxiety (Broqua, Wettstein, Rocher, Gauthier-Martin, & Junien, 1995). Animal models of PTSD have shown that rats with PTSD-like symptoms have lower levels of central nervous system NPY. In addition, these PTSD symptoms can be reduced through central administration of NPY (Cohen et al., 2012).

The anxiolytic effects of NPY appear to be mediated by NPY binding to the Y1 NPY receptor. Central administration of Y1 receptor antagonists induces anxiety-like behaviors in rats (Sajdyk, Vandergriff, & Gehlert, 1999). Furthermore, Y1 knockout mice do not experience reductions in anxiety-like symptoms after NPY administration, demonstrating that the Y1 receptor is crucial for NPY's anxiolytic effect (Karlsson et al., 2008). The Y2 receptor is another NPY receptor that is believed to be involved in modulating anxiety; however, its role is incompletely understood.

Multiple clinical studies have helped to elucidate NPY's role in the pathophysiology of anxiety disorders. Patients with PTSD have been shown to possess lower plasma NPY levels and, more recently, lower cerebrospinal fluid NPY levels than healthy controls (Sah et al., 2009). Higher plasma NPY levels have also been found in combat-exposed veterans without PTSD than in other combat-exposed veterans with PTSD (Yehuda & Seckl, 2011). This finding not only highlights the role of NPY in anxiety but also suggests its involvement in resilience to anxiety and possibly recovery from psychiatric illness. Finally, evidence of lower levels of NPY in prior trauma exposure in soldiers has led to the hypothesis that neurobiological differences in NPY may predispose some individuals to developing anxiety disorders (Morgan, 2001).

Serotonin

Serotonin (5-hydroxytryptamine, 5-HT) is a monoamine neurotransmitter found throughout the body, such as in the gastrointestinal tract, blood platelets, and the central nervous system. Multiple lines of evidence suggest that 5-HT possesses both anxiogenic and anxiolytic properties (Graeff, 2004). The differential effect of 5-HT is dependent upon the brain region and the receptor subtype that it affects. In response to stress, 5-HT's turnover rate increases in the amygdala, hypothalamus, nucleus accumbens, and prefrontal cortex (Amiel et al., 2009). It is hypothesized that in the amygdala and prefrontal cortex, 5-HT augments learned responses to threatening stimuli, and in the midbrain it inhibits unconditioned response threat (Graeff, 2004). The role of 5-HT in the development of anxiety disorders is not well understood; however, it appears that dysfunction of 5-HT modifies the function of related neurotransmitters, which may contribute to the pathogenesis of anxiety disorders.

With regard to receptor function, stimulation of the 5-HT_{2A} receptor is considered to be anxiogenic and stimulation of the 5-HT_{1A} receptor is anxiolytic (Graeff, 2004). 5-HT_{1A} receptor knockout mice display more anxious behaviors compared to control mice, indicating that this receptor plays a critical role in mediating an appropriate response to fear (Olivier et al., 2001). As in animal models of anxiety, clinical studies have demonstrated altered 5-HT receptor expression that is related to anxious behaviors (Akimova, Lanzenberger, & Kasper, 2009). Specifically, PET receptor imaging revealed lower 5-HT_{1A} receptor density in the amygdala and anterior cingulate gyrus of patients with panic disorder and social anxiety disorder (Nash et al., 2008; Neumeister et al., 2004).

There is also strong evidence that the 5-HT transporter (5-HTT) also plays a crucial role in the pathophysiology of anxiety disorders. Polymorphisms exist in the promoter region of the gene that encodes the 5-HTT. This polymorphism has traditionally been recognized as existing in two variations: either a short (S) or long (L) allele (reviewed by Daniele et al., 2011). The S carriers exhibit lower expression of the 5-HTT, reduced reuptake of 5-HT and exaggerated amygdala activation in response to fearful stimuli (Hariri et al., 2005). In addition, S carriers are hypothesized to be more vulnerable to developing depression and anxiety disorders, especially if they are exposed to early-life stressors, and a higher occurrence of anxious phenotype (Caspi et al., 2003).

Reduced 5-HTT binding and reuptake of 5-HT in the amygdala, resulting from the S allele polymorphism, may play a role in the pathophysiology of PTSD. Specifically, altered 5-HTT functioning in the amygdala is hypothesized to lead to an increased acquisition of conditioned fears and decreased extinction (Lonsdorf et al., 2009). Recently, PET receptor imaging work has supported this hypothesis, revealing reduced amygdala 5-HTT binding in PTSD patients (Murrough et al., 2011). Some studies have presented conflicting evidence indicating a lack of any association between the S allele and anxiety (Gustavsson et al., 1999). However, it should be no surprise that consensus has not been reached on the role of the S allele in anxiety, because of the complexity and tremendous variability in the pathophysiology, presentation, and individual risk factors for developing anxiety disorders (Margoob & Mustaq, 2011).

SOCIAL RISK FACTORS

Individual Differences in Children

Anxiety disorders represent the most common psychiatric disorders in children and adolescents, with prevalence rates ranging from 2% to 17% (Rapee, Schniering, & Hudson, 2009). Once diagnosed, anxiety tends to persist throughout development and impacts children's psychosocial, academic, and vocational trajectories. A major focus of contemporary research on anxiety in children and adolescents is to identify the mechanisms that precede or maintain anxiety in order to develop effective prevention and treatment programs (Degnan, Almas, & Fox, 2010).

Behavioral inhibition

Behavioral inhibition is a component of temperament that concerns an individual's responsiveness to novelty and threat, negative emotionality, vigilant behavior in response to unfamiliar situations, and social withdrawal or reticence (Hane, Fox, Henderson, & Marshall, 2008; Calkins, Fox, & Marshall, 1996; Fox, Henderson, Rubin, Calkins, & Schmidt, 2001). Inhibition in early childhood has been linked to anxiety symptoms or a diagnosis of an anxiety disorder later in life (Biederman et al., 1990; Gladstone & Parker, 2005; Hirshfeld-Becker et al., 2007).

Though behavioral inhibition is generally a social quality, consistent inhibited behaviors can have biological implications. For example, fMRI studies of adolescents and adults with current or past patterns of behavioral inhibition revealed perturbations in amygdala functioning in response to emotionally relevant stimuli (Pérez-Edgar et al., 2007). In addition, inhibited children have been shown to display heightened autonomic activity in anxiety-inducing situations compared to uninhibited children (Schmidt, Fox, Schulkin, & Gold 1999).

Intuitively, it might seem that inhibited behaviors such as avoidance would decrease the fear response, but in fact they reinforce the associated physiological responses, perpetuating inhibition and social wariness (Degnan et al., 2010). These qualities, as components of the larger constellation of traits associated with behavioral inhibition, have significant implications for psychosocial functioning and could ultimately contribute to the development of anxiety-related psychopathology.

Parent–child attachment

In the mid 20th century, psychologist Mary Ainsworth devised the strange situation paradigm to evaluate children's attachment patterns with their primary caregivers (Ainsworth & Bell, 1970). In the strange situation, a child is placed in a room with the mother and a female stranger. The mother then leaves the child alone with the stranger and returns several moments later. The way the child interacts with the mother when she returns reveals the child's style of attachment, which can fall into one of three categories: secure, anxious/resistant, and anxious/avoidant. The latter two categories are classified as insecure attachment and have been shown to contribute to anxiety later in life (Colonnesi et al., 2011).

Children who have insecure attachment styles perceive their caregivers as inconsistent or unpredictable, and might overreact to distressing situations in order to safeguard the attention of their caregivers (Colonnesi et al., 2011). They might then transfer this pattern of behavior to different settings, reacting inappropriately in social interactions with adults or peers. While insecure attachment does not categorically determine later anxiety, it does influence patterns of social functioning in ways that can make individuals more vulnerable to anxiety symptoms. For example, children with insecure attachment patterns tend to experience more difficulty initiating friendships and resolving social issues compared to children with secure attachment patterns (Sroufe, Carlson, & Shulman, 1993). Insecurely attached children are more likely to be perceived as shy or aggressive and are more likely to be victimized or rejected by peers; girls in particular are more likely to be neglected by peers (Dykas, Ziv, & Cassidy, 2008). Childhood attachment patterns can also influence individuals later in life; adults who had insecure attachment patterns as children tend to have more negative self-esteem and difficulties in friendships and romantic relationships (McCarthy, 1999).

Negative life events

Traumatic life events in childhood, such as witnessing violence or experiencing physical abuse or neglect, are linked to the development of anxiety later in life. For example, child sexual abuse, a problem that affects tens of thousands of children in the United States annually, often results in the development of PTSD (Hornor, 2010). Negative social events, including peer rejection and bullying, have also been identified as a risk factors for anxiety (van Oort, Greaves-Lord, Ormel, Verhulst, & Huizink, 2011). Trauma exposure in adulthood is also correlated with the development anxiety.

CONCLUSION

Anxiety is a spectrum of intricate psychological, biological, and social processes that all must be considered when investigating its pathophysiology, risk factors, and treatment. Though research into anxiety has produced a vast array of knowledge about discrete phenomena, the challenge of developing a comprehensive and integrative view of anxiety is ongoing. While many unanswered questioned still remain, it is important to acknowledge the tremendous growth of new information that has resulted from diverse research approaches in only the past few decades. We hope that this introduction has provided a framework to organize our current psychological, biological, and social theories of anxiety, piece together common themes within each field, and identify topics of interest that warrant further research.

Clinical Points to Remember

1. Fear conditioning, a type of classical conditioning whereby organisms learn relationships between stimuli and aversive events, forms the basis for much of contemporary research on anxiety in humans.
2. To interact successfully with its environment, an organism must acquire and store memories of various stimuli and the outcomes they predict. The amygdala and hippocampus are key brain structures where memory consolidation is localized.
3. The amygdalocentric model hypothesizes that the amygdala is hyperresponsive and lacks control by ventral/medial PFC and hippocampus in an anxious individual when they are presented with threatening or fearful stimuli, resulting in symptoms of hyperarousal.
4. Many neurochemical systems play a role in the pathophysiology of anxiety disorders. These systems respond to stressful stimuli by releasing a variety of neurochemicals that mediate various intricate interactions between anxiety-processing neurocircuitry.
5. Several lines of research, including imaging studies, indicate a relationship between dysregulation in neural fear-processing circuits and pathological anxiety.
6. Both biological and environmental factors are implicated in the development of pathological anxiety. The diathesis–stress model describes anxiety as the product of dispositional vulnerabilities and negative environmental circumstances or internal stressors.
7. Anxiety disorders represent the most common group of psychiatric disorders in children. Once diagnosed in childhood, pathological anxiety tends to persist throughout development.
8. Reconsolidation and extinction are critical concepts in understanding how and why anxiety disorders develop and persist.

REFERENCES

Acheson, D. T., Forsyth, J. P., & Moses, E. (2012). Interoceptive fear conditioning and panic disorder: The role of conditioned stimulus-unconditioned stimulus predictability. *Behavior Therapy, 43*(1), 174–189.

Ainsworth, M. D. S., & Bell, S. M. (1970). Attachment, exploration, and separation: Illustrated by the behavior of one-year-olds in a strange situation. *Child Development, 41,* 49–67.

Akimova, E., Lanzenberger, R., & Kasper, S. (2009). The serotonin-1A receptor in anxiety disorders. *Biological Psychiatry, 66,* 627–635.

Akirav, I. (2007). NMDA partial agonist reverses blocking of extinction of aversive memory by GABA(A) agonist in the amygdala. *Neuropsychopharmacology, 32*(3), 542–550.

Amaral, O. B., & Roesler, R. (2008). Targeting the NMDA receptor for fear-related disorders. *Recent Patents in CNS Drug Discovery, 3*(3), 166–178.

American Psychiatric Association (APA). (2000). *Diagnostic and statistical manual of mental disorders* (4th ed., text revision). Washington, DC: APA.

Amiel, J. M., Mathew, S. J., Garakani, A., Neumeister, A., & Charney, D. S. (2009). Neurobiology of anxiety disorders. In C. B. Nemiroff & A. F. Schatzberg (Eds.), *The American Psychiatric Publishing textbook of psychopharmacology* (4th ed.). Washington, DC: American Psychiatric Publishing.

Bale, T. L., Contarino, A., Smith, G. W., Chan, R., Gold, L. H., Sawchenko, P. E., et al. (2000). Mice deficient for corticotropin-releasing hormone receptor-2 display anxiety-like behaviour and are hypersensitive to stress. *Nature Genetics, 24,* 410–414.

Bechara, A., Tranel, D., Damasio, H., Adolphs, R., Rockland, C., & Damasio, A. R. (1995). Double dissociation of conditioning and declarative knowledge relative to the amygdala and hippocampus in humans. *Science, 269*(5227), 1115–1118.

Beckers, T., Krypotos, A. M., Boddez, Y., Effting, M., & Kindt, M. (in press). What's wrong with fear conditioning? *Biological Psychology.*

Biederman, J., Rosenbaum, J. F., Hirshfeld, D. R., Faraone, S. V., Bolduc, E. A., Gersten, M., et al. (1990). Psychiatric correlates of behavioral inhibition in young children of parents with and without psychiatric disorders. *Archives of General Psychiatry, 47,* 21–26.

Bonfiglio, J., Inda, C., Refojob, D., Holsboerb, F., Arzta, E., & Silberstain, S. (2011). The corticotropin-releasing hormone network and the hypothalamic–pituitary–adrenal axis: Molecular and cellular mechanisms involved. *Neuroendocrinology, 94,* 12–20.

Bonne, O., Vythilingam, M., Inagaki, M., Wood, S., Neumeister, A., Nugent, A. C., et al. (2008). Reduced posterior hippocampal volume in posttraumatic stress disorder. *Journal of Clinical Psychiatry, 69*(7), 1087–1091.

Bremner, J. D., Vythilingam, M., Vermetten, E., Southwick, S. M., McGlashan, T., Nazeer, A., et al. (2003). MRI and PET study of deficits in hippocampal structure and function in women with childhood sexual abuse and posttraumatic stress disorder. *American Journal of Psychiatry, 160,* 924–932.

Bremner, J. D., Mletzko, T., Welter, S., Siddiq, S., Reed, L., Williams, C., et al. (2004). Treatment of post-traumatic stress disorder with phenytoin: An open label pilot study. *Neuropsychopharmacology, 29,* S91.

Broqua, P., Wettstein, J. G., Rocher, M. N., Gauthier-Martin, B., & Junien, J. L. (1995). Behavioral effects of neuropeptide Y receptor agonists in the elevated plusmaze and fear-potentiated startle procedures. *Behavioural Pharmacology, 6*, 215–222.

Büchel, C., Dolan, R. J., Armony, J. L., & Friston, K. J. (1999). Amygdala–hippocampal involvement in human aversive trace conditioning revealed through eventrelated functional magnetic resonance imaging. *Journal of Neuroscience, 19*(24), 10869–10876.

Calkins, S. D., Fox, N. A., & Marshall, T. R. (1996). Behavioral and physiological antecedents of inhibited and uninhibited behavior. *Child Development, 67*(2), 523–540.

Calkins, A. W., Otto, M. W., Cohen, L. S., Soares, C. N., Vitonis, A. F., Hearon, B. A., & Harlow, B. L. (2009). Psychosocial predictors of the onset of anxiety disorders in women: Results from a prospective 3-year longitudinal study. *Journal of Anxiety Disorders, 23*(8), 1165–1169.

Cannon, W. B. (1929). *Bodily changes in pain, hunger, fear, and rage*. New York: D. Appleton.

Caspi, A., Sugden, K., Moffitt, T. E., Taylor, A., Craig, I. W., Harrington, H., et al. (2003). Influence of life stress on depression: Moderation by a polymorphism in the 5-HTT gene. *Science, 301*, 386–389.

Chambless, D. L., Hunter, K., & Jackson, A. (1982). Social anxiety and assertiveness: A comparison of the correlations in phobic and college student samples. *Behaviour Research and Therapy, 20*(4), 403–404.

Cohen, H., Liu, T., Kozlovsky, N., Kaplan, Z., Zohar, J., & Mathé, A. (2012). The neuropeptide Y (NPY)-ergic system is associated with behavioral resilience to stress exposure in an animal model of post-traumatic stress disorder. *Neuropsychopharmacology, 37*, 350–363.

Colonnesi, C., Draijer, E. M., Jan, J. M., Stams, G., Van der Bruggen, C. O., Bögels, S. M., & Noom, M. J. (2011). The relation between insecure attachment and child anxiety: A meta-analytic review. *Journal of Clinical Child and Adolescent Psychology, 40*, 630–645.

Coric, V., Taskiran, S., Pittenger, C., Wasylink, S., Mathalon, D. H., Saksa, J., et al. (2005). Riluzole augmentation in treatment-resistant obsessive-compulsive disorder: An open-label trial. *Biological Psychiatry, 58*, 424–428.

Cowan, N. (2001). The magical number 4 in short-term memory: A reconsideration of mental storage capacity. *Behavioral and Brain Sciences, 24*(1), 87–114.

Daniele, A., Divella, R., Paradiso, A., Mattioli, V., Romito, F., Giotta, F., et al. (2011). Serotonin transporter polymorphism in major depressive disorder (MDD), psychiatric disorders, and in MDD in response to stressful life events: Causes and treatment with antidepressant. *In Vivo, 25*, 895–901.

Debiec, J., & Ledoux, J. E. (2004). Disruption of reconsolidation but not consolidation of auditory fear conditioning by noradrenergic blockade in the amygdala. *Neuroscience, 129*(2), 267–272.

Degnan, K. A., Almas, A. N., & Fox, N. A. (2010). Temperament and the environment in the etiology of childhood anxiety. *Journal of Child Psychology and Psychiatry, 51*, 497–517.

Demirkan, A., Penninx, B. W., Hek, K., Wray, N. R., Amin, N., Aulchenko, Y. S., et al. (2011). Genetic risk profiles for depression and anxiety in adult and elderly cohorts. *Molecular Psychiatry, 16*(7), 773–783.

DeSantis, S. M., Baker, N. L., Back, S. E., Spratt, E., Ciolino, J. D., Moran-Santa Maria, M., et al. (2011). Gender differences in the effect of early life trauma on hypothalamic–pituitary–adrenal axis functioning. *Depression and Anxiety, 28,* 383–392.

De Young, A. C., Kenardy, J. A., & Cobham, V. E. (2011). Trauma in early childhood: A neglected population. *Clinical Child and Family Psychology Review, 14,* 231–250.

Dykas, M. J., Ziv, Y., & Cassidy J. (2008). Attachment and peer relations in adolescence. *Attachment and Human Development, 10,* 123–141.

Enns, M. W., & Cox, B. J. (2002). The nature and assessment of perfectionism: A critical analysis. In G. L. Flett & P. L. Hewitt (Eds.), *Perfectionism: Theory, research and treatment* (pp. 33–63). Washington, DC: American Psychological Association.

Falls, W. A., Miserendino, M. J., & Davis, M. (1992). Extinction of fear-potentiated startle: blockade by infusion of an NMDA antagonist into the amygdala. *Journal of Neuroscience, 12(3),* 854–863.

Fox, N. A., Henderson, H. A., Rubin, K. H., Calkins, S. D., & Schmidt, L. A. (2001). Continuity and discontinuity of behavioral inhibition and exuberance: Psychophysiological and behavioral influences across the first four years of life. *Child Development, 72(1),* 1–21.

Fricks-Gleason, A. N., Khalaj, A. J., & Marshall, J. F. (2012). Dopamine D1 receptor antagonism impairs extinction of cocaine-cue memories. *Behavioural Brain Research, 226,* 357–360.

Gladstone, G., & Parker, G. (2005). Measuring a behaviorally inhibited temperament style: Development and initial validation of new self-report measures. *Psychiatry Research, 135,* 133–143.

Graeff, F. G. (2004). Serotonin, the periaqueductal gray and panic. *Neuroscience and Biobehavioral Reviews, 28,* 239–259.

Gustavsson, J. P., Nöthen, M. M., Jönsson, E. G., Neidt, H., Forslund, K., Rylander, G., et al. (1999). No association between serotonin transporter gene polymorphisms and personality traits. *American Journal of Medical Genetics, 88,* 430–436.

Guyton, A., & Hall, J. (2006). Chapter 10: Rhythmical excitation of the heart. In R. Gruliow (Ed.), *Textbook of medical physiology* (11th ed., p. 122). Philadelphia: Elsevier.

Hane, A. A., Fox, N. A., Henderson, H. A., & Marshall, P. J. (2008). Behavioral reactivity and approach-withdrawal bias in infancy. *Developmental Psychology, 44(5),* 1491–1496.

Hariri, A. R., Drabant, E. M., Munoz, K. E., Kolachana, B. S., Mattay, V. S., Egan, M. F., & Weinberger, D. R. (2005). A susceptibility gene for affective disorders and the response of the human amygdala. *Archives of General Psychiatry, 62,* 146–152.

Hartley, C. A., & Phelps, E. A. (2010). Changing fear: The neurocircuitry of emotional regulation. *Neuropsychopharmacology, 35(1),* 136–146.

Heinrichs, S. C., & Koob, G. F. (2004). Corticotropin-releasing factor in brain: A role in activation, arousal, and affect regulation. *Journal of Pharmacology and Experimental Therapeutics, 311,* 427–440.

Hirshfeld-Becker, D. R., Biederman, J., Henin, A., Faraone, S. V., Davis, S., Harrington, K., & Rosenbaum, J. F. (2007). Behavioral inhibition in preschool children at risk is a specific predictor of middle childhood social anxiety: A five-year follow-up. *Journal of Developmental and Behavioral Pediatrics, 28,* 225–233.

Holsboer, F., & Ising, M. (2008). Central CRH system in depression and anxiety: Evidence from clinical studies with CRH1 receptor antagonists. *European Journal of Pharmacology, 583,* 350–357.

Hornor, G. (2010). Child sexual abuse: Consequences and implications. *Journal of Pediatric Health Care, 24,* 358–364.

Ising, M., & Holsboer, F. (2007). CRH1 receptor antagonists for the treatment of depression and anxiety. *Experimental and Clinical Psychopharmacology, 15,* 519–528.

Kahn, R. S., van Praag, H. M., Wetzler, S., Asnis, G. M., & Barr, G. (1988). Serotonin and anxiety revisited. *Biological Psychiatry, 23,* 189–208.

Karlamangla, A. S., Singer, B. H., McEwen, B. S., Rowe, J. W., & Seeman, T. E. (2002). Allostatic load as a predictor of functional decline: MacArthur studies of successful aging. *Journal of Clinical Epidemiology, 55,* 696–710.

Karlsson, R. M., Choe, J. S., Cameron, H. A., Thorsell, A., Crawley, J. N., Holmes, A., & Heilig, M. (2008). The neuropeptide Y Y1 receptor subtype is necessary for the anxiolytic-like effects of neuropeptide Y, but not the antidepressant-like effects of fluoxetine, in mice. *Psychopharmacology, 195,* 547–557.

Kent, J. M., & Rauch, S. L. (2003). Neurocircuitry of anxiety disorders. *Current Psychiatry Reports, 5*(4), 266–273.

Kindt, M., Soeter, M., & Vervliet, B. (2009). Beyond extinction: Erasing human fear responses and preventing the return of fear. *Nature Neuroscience, 12*(3), 256–258.

Korte, S. M., Koolhaas, J. M., Wingfield, J. C., & McEwen, B. S. (2005). The Darwinian concept of stress: Benefits of allostasis and costs of allostatic load and the trade-offs in health and disease. *Neuroscience and Biobehavioral Reviews, 29,* 3–38.

Langton, J. M., & Richardson, R. (2008). D-Cycloserine facilitates extinction the first time but not the second time: An examination of the role of NMDA across the course of repeated extinction sessions. *Neuropsychopharmacology, 33*(13), 3096–3102.

LeDoux, J. (2003). The emotional brain, fear, and the amygdala. *Cellular and Molecular Neurobiology, 23,* 727–738.

Lee, Y., & Davis, M. (1997). Role of the hippocampus, the bed nucleus of the stria terminalis, and the amygdala in the excitatory effect of corticotropin-releasing hormone on the acoustic startle reflex. *Journal of Neuroscience, 17,* 6434–6445.

Lewis, D. J., Bregman, N. J., & Mahan, J. J. (1972). Cue-dependent amnesia in rats. *Journal of Comparative and Physiological Psychology, 81*(2), 243–247.

Linnman, C., Zeidan, M. A., Furtak, S. C., Pitman, R. K., Quirk, G. J., & Milad, M. R. (2012). Resting amygdala and medial prefrontal metabolism predicts functional activation of the fear extinction circuit. *American Journal of Psychiatry, 169*(4), 415–423.

Lonsdorf, T. B., Weike, A. I., Nikamo, P., Schalling, M., Hamm, A., & Ohman, A. (2009). Genetic gating of human fear learning and extinction: Possible implications for gene–environment interaction in anxiety disorder. *Psychological Science, 20,* 198–206.

Malenka, R. C., & Bear, M. F. (2004). LTP and LTD: An embarrassment of riches. *Neuron, 44*(1), 5–21.

Malizia, A. L., Cunningham, V. J., Bell, C. J., Liddle, P. F., Jones, T., & Nutt, D. J. (1998). Decreased brain GABA(A)–benzodiazepine receptor binding in panic disorder: Preliminary results from a quantitative PET study. *Archives of General Psychiatry, 55,* 715–720.

Margoob, M. A., & Mushtaq, D. (2011). Serotonin transporter gene polymorphism and psychiatric disorders: Is there a link? *Indian Journal of Psychiatry, 53,* 289–299.

McCarthy, G. (1999). Attachment style and adult love relationships and friendships: A study of a group of women at risk of experiencing relationship difficulties. *British Journal of Medical Psychology, 72,* 305–321.

McDonald, A. J. (1996). Glutamate and aspartate immunoreactive neurons of the rat basolateral amygdala: Colocalization of excitatory amino acids and projections to the limbic circuit. *Journal of Comparative Neurology, 365*, 367–379.

McGrath, M., Kawachi, I., Ascherio, A., Colditz, G. A., Hunter, D. J., & De Vivo, I. (2004). Association between catechol-O-methyltransferase and phobic anxiety. *American Journal of Psychiatry, 161*, 1703–1705.

Merali, Z., Du, L., Hrdina, P., Palkovits, M., Faludi, G., Poulter, M. O., & Anisman, H. (2004). Dysregulation in the suicide brain: mRNA expression of corticotropin-releasing hormone receptors and GABA$_A$ receptor subunits in frontal cortical brain region. *Journal of Neuroscience, 24*, 1478–1485.

Miller, G. (1956). The magical number seven plus or minus two: Some limits on our capacity for processing information. *Psychological Review, 101*(2), 81–97.

Mineka, S., & Oehlberg, K. (2008). The relevance of recent developments in classical conditioning to understanding the etiology and maintenance of anxiety disorders. *Acta Psychologia (Amsterdam), 127*(3), 567–580.

Morgan, C. A. (2001). Relationship among plasma cortisol, catecholamines, neuropeptide Y, and human performance during exposure to uncontrollable stress. *Psychosomatic Medicine, 63*, 412–422.

Morrow, B. A., Elsworth, J. D., Rasmusson, A. M., & Roth, R. H. (1999). The role of mesoprefrontal dopamine neurons in the acquisition and expression of conditioned fear in the rat. *Neuroscience, 92*, 553–564.

Moser, J. S., Slane, J. D., Alexandra, B. S., & Klump, K. L. (2012). Etiologic relationships between anxiety and dimensions of maladaptive perfectionism in young adult female twins. *Depression and Anxiety, 29*(1), 47–53.

Munck, A., Guyre, P. M., & Holbrook, N. J. (1984). Physiological functions of glucocorticoids in stress and their relations to pharmacological actions. *Endocrine Reviews, 5*, 25–44.

Murrough, J. W., Huang, Y., Hu, J., Henry, S., Williams, W., Gallezot, J. D., et al. (2011). Reduced amygdala serotonin transporter binding in posttraumatic stress disorder. *Biological Psychiatry, 70*, 1033–1038.

Nash, J. R., Sargent, P. A., Rabiner, E. A., Hood, S. D., Argyropoulos, S. V., Potokar, J. P., et al. (2011). Serotonin 5-HT1A receptor binding in people with panic disorder: Positron emission tomography study. *British Journal of Psychiatry, 193*, 229–234.

National Institute of Mental Health. (2008). *Posttraumatic stress disorder.* DHHS Publication No. ADM 08-3561. Washington, DC: U.S. Government Printing Office.

Nemeroff, C. B. (2003). Anxiolytics: Past, present, and future agents. *Journal of Clinical Psychiatry, 64*, 3–6.

Nemeroff, C. B. (2003). The role of GABA in the pathophysiology and treatment of anxiety disorders. *Psychopharmacology Bulletin, 37*(4), 133–146.

Neumeister, A., Bain, E., Nugent, A. C., Carson, R. E., Bonne, O., Luckenbaugh, D. A., et al. (2004). Reduced serotonin type 1A receptor binding in panic disorder. *Journal of Neuroscience, 24*, 589–591.

Neumeister, A., Charney, D. S., Belfer, I., Geraci, M., Holmes, C., Sharabi, Y., et al. (2005). Sympathoneural and adrenomedullary functional effects of alpha2C-adrenoreceptor gene polymorphism in healthy humans. *Pharmacogenetics and Genomics, 15*, 143–149.

Neumeister, A., Drevets, W. C., Belfer, I., Luckenbaugh, D. A., Henry, S., Bonne, O., et al. (2006). Effects of a alpha2C-adrenoreceptor gene polymorphism on neural responses to facial expressions in depression. *Neuropsychopharmacology,* *31*, 1750–1756.

O'Connor, R., Rasmussen, S., & Hawton, K. (2010). Predicting depression, anxiety and self-harm in adolescents: The role of perfectionism and acute life stress. *Behaviour Research and Therapy, 48*(1), 52–59.

O'Donnell, T., Hegadoren, K. M., & Coupland, N. C. (2004). Noradrenergic mechanisms in the pathophysiology of post-traumatic stress disorder. *Neuropsychobiology, 50*, 273–283.

Olivier, B., Pattij, T., Wood, S. J., Oosting, R., Sarnyai, Z., & Toth, M. (2001). The 5-HT(1A) receptor knockout mouse and anxiety. *Behavioural Pharmacology, 12*, 439–450.

Pavlov, I. P. (1927). *Conditioned reflexes: An investigation of the physiological activity of the cerebral cortex* (translated by G. V. Anrep). London: Oxford University Press.

Pérez-Edgar, K., Roberson-Nay, R., Hardin, M. G., Poeth, K., Guyer, A. E., Nelson, E. E., et al. (2007). Attention alters neural responses to evocative faces in behaviorally inhibited adolescents. *Neuroimage, 35*, 1538–1546.

Radley, J. J., Kabbaj, M., Jacobson, L., Heydendael, W., Yehuda, R., & Herman, J. P (2011). Stress risk factors and stress-related pathology: Neuroplasticity, epigenetics and endophenotypes. *Stress, 14*, 481–497.

Rapee, R. M., Schniering, C. A., & Hudson, J. L. (2009). Anxiety disorders during childhood and adolescence: Origins and treatment. *Annual Review of Clinical Psychology, 5*, 311–341.

Rauch, S. L., Shin, L., & Phelps, E. (2006). Neurocircuitry models of posttraumatic stress disorder and extinction: Human neuroimaging research—past, present, and future. *Biological Psychiatry, 60*(4), 376.

Reiter, S. R., Otto, M. W., Pollack, M. H., & Rosenbaum, J. F. (1991). Major depression in panic disorder patients with comorbid social phobia. *Journal of Affective Disorders, 22*(3), 171–177.

Rosen, J. B., & Schulkin, J. (1998). From normal fear to pathological anxiety. *Psychology Review, 105*(2), 325–350.

Rothe, C., Koszycki, D., Bradwejn, J., King, N., Deluca, V., Tharmalingam, S., et al. (2006). Association of the Val158Met catechol O-methyltransferase genetic polymorphism with panic disorder. *Neuropsychopharmacology, 31*, 2237–2242.

Sah, R., Ekhator, N. N., Strawn, J. R., Sallee, F. R., Baker, D. G., Horn, P. S., & Geracioti, T. D. Jr. (2009). Low cerebrospinal fluid neuropeptide Y concentrations in post-traumatic stress disorder. *Biological Psychiatry, 66*(7), 705–707.

Sajdyk, T. J., Vandergriff, M. G., & Gehlert, D. R. (1999). Amygdalar neuropeptide Y Y1 receptors mediate the anxiolytic-like actions of neuropeptide Y in the social interaction test. *European Journal of Pharmacology, 368*, 143–147.

Sapolsky, R. M. (2003). Stress and plasticity in the limbic system. *Neurochemical Research, 28*, 1735–1742.

Schiller, D., Monfils, M.-H., Raio, C. M., Johnson, D. C., LeDoux, J. E., & Phelps, E. A. (2010). Preventing the return of fear in humans using reconsolidation update mechanisms. *Nature, 463*(7277), 49–53.

Schmidt, L. A., Fox, N. A., Schulkin, J., & Gold, P. W. (1999). Behavioral and psychophysiological correlates of self-presentation in temperamentally shy children. *Developmental Psychobiology, 35*, 119–135.

Schwartz, R. D. (1988). The GABA-A receptor-gated ion channel: Biochemical and pharmacological studies of structure and function. *Biochemical Pharmacology, 27,* 3369–3378.

Scoville, W. B., & Milner, B. (1957). Loss of recent memory after bilateral hippocampal lesions. *Journal of Neurology, Neurosurgery and Psychiatry, 20*(1), 11–21.

Simson, P. E., & Weiss, J. M. (1988). Altered activity of the locus coeruleus in an animal model of depression. *Neuropsychopharmacology, 1,* 287–295.

Southwick, S. M., Bremner, J. D., Rasmusson, A., Morgan, C. A., Arnsten, A., & Charney, D. S. (1999) Role of norepinephrine in the pathophysiology and treatment of posttraumatic stress disorder. *Biological Psychiatry, 46,* 1192–1204.

Sroufe, L. A., Carlson, E., & Shulman, S. (1993). Individuals in relationships: Development from infancy through adolescence. In D. Funder, R. Parke, C. Tomlinson-Keasey, & K. Widaman (Eds.), *Studying lives through time: Personality and development* (pp. 315–342). Washington, DC: American Psychological Association.

Stanton, P. K. (1996). LTD, LTP, and the sliding threshold for long-term synaptic plasticity. *Hippocampus, 6,* 35–42.

Starkman, M. N., Gebarski, S. S., Berent, S. S., & Schteingart, D. E. (1992). Hippocampal formation volume, memory dysfunction, and cortisol levels in patients with Cushing's syndrome. *Biological Psychiatry, 32,* 756–765.

Tang, J. I., Kenyon, C. J., Seckl, J. R., & Nyirenda, M. J. (2011). Prenatal overexposure to glucocorticoids programs renal 11β-hydroxysteroid dehydrogenase type 2 expression and salt-sensitive hypertension in the rat. *Journal of Hypertension, 29,* 282–289.

van Oort, F. V., Greaves-Lord, K., Ormel, J., Verhulst, F. C., & Huizink, A. C. (2011). Risk indicators of anxiety throughout adolescence: The TRAILS study. *Depression and Anxiety, 6,* 485–494.

Ventura, R., Cabib, S., & Puglisi-Allegra S. (2002). Genetic susceptibility of mesocortical dopamine to stress determines liability to inhibition of mesoaccumbens dopamine and to behavioral "despair" in a mouse model of depression. *Neuroscience, 115,* 999–1007.

Watanabe, M., Maemura, K., Kanbara, K., Tamayama, T., & Hayasaki, H. (2002). GABA and GABA receptors in the central nervous system and other organs. *International Review of Cytology, 213,* 1–47.

Watson, J. B., & Rayner, R. (1920). Conditioned emotional reactions. *Journal of Experimental Psychology, 3*(1), 1–14.

Weinstock, L. M., & Whisman, M. A. (2006). Neuroticism as a common feature of the depressive and anxiety disorders: A test of the revised integrative hierarchical model in a national sample. *Journal of Abnormal Psychology, 115,* 68–74.

Whitlock, J. R, Heynen, A. J., Shuler, M. G., & Bear, M. F. (2006). Learning induces long-term potentiation in the hippocampus. *Science, 5790,* 1093–1097.

Wu, G., Feder, A., Wegener, G., Bailey, C., Saxena, S., Charney, D., & Mathé, A. A. (2011). Central functions of neuropeptide Y in mood and anxiety disorders. *Expert Opinion on Therapeutic Targets, 15,* 1317–1331.

Yehuda, R., & Seckl, J. (2011). Minireview: Stress-related psychiatric disorders with low cortisol levels: A metabolic hypothesis. *Endocrinology, 152,* 4496–4503.

CHAPTER 3

Pharmacological Treatment of Anxiety Disorders Across the Lifespan

Robert M. Julien

HISTORY OF THE PHARMACOLOGICAL TREATMENT OF ANXIETY

The history of the pharmacological treatment of anxiety is both long (millennia), incredibly short, and continuing. For millennia, naturally occurring herbal substances (e.g., valerian, laudanum, and kava kava) and fermentation-derived alcohols (ethanol) have been used for amelioration of anxiety. For example, in Genesis (9:20–21) Noah planted a vineyard, drank of the fermented wine, became drunk, and was lying uncovered in his tent. While drunkenness was a "sin," moderate doses were anxiolytic and presumably socially acceptable. Thus, alcohol, along with several bromide preparations, chloral hydrate, and paraldehyde, was classically used to treat anxiety; however, the adverse societal and medical consequences of such use no longer support this as a medical approach. Self-medication with alcohol as an anxiolytic continues, however.

The next step in the pharmacological treatment of anxiety was the development of the barbiturates in the early 20th century and the marketing of phenobarbital in 1914. All the marketed barbiturates (there were at least 50) were used from about 1915 to 1960 as anxiolytics as well as sedatives, hypnotics, anticonvulsants, and anesthetics. All barbiturates induce sedation as well as profound psychomotor impairments. They are also lethal in overdose, leading to remaining and very controversial medical uses in physician-assisted suicide and in lethal injection procedures.

In the early 1950s, attempts were made to identify sedative drugs that were safer (less lethal in overdosage) than the barbiturates. This led in two directions: first were the less sedating anticonvulsants (e.g., diphenylhydantoin and others) and second were the non-barbiturate anxiolytics/hypnotics. The latter included meprobamate (Equanil, Miltown), carisoprodol (Soma), glutethamide (Doriden), methyprylon (Noludar), etchlorvynol (Placidyl), and, in the early 1970s, methaqualone (Quaalude). These drugs all attempted to provide anxiolysis with less hypnotic action, less lethality in overdose, and less potential for psychomotor impairment and physical dependence. In general, such goals were not met and their use today is rare. One exception is carisoprodol (which is metabolized to meprobamate), which is frequently prescribed, yet somewhat inappropriately, as a "muscle relaxant"; it is also a commonly encountered drug of abuse and intoxicant.

A landmark in anxiolytic history was the introduction of the *benzodiazepine tranquilizers* such as diazepam (Valium) and chlordiazepoxide (Librium) in the early 1960s, followed by many others throughout that decade. Their claim to fame was that they were relatively non-fatal in overdosage, and presumably less sedating. This enhanced safety led to incredible popularity and widespread use that continues today. Uses include treatment of anxiety, epilepsy, alcohol withdrawal, insomnia, agitation, and muscle tension, and even to provide amnesia for certain types of medical and dental procedures under the term "conscious sedation." Unfortunately, benzodiazepines retain the cognitive-impairing effects, the psychomotor impairments, and the dependence-inducing and "addicting" characteristics of the barbiturates. Because of the adverse cognitive effects of the benzodiazepines, their use in the young and the elderly has become relatively contraindicated (because of learning impairments in the young and dementing and extreme psychomotor effects in the elderly).

At about the same time that the benzodiazepines were being introduced into medicine, chlorpromazine (Thorazine) and several other *phenothiazine tranquilizers* were identified and introduced for the treatment of schizophrenia. The phenothiazines induced a state of neuroleptic tranquilization and anxiolysis, but this was accompanied by serious side effects, including Parkinsonian-like movements and a "neuroleptic state" characterized by reduced activity, lethargy, and impaired motor control. These neuroleptic tranquilizers reduced confusion, delirium, delusions, hallucinations, anxiety, and psychomotor agitation in psychotic persons.

To differentiate the phenothiazines from the benzodiazepines, the former were referred to as *major tranquilizers* and the latter as *minor tranquilizers*. The major tranquilizers were not clinically used to treat anxiety (except in schizophrenic patients), so the minor tranquilizers dominated the treatment of anxiety until the late 1980s, when fluoxetine (Prozac), the first serotonin-specific reuptake inhibitor (SSRI), was marketed as an antidepressant/anxiolytic. Fluoxetine (and five additional SSRIs to follow in the 1990s) differentiated themselves from the barbiturates and the benzodiazepines in that they were not fatal in overdosage and exerted a much lower degree of cognitive inhibition. Indeed, as depression and anxiety are relieved, a degree of cognitive enhancement can be observed.

Importantly, as the SSRIs were being marketed as antidepressants/anxiolytics, the "atypical antipsychotic" drugs were almost simultaneously being developed for treating schizophrenia and bipolar disorder; these drugs were relatively devoid of the neuroleptic properties displayed by the older "major tranquilizers," at least at therapeutic doses. Among their many clinical uses, the atypical antipsychotic drugs possess useful anxiolytic properties for use in "resistant" anxiety states (Julien, Advokat, & Comaty, 2011). Indeed, atypical antipsychotics have been utilized in the treatment of multiple types of anxiety disorders, including treatment-resistant posttraumatic stress disorder (PTSD) (Ahern, Juergens, Cordes, Becker, & Krahn, 2011). However, the evidence is less clear for military service-related PTSD (Krystal et al., 2011).

Next, several of the newer antiepileptic drugs (in addition to possessing anti-convulsant properties) have been shown to possess important anxiolytic properties. Specifically, they have been shown to be useful in the treatment of such disorders as social anxiety (Feltner, Liu-Dumaw, & Schweizer, 2011) and the nightmares and sleep disruptions associated with PTSD (Ahern et al., 2011).

Finally, certain medications used clinically to lower blood pressure in patients with hypertension are successfully used for certain anxiety states. For example, propranolol (Inderal) has long been used to reduce performance anxiety, and prazosin (Minipres) has been recommended for the treatment of PTSD-associated nightmares (Aurora et al., 2010).

In summary, anxiety disorders today are being medically treated with drugs of many classes, including:

- benzodiazepines, such as alprazolam (Xanax), lorazepam (Ativan), clonazepam (Klonopin), and diazepam (Valium);
- antidepressant/anxiolytic SSRIs and the serotonin–norepinephrine reuptake inhibitors (SNRIs) such as venlafaxine (Effexor) and duloxetine (Cymbalta);
- atypical antipsychotics, such as quetiapine (Seroquel), risperidone (Risperdal), and aripiprazole (Abilify);
- antiepileptic drugs, such as gabapentin (Neurontin), pregabalin (Lyrica), lamotrigine (Lamictal), and topiramate (Topamax);
- certain antihypertensive medications that either slow heart rate (e.g., propranolol) or relax arterial blood vessels (prazosin).

All of this allows the treatment provider a range of prescription options never before available with which to tailor medication to an individual's particular needs and to balance therapeutic efficacy with potential side effects that might be inappropriate for individual patients. The remainder of this chapter will focus on medication selection for the treatment of anxiety disorders in persons from the intrauterine state, through childhood and adulthood, and into their elderly years.

TREATMENT OF ANXIETY IN THE NEONATE

There is increasing evidence that untreated anxiety and depressive disorders in pregnant women are associated with adverse outcomes in the newborn infant. This link between maternal disease and early appearance of symptomatology in the newborn seems to be due to environmental processes, independent of inherited effects (Gleason et al., 2010; Lewis, Rice, Harold, Collishaw, & Thapar, 2011). By inference, treating anxiety during pregnancy should lead to improvements in pregnancy outcomes, benefiting the longer-term mental health of the offspring. Therefore, the susceptibility to future states of anxiety (and depression) begins even before birth. The overall goal of treating early-onset anxiety (even neonatal) is to reduce the severity of current anxiety symptoms in the pregnant female, and ultimately to prevent the long-term consequences of untreated anxiety in offspring. Obviously, we do not know whether or not a neonate can experience anxiety symptoms; but we are learning that untreated maternal anxiety disorders have profound effects on the developing brain of a neonate.

Multiple approaches are needed to reduce anxiety in pregnant women. Treatments involve resolving nutritional deficiencies, to psychosocial interventions, to pharmacological intervention. Here I focus on pharmacological interventions, although nutrition will be briefly addressed.

Can a neonate suffer from anxiety? No one knows; but untreated maternal anxiety sets the stage for reduced developmental scores in the newborn, slowed mental development, and potentially the future development of anxiety and depressive disorders in the young child. This is consistent with the work of Luby (2009; 2010), Luby, Si, Belden, Tandon, and Spitznagel (2009), and U. Rao and colleagues (2010), who demonstrated that depression in preschool children (as young as three years of age) is correlated with untreated depression and anxiety in the pregnant mother and is associated with abnormal development of neurons within the hippocampus of the newborn. This may potentially increase their susceptibility to early-age depressive and anxiety disorders.

Why might the prenatal infant brain be so vulnerable during prenatal development? As stated by Agin (2010, p. 57), "It is estimated that in the developing brain and nervous system of the prenatal human, about 250,000 new neurons are generated each minute at the peak of cell proliferation during gestation." Therefore, the prenatal treatment of the long-term childhood anxiety outcomes lies in treating anxiety in the pregnant mother. Such stress can result in poor compliance with prenatal care, exposure to drugs of abuse, alcohol, and cigarettes, and disruptions in the home environment. All adversely affect the fetal environment. The overall goal is to reduce the mother's levels of stress hormones and restore nutritional deficiencies necessary for normal development of the fetal brain. In the developing fetal brain, stress hormones, certain vitamin deficiencies, and deficiencies in omega-3-fatty acids all adversely affect neurogenesis and migration programming.

Pharmacological treatment of anxiety in the mother involves consideration of adverse effects of medications on organ development (teratogenesis) in the infant and in long-term medication-related neurobehavioral outcomes. Despite decades of study, data remain controversial and conflicting. However, with some positive reports of adverse structural deficits, most hold that benzodiazepines should likely be avoided during the first trimester of pregnancy. Since pregnancy is unplanned in about 50% of pregnancies, these women are unaware that they are pregnant for several weeks following conception. It is therefore wise to avoid benzodiazepine therapy in women who could potentially become pregnant and therefore expose a young fetus to undesired drug effects. Also of consideration are residual drug effects and withdrawal symptoms in children born of a female taking benzodiazepines until the time of delivery.

Regarding SSRI-type antidepressants/anxiolytics, these medications in humans do not appear to increase the risk of congenital anomalies. One possible exception is paroxetine (Paxil), which has been associated with a slight increase in cardiac anomalies. Importantly, the mother should likely be exposed to only one medication, as polypharmacy increases risk substantially (Kornum, Nielsen, Pedersen, Mortensen, & Norgaard, 2010). Fluoxetine has perhaps the widest margin of safety, but probably should be withdrawn several weeks before delivery to minimize SSRI withdrawal signs in the newborn.

Neurodevelopmental effects in children exposed to SSRIs *in utero* remain controversial. No major adverse effects have been reported, although recent research (Croen, Grether, Yoshida, Odouli, & Hendrick, 2011) indicates a potentially small increase in the incidence of autism spectrum disorders. It is agreed, however, that if such a risk occurs, it is unlikely to be a major risk factor for these disorders.

Regarding anticonvulsant drugs as anxiolytics during pregnancy, in general these should be avoided, as they pose a much more serious teratogenic risk (Grover, Avasthi, & Sharma, 2006). If necessary, lamotrigine (Lamictal) appears to have the greatest safety ratio of available anticonvulsants.

Atypical antipsychotic drugs are widely used by women of childbearing age for multiple disorders, including treatment of bipolar disorder, depression, and anxiety. Exposure to one of these drugs is therefore quite likely in many women who may become pregnant. While much remains to be learned, in February 2011 the U.S. Food and Drug Administration (FDA) issued class warnings for atypical antipsychotic use during pregnancy, advising of abnormal muscle movements and withdrawal signs in offspring whose mothers received these drugs during pregnancy. The potential teratogenicity of atypical antipsychotic drugs taken by women during pregnancy is little studied.

In summary, at this point SSRIs appear to be among the safest medications for treatment of anxiety during pregnancy (although perhaps paroxetine should be avoided in the first trimester).

TREATMENT OF PRESCHOOL ANXIETY

Anxiety disorders during the preschool period (ages 3–5 years) are common, with social anxiety, generalized anxiety, separation anxiety, and specific fears leading the list of such disorders (Edwards, Rapee, Kennedy, & Spence, 2010). Further, these disorders have a years-long stability, potentially leading the developing person to have a predisposition to anxiety disorders as a young adult. Therefore, aggressive treatment of preschool-aged children is necessary, not only to control current problems but also to prevent progression to disorders in subsequent years. These youngsters will not "grow out" of their disorder (Fanton & Gleason, 2009).

For non-PTSD and non-OCD anxiety disorders in preschoolers, behavioral therapy techniques and cognitive therapies are valuable (Hirshfeld-Becker, Micco, Mazursky, Bruett, & Henin, 2011). Treatment is continued for at least 3 months before considering medication. Parental psychiatric assessment may be valuable and necessary. For non-PTSD and non-OCD anxiety disorders in preschoolers, the entire pharmacological literature comprises only a handful of case reports. Fluoxetine may be the first choice for pharmacological treatment of preschool anxiety, but this is based only on empirical evidence. A discontinuation trial after 6–9 months of therapy has been recommended. Benzodiazepines are not recommended, because of possible cognitive impairments and subsequent learning difficulties. The only exception to this might be for ultra-short-term treatment of dental anxiety.

PTSD is common in preschoolers and difficult to treat. Psychotherapeutic interventions are the treatments of choice. As stated by Julien et al. (2011, p. 604), "The experts do not endorse medication; however, according to surveys, only 11% of providers reported that they *did not* use medication for preschool PTSD. Here, experts differ from practitioners. Again, benzodiazepines are not recommended." There is little research on OCD in preschoolers. Psychoeducation, cognitive therapies, and exposure therapies are effective. SSRIs may be effective and can be combined with cognitive therapies. SSRI therapy probably should be considered as the treatment of last resort, and SSRI treatment should always occur in the context of ongoing cognitive and/or behavioral interventions.

It is important to note that certain preschool disorders (such as ADHD) may be treated with dopaminergic compounds such as amphetamine (Adderall) and methylphenidate (Ritalin). Any medications that act by increasing brain dopamine levels may induce or worsen anxiety disorders. Often such anxiety is treated by adding an anxiolytic, rather than discontinuing the stimulant and reevaluating the situation. In its use in adults with depression, bupropion (Wellbutrin) can cause an identical effect.

TREATMENT OF ANXIETY IN SCHOOL-AGE CHILDREN AND ADOLESCENTS

Anxiety disorders are common in school-aged children and adolescents, and cause substantial impairments in school, in family relationships, and in social functioning. Such disorders are among the earliest psychiatric conditions to manifest, with a median age of onset of 11 years (Ramsawh, Chavira, & Stein, 2010). Anxiety disorders in youth also predict adult anxiety disorders, substance abuse, and major depression. A reasonable estimate of the occurrence of any anxiety disorder during adolescence is about 13%, with a prevalence rate in children under 18 years at 5.7–12.8%. Bridge and coworkers (2007), in a large meta-analysis, found considerable therapeutic efficacy of antidepressant medications in treating anxiety disorders in children and adolescents. Indeed, it is now generally agreed that psychotherapy and pharmacotherapy are effective in improving clinical impairments from anxiety disorders and maintaining these improvements (Kodish, Rockhill, Ryan, & Varley, 2011; Rynn et al., 2011).

With increasing recognition of childhood anxiety as a serious illness with potentially lifelong consequences, interest has risen about the use of psychopharmacologic interventions. On the other hand, this has been accompanied by concern over potential overdiagnosis and overtreatment of youths (Correll, Kratochvil, & March, 2011), and potential for medication-induced suicidal thoughts or actual suicides. Regarding suicidality with SSRIs, anxiety alone does not appear to be a predictive factor; however, these medications can at the beginning of administration as monotherapy have pro-suicidal effects in patients with hints of suicidality or suicidal behavior, by increasing the intensity of already present suicidal predictors, such as dysphoria, impulsiveness, agitation, and so forth. If depression is suspected, appropriate diagnosis and interventions should be undertaken before SSRI treatment is initiated.

In clinical trials, generalized anxiety disorder, separation anxiety, and social phobia are often grouped together because of a high degree of symptom overlap, their distinction from other anxiety disorders, and their similar response rates compared with OCD and PTSD. Research suggests that both cognitive-behavioral therapy (CBT) and SSRIs are effective in the treatment of these anxiety disorders in children and adolescents. Indeed, CBT and SSRIs seem to be equally efficacious in treatment. Furthermore, combination treatment (CBT plus an SSRI) may be more efficacious than either treatment alone. For example, Walkup and coworkers (2008) found that 81% of children with anxiety disorders receiving both sertraline (Zoloft) and CBT were classified as responders, versus 60% with CBT alone, 55% for sertraline alone, and 23% for placebo medication. The authors concluded that

> CBT alone, sertraline alone, and the combination are all efficacious short-term treatments. Combination therapy is the most efficacious and provides the best chance for a positive outcome. Any of the three can be recommended, taking into consideration the family's treatment preferences, treatment availability, cost, and time burden.

(p. 2762)

As reviewed by Connolly, Suarez, and Sylvester (2011, p. 99):

> CBT has been extensively studied and has shown good efficacy in the treatment of childhood anxiety disorders. A combination of CBT and medication may be required for moderate to severely impairing anxiety disorders and may improve functioning better than either intervention alone. SSRIs are currently the only medications that have consistently shown efficacy. Despite this, the availability of CBT in the community is limited. Current research is focusing on early identification of anxiety disorders in community settings, increasing the availability of evidence-based interventions, and modification of interventions for specific populations.

Obsessive-compulsive disorder (OCD) is now estimated as the fourth most common psychiatric disorder in adolescents, with an incidence of 2–3.6%. Pharmacotherapy with SSRIs is usually indicated as part of multimodal therapy. As stated in a recent POTS II study (Pediatric OCD Treatment Study II; Franklin et al., 2011, p. 1224),

> Partial response to SSRIs is the norm and augmentation with short-term OCD-specific CBT provides additional benefit (Franklin et al., 2011); 68% of OCD youths receiving medication management plus CBT strategy were considered responders, which was superior to 34% in the CBT group and 30% in the medication-only group.

From the earlier POTS I study, only about 3.6% would be expected to respond to placebo therapy (Pediatric OCD Treatment Study (POTS) Team, 2004).

Despite these positive results, perhaps 30% of youth with OCD will be resistant to SSRI plus CBT therapy. Augmentation strategies are therefore necessary. Here, a focus has been on the use of atypical antipsychotics in such youth. At this early stage of research, both quetiapine (Seroquel) and aripiprazole (Abilify) have reported efficacy (Mohr, Vythilingum, Emsley, & Stein, 2002; Masi, Pfanner, Millepiedi, & Berloffa, 2010). In the study by Masi and coworkers, 39 adolescents (mean age 12 years) were titrated to a final dose of 12 mg of aripiprazole per day and the drug was effective in more than 50% of patients resistant to continuing SSRI therapy. For a recent analysis of this literature, see the Brown University Child and Adolescent Psychopharmacology Update (2011).

Posttraumatic stress disorder (PTSD) is relatively common in children and adolescents, often as a result of early-age traumas. Despite this, little has been reported on the efficacy of pharmacological interventions. A recent practice parameter for child and adolescent PTSD includes little on psychopharmacologic treatment. Strawn, Keeshin, DelBello, Geracioti, and Putnam (2010), performing a meta-analysis of published literature, noted that the data do not support the use of SSRIs as first-line treatments for PTSD in children and ado-lescents. For example, sertraline (Zoloft) was ineffective in a placebo-controlled study in 131 youths (aged 6–17 years) with PTSD (Robb, Cueva, Sporn, Yang, & Vanderburg, 2010). Limited evidence notes that atypical antipsychotics and several mood stabilizers may attenuate some symptoms, such as intrusive thoughts. Antiadrenergic agents (e.g., clonidine, guanfacine, prazosin) can reduce symptoms such as hyperarousal, intrusive symptoms, and impulsivity. Other medications may be needed to target various associated PTSD symp-toms such as depression, affect instability, disruptive behavior, and dysregu-lated attachment.

Again, it must be stated that cognitive inhibitors are not indicated for use in children and adolescents. This greatly limits the use of benzodiazepines and tri-cyclic antidepressants.

TREATMENT OF ANXIETY IN ADULTS

As listed above, multiple classes of medications are used to treat anxiety disor-ders in adults. These include benzodiazepines, antidepressant/anxiolytic SSRIs, serotonin–norepinephrine reuptake inhibitors (SNRIs), atypical antipsychotics, and certain antiepileptic drugs. Other compounds occasionally encountered include medications that blunt the tachycardic response to anxiety (beta-blockers and calcium channel blockers), antihypertensive drugs that dilate blood vessels (prazosin) and certain antihistamines such as hydroxyzine (Vistaril).

Benzodiazepines

For 50 years, benzodiazepines formed the mainstay of anxiety treatment. Their efficacy and immediacy of response is their primary advantage. This, however, is offset by cognitive impairments (ranging from tolerable to debilitating), addicting properties, and withdrawal complications (sleep disruptions to fatal seizures). Other side effects include sedation, hypnosis, and anterograde amne-sia (the extreme of cognitive dysfunction).

Because of these side effects, benzodiazepines today may be more properly classified as sedative-hypnotic drugs rather than anxiolytics, the latter term implying some sort of specific effect to ameliorate anxiety separate from gen-eral depression of the CNS. Of note, the depressant effects of benzodiazepines are additive with the action of ethanol, causing further impairment in psycho-motor skills.

The adverse cognitive effects of benzodiazepines are insidious and often missed in clinical practice. The reason for this is the long half-lives of these drugs, almost all of which exceed the usually prescribed dose intervals. For example, several benzodiazepines are metabolized to a long-acting active intermediate (nordiazepam) that has a half-life of several days. Others considered to be shorter-acting have half-lives of 12–14 hours (alprazolam, temazepam, lorazepam) or more than 24 hours (clonazepam). Only triazolam (half-life of 2.5 hours) and midazolam (half-life of about 1.5 hours) have a rapid onset and noticeable cessation of action. When a drug with a half-life of greater than 12 hours is administered every 6–8 hours, one is never "drug-free." As a result, even professionals seeing these persons rarely notice drug-induced impairments. Even if the benzodiazepine is taken only at bedtime for sleep, residual daytime impairment will persist and some drug remains when the next bedtime dose is taken (leading to drug accumulation and even more impairment).

Clinical uses still appropriate for benzodiazepines may include: (1) intentional anterograde amnesia [midazolam (Versed)]; rapid onset of sleep [triazolam (Halcion)]; perhaps the short-term treatment of debilitating anxiety [alprazolam (Xanax), clonazepam (Klonopin), lorazepam (Ativan)]; perhaps short-term use in event-driven emotional distress; and the prevention of seizures in alcohol withdrawal [chlordiazepoxide (Librium)]. Regarding the latter, antiepileptic drugs such as gabapentin (Neurontin) and pregabalin (Lyrica) may be viable options. Clonazepam, alprazolam, and lorazepam are commonly prescribed today for the treatment of anxiety; however, their efficacy is limited, tolerance and dependence are problematic, and cognitive dysfunction is often underappreciated and poorly recognized.

Antidepressants

Most antidepressants (with the notable exception of bupropion) exert anxiolytic actions as well as antidepressant actions. This is fortunate, because of the common occurrence and comorbidity of depression with one or more anxiety disorders. Whether such common actions are a result of potentiation of either (or both) serotonin and norepinephrine neurotransmission (by reuptake blockade) remains unclear. The *tricyclic antidepressants* (TCAs) were introduced into medicine about 50 years ago, blocking both norepinephrine and serotonin reuptake (the original *dual-action* antidepressants). These drugs have anxiolytic properties, but side effects limit their use. Such side effects include sedation, cognitive impairments, delirium, and other signs of histaminic and cholinergic receptor blockade. These medications are also potentially fatal in overdose. Today, their use is generally restricted to situations where other, safer medications are unaffordable. Clomipramine (Anafranil) is a TCA approved long ago for the treatment of OCD (the first FDA approval of an antidepressant for treatment of an anxiety disorder). Its use for treatment of OCD remains.

Modern versions of dual-acting antidepressants that block norepinephrine and serotonin reuptake include venlafaxine (Effexor), desvenlafaxine (Pristiq, the active metabolite of venlafaxine), duloxetine (Cymbalta), and milnacepram (Savella). In general, these three medications act through the same mechanisms of action as the TCAs except that they lack the antihistaminic and anticholinergic properties of the TCAs. All three share antidepressant/anxiolytic/analgesic actions, making them particularly useful in the treatment of disorders where two or all three actions are desired (e.g., in the treatment of fibromyalgia and chronic pain conditions). Of particular note, these medications are useful in the treatment of generalized anxiety disorder (venlafaxine is FDA-approved for such use), panic disorder (Serretti et al., 2011), panic disorder with agoraphobia (M. H. Chen & Liou, 2011), and as an alternative to SSRIs in the treatment of obsessive-compulsive disorder (Sansone & Sansone, 2011). Duloxetine may be more effective in reducing anxiety than is venlafaxine (Serafini et al., 2010), although no definitive explanation can be offered for this observation. With these three medications, one must be aware of potential "switching" from depression to hypomania and mania, with adverse consequences (Gao et al., 2008; J. Chen et al., 2010).

Anticonvulsants

Certain anticonvulsants have long been utilized in the management of chronic pain syndromes, including the pain associated with peripheral neuropathies. More recently, their anxiolytic properties have been elucidated, reducing the amygdalar activation during anticipation of emotional images (Aupperle et al., 2011). Most studied is the use of pregabalin (Lyrica) for generalized anxiety disorder (Boschen, 2011) and social anxiety disorder (Feltner et al., 2011). An older and closely related drug, gabapentin, is less expensive and most likely similarly effective. The less sedating anticonvulsant/antidepressant medication lamotrigine (Lamictal) may similarly reduce anxiety (Sepić-Grahovac, Grahovac, Ružić-Baršić, & Dadić-Hero, 2011). Topiramate (Topamax) also has anxiolytic properties, but its use is limited by clinically significant cognitive difficulties. Anastassiou and coworkers (2011) recently wrote, "Significant reductions in mean pain and pain-related sleep interference, combined with reductions in feelings of anxiety and depression, suggest that pregabalin under real-world conditions improves the overall health and well-being of patients with neuropathic pain" (p. 417).

Atypical Antipsychotics

As stated earlier, traditional (first-generation) antipsychotic drugs reduce the symptoms of schizophrenia accompanied by emotional tranquilization, calming, and anxiolysis. Adversely, these effects could not be achieved without the accompanying movement disorders and induction of the "neuroleptic state." The claim to fame of newer, second-generation or "atypical" antipsychotics is that relief of symptoms of schizophrenia could be achieved at doses that did not necessarily have these accompanying movement and neuroleptic side effects. These properties rapidly led to exploration of their uses outside of the treatment of schizophrenia. Such uses included treatment of bipolar disorder, autism spectrum disorders, behavioral agitation and aggressive disorders, anger disorders, and (more recently) depression and anxiety disorders. Indeed, two of these atypical antipsychotics, aripiprazole (Abilify) and quetiapine (as Seroquel-XR), are FDA-approved as either monotherapy or as augmenting agents in the treatment of depression. "Off-label," these medications (especially quetiapine and aripiprazole) are being widely used as effective medication in either monotherapy or combination therapy in the treatment of generalized anxiety disorder, OCD (Katzman, 2011; Maher et al., 2011; Vulink, Figee, & Denys, 2011), and PTSD (Ahearn et al., 2011; Krystal et al., 2011).

Side effects of atypical antipsychotics are significant and can limit their therapeutic utility. These effects include weight gain (with risperidone and occasionally with quetiapine), a potential for early-onset diabetes mellitus, sedation (with risperidone and quetiapine), elevated blood lipids, akathisia (with aripiprazole), and occasional extrapyramidal signs. Because of this potential, most practitioners begin therapy of anxiety disorders with an SSRI, reserving atypical antipsychotics for "failed" or SSRI-resistant cases. Atypical antipsychotics have the advantage of more rapid onset of effect, less sexual dysfunction, and improved mood stability, for example in anxious depression (S. Rao & Zisook, 2009; Gao, Sheehan, & Calabrese, 2009).

TREATMENT OF ANXIETY IN THE ELDERLY

There is a paucity of research on the treatment of anxiety in older people, although the availability of several new assessment scales suggests increased interest in this topic. Indeed, anxiety disorders are common. Likely, such anxiety is disruptive, and frequently overmedicated in order to achieve behavioral control. There is also a potential for worsening of any existing cognitive impairment. This applies especially to the administration of benzodiazepines to elderly persons.

Benzodiazepines

One-quarter of the prescription drugs sold in the United States are used by the elderly, often for chronic pain, insomnia, and anxiety. Of available drugs, benzodiazepines continue to be used in this population, both for treating anxiety and for treating insomnia. While such use was perhaps condoned in past years, today it is felt that benzodiazepines should be rarely, if ever, prescribed in this population (Manthey et al., 2011). Many patients treated with benzodiazepines should be withdrawn, and therapeutic strategies other than benzodiazepines should be considered to treat anxiety and insomnia in these patients (Bourin, 2010). Why such strong words?

- First, benzodiazepines have well-described adverse cognitive effects, either worsening preexisting dementia or inducing *de novo* dementia that is reversible with drug discontinuation.
- Second, benzodiazepine use in the elderly is associated with an increased incidence of falls with debilitating hip fractures.
- Third, problems posed by the elderly operating motor vehicles are potentiated if they are using benzodiazepines.
- Fourth, many elderly people consume alcohol, and benzodiazepine use with alcohol produces remarkable cognitive dysfunction and behavioral risks.
- Fifth, withdrawal is difficult, with a risk of seizures, insomnia, and rebound increases in anxiety and agitation.

Antidepressants

SSRIs are currently the drugs of choice for treating anxiety in the elderly. Use of the tricyclics (TCAs) is severely limited by cognitive impairments and possibly anticholinergic delirium. Lenze and coworkers (2011) studied escitalopram (Lexapro) in the treatment of generalized anxiety disorder in adults older than 60 years. They noted that the drug reduced peak and total cortisol levels in the brain and that these reductions paralleled reductions in anxiety. It is likely that all SSRIs share these actions. Doses should likely be started at low levels and advanced slowly.

Since elderly people frequently take multiple prescribed medications (20–40% of the elderly take eight or more medications), the potential for drug interactions is real. SSRIs inhibit the activity of multiple drug-metabolizing enzyme systems. The result of such inhibition is reduced metabolic breakdown of other medicines taken by these patients. This reduced metabolism results in marked increases in the blood concentrations of other drugs, sometimes even doubling these concentrations, often resulting in dangerous situations. For example, increasing the blood concentration of blood thinners (anticoagulants such as warfarin) may lead to fatal hemorrhage. SSRIs can also inhibit the breakdown of many opioid analgesics, with methadone being the most susceptible (Tennant, 2010).

Recently, duloxetine (Cymbalta) has been reported to be effective in treating elderly patients suffering from comorbid depression, anxiety, and chronic low back pain (Karp et al., 2010).

For elderly people suffering from comorbid insomnia, anxiety, and depression, mirtazapine (Remeron) has proved very effective. It is as effective as the SSRIs, and improves sleep quality with bedtime use (Croom, Perry, & Plosker, 2009). Its side effect of increasing appetite, with modest weight gain, may be of benefit in this population. Its use as a nighttime sleep aid has not been accompanied by an increase in falls and fractures (Coupland et al., 2011).

Atypical Antipsychotics

For as long as the traditional antipsychotics have been available, they have been used to calm agitated and aggressive behaviors in the elderly. This type of chemically induced behavioral control has always been ethically controversial, often appropriately so. A need has remained for superior medications to treat this common disorder in elderly people who exhibit difficult behaviors.

Since their introductions in the 1990s, the atypical antipsychotic medications have become the standard of care for behavioral and psychological symptoms of dementia, and to control agitated, anxious, and aggressive behaviors in the elderly. This is said despite warnings from the FDA about potential adverse reactions possibly associated with such use (discussed in what follows). Today, following increases in such use, reductions to more acceptable and reasonable levels of use are perhaps occurring (Dorsey, Rabbani, Gallagher, Conti, & Alexander, 2010).

Atypical antipsychotics can relieve symptoms that arise in elderly patients with dementia:

- anxiety and confusion;
- agitation with pacing, wandering, and restlessness;
- aggression (verbal and physical);
- physical resistance and non-compliance with care;
- psychosis (hallucinations and delusions);
- depressive symptoms;
- sleep disturbances (day/night reversal, wandering behaviors).

Used appropriately and at low doses, anxiety, sleep disturbances, agitation, and aggression can be moderated without undue and adverse behavioral control. Some atypical antipsychotics are associated with weight gain, diabetes mellitus, and undue sedation (e.g., risperidone). Quetiapine (Seroquel) is associated with somewhat lower degrees of sedation, weight gain, and diabetes and therefore became preferred over risperidone. More recently, aripiprazole (Abilify) has been studied and is associated with even less sedation, little or no weight gain, presumably a lower propensity to diabetes, improvements in cognitive functioning, and a clinically significant antidepressant action. Used in low doses, these two newer agents confer anxiolytic effects with calming of agitated and aggressive behaviors, all with a reasonable degree of safety (Madhusoodanan & Shah, 2008; Kohen, Lester, & Lam, 2010).

In 2005 the FDA issued a public health advisory indicating a 1.7-fold increased risk of all-cause mortality from these drugs (all atypical antipsychotics) compared to placebo. Other researchers have failed to verify any increased risk of death. Indeed, while traditional antipsychotics likely carry some increased risk of cardiac mortality, this does not appear to extend to the atypical agents (Laredo et al., 2011; Mehta, Chen, Johnson, & Aparasu, 2011). Nevertheless, careful decision making is warranted in the use of atypical antipsychotic medicines in this vulnerable population of persons.

An individualized, carefully monitored trial of these medications in anxious, aggressive, agitated elderly people with dementia may result in improvements in quality of life both for the patient and for the caregivers. In these patients, benefits of medication may allow the patient to remain in a less structured and less confining environment than otherwise would be possible. Thus, the humanitarian benefits may outweigh any postulated increased risk associated with such use. These agents should be used with discretion and only as part of non-pharmacological environmental and behavioral interventions (Julien et al., 2011, p. 651)

Clinical Points to Remember

1. Man has sought medicinal relief from anxiety for millennia, using remedies ranging from alcohols to barbiturates, benzodiazepines, benzodiazepine alternatives, to "tranquilizers," and even to atypical antipsychotics.

2. Consistently, the major side effects associated with many anxiolytics include sedation, cognitive impairments, and psychomotor impairment.

3. The terms *major tranquilizer* and *minor tranquilizer* are classic. "Major tranquilizers" are sedating drugs used to treat schizophrenia (e.g., phenothiazines and haloperidol).

4. Proneness to future anxiety disorders may begin in the neonate; reductions in maternal affective disorders may reduce anxiety risk in the newborn.

5. Preschool anxiety disorders are common; pharmacological intervention is secondary to psychological interventions and should not be used with concomitant psychological therapy. Benzodiazepines (because of adverse learning effects) are not recommended; SSRIs are the pharmacological therapy of first choice.

6. Anxiety disorders in school-aged children and adolescents are common, disabling, and persistent into adulthood, with lifelong implications. If medications are necessary, those with adverse effects on learning and memory should be avoided when possible.

7. In adult anxiety disorders, benzodiazepines remain widely used despite adverse addictive and cognitive side effects. SSRIs are widely chosen as initial agents, but their efficacy is often incomplete. Therefore, knowledge of medications (e.g., anticonvulsants and atypical antipsychotics) for SSRI-resistant anxiety is essential.

8. In the elderly, anxiety disorders are common and often underrecognized and undertreated. Any agent that impairs mental functioning should be avoided. SSRI-type antidepressants may treat comorbid anxiety and depression.

9. Finally, in the elderly, certain atypical antipsychotic medications (e.g., risperidone and quetiapine) may calm anxious, aggressive, confused, and agitated patients. Weighing the positive effects in light of potential adverse reactions is essential. These drugs should not be used solely for behavioral calming.

REFERENCES

Agin, D. (2010). *More than genes: What science can tell us about toxic chemicals, development, and the risk to our children.* Oxford: Oxford University Press.

Ahern, E. P., Juergens, T., Cordes, T., Becker, T., & Krahn, D. (2011a). A review of atypical antipsychotic medications for posttraumatic stress disorder. *International Clinical Psychopharmacology, 26*(4), 193–200.

Anastassiou, E., Iatrou, C. A., Vlaikidis, N., Vafiadou, M., Stamatiou, G., Plesia, E., et al. (2011). Impact of pregabalin treatment on pain, pain-related sleep interference and general well-being in patients with neuropathic pain: A non-interventional, multicentre, post-marketing study. *Clinical Drug Investigations, 31*(6), 417–426.

Aupperle, R. L., Ravindran, L., Tankersley, D., Flagan, T., Stein, N. R., Simmons, A. N., et al. (2011). Pregabalin influences insula and amygdala activation during anticipation of emotional images. *Neuropsychopharmacology, 36*(7), 1466–1477.

Aurora, R. N., Zak, R. S., Auerbach, S. H., Casey, K. R., Chowdhuri, S., Karippot, A., et al. (2010). Best practice guide for the treatment of nightmare disorder in adults. *Journal of Clinical Sleep Medicine, 6*(4), 389–401.

Boschen, M. J. (2011). A meta-analysis of the efficacy of pregabalin in the treatment of generalized anxiety disorder. *Canadian Journal of Psychiatry, 56*(9), 558–566.

Bourin, M. (2010). The problems with the use of benzodiazepines in elderly patients. *Encephale, 36*(4), 340–347.

Bridge, J. A., Iyengar, S., Salary, C. B., Barbe, R. P., Birmaher, B., Pincus, H. A., et al. (2007). Clinical response and risk for reported suicidal ideation and suicide attempts in pediatric antidepressant treatment: A meta-analysis of randomized controlled trials. *JAMA: Journal of the American Medical Association, 297*(15), 1683–1696.

Brown University Child and Adolescent Psychopharmacology Update (2011, November). Adding full CBT shows best response in pediatric SRI-partial responders with OCD. *Brown University Child and Adolescent Psychopharmacology Update, 13*(11), 1–4.

Chen, J., Fang, Y., Kemp, D. E., Calabrese, J. R., & Gao, K. (2010). Switching to hypomania and mania: Differential neurochemical, neurppsychological, and pharmacologic triggers and their mechanisms. *Current Psychiatry Reports, 12*(6), 512–521.

Chen, M. H., & Liou, Y. J. (2011). Milnacepram in panic disorder with agoraphobia and major depressive disorder: A case report. *Clinical Neuropharmacology, 34*(5), 201–202.

Connolly, S. D., Suarez, L., & Sylvester, C. (2011). Assessment and treatment of anxiety disorders in children and adolescents. *Current Psychiatric Reports, 13*(2), 99–110.

Correll, C. U., Kratochvil, C. J., & March, J. S. (2011). Developments in pediatric psychopharmacology: Focus on stimulants, antidepressants, and antipsychotics. *Journal of Clinical Psychiatry, 72*(5), 655–670.

Coupland, C., Dhiman, P., Morriss, R., Arthur, A., Barton, G., & Hippisley-Cox, J. (2011). Antidepressant use and risk of adverse outcomes in older people: Population based cohort study. *BMJ: British Medical Journal, 343*:d4551. doi: 10.1136/bmj.d4551

Croen, L. A., Grether, J. K., Yoshida, C. K., Odouli, R., & Hendrick, V. (2011). Antidepressant use during pregnancy and childhood autism spectrum disorders. *Archives of General Psychiatry, 68*(11), 1104–1112.

Croom, K. F., Perry, C. M., & Plosker, G. L. (2009). Mirtazepine: A review of its use in major depression and other psychiatric disorders. *CNS Drugs, 23*(5), 427–452.

Dorsey, E. R., Rabbani, A., Gallagher, S. A., Conti, R. M., & Alexander, G. C. (2010). Impact of FDA black box advisory on antipsychotic medication use. *Archives of Internal Medicine, 170*(1), 96–103.

Edwards, S. L., Rapee, R. M., Kennedy, S. J., & Spence, S. H. (2010). The assessment of anxiety symptoms in preschool-aged children: The revised preschool anxiety scale. *Journal of Clinical Child and Adolescent Psychology, 39*(3), 400–409.

Fanton, J., & Gleason, M. M. (2009). Psychopharmacology and preschoolers: A critical review of current conditions. *Child and Adolescent Psychiatric Clinics of North America, 18*(3), 753–771.

Feltner, D. E., Liu-Dumaw, M., & Schweizer, E. (2011). Efficacy of pregabalin in generalized social anxiety disorder: Results of a double-blind, placebo-controlled, fixed-dose study. *International Clinical Psychopharmacology, 26*(4), 213–220.

Franklin, M. E., Saptya, J., Freeman, J. B., Khanna, M., Compton, S., Almirall, D., et al. (2011). Cognitive behavior therapy augmentation of pharmacotherapy in pediatric obsessive-compulsive disorder: The Pediatric OCD Treatment Study II (POTS II) randomized controlled trial. *JAMA: Journal of the American Medical Association, 306*(11), 1224–1232.

Gao, K., Kemp, D. E., Ganocy, S. J., Muzina, D. J., Xia, G., Findling, R. L., & Calabrese, J. R. (2008). Treatment-emergent mania/hypomania during antidepressant monotherapy in patients with rapid cycling bipolar disorder. *Bipolar Disorder, 10*(8), 907–915.

Gao, K., Sheehan, D. V., & Calabrese, J. R. (2009). Atypical antipsychotics in primary generalized anxiety disorder or comorbid with mood disorders. *Expert Reviews in Neurotherapy, 9*(8), 1147–1158.

Gleason, G., Liu, B., Bruening, S., Zupan, B., Auerbach, A., Mark, W., et al. (2010). The serotonin$_{1A}$ receptor gene as a genetic and prenatal maternal environmental factor in anxiety. *Proceedings of the National Academy of Sciences of the United States of America, 107*(16), 7592–7597.

Grover, S., Avasthi, A., & Sharma, Y. (2006). Psychotropics in pregnancy. *Indian Journal of Medical Research, 123*(4), 497–512.

Hirshfeld-Becker, D. R., Micco, J. A., Mazursky, H., Bruett, L., & Henin, A. (2011). Applying cognitive-behavioral therapy for anxiety to the younger child. *Child and Adolescent Psychiatric Clinics of North America, 20*(2), 349–368.

Julien, R. M., Advokat, C. D., & Comaty, J. E. (2011). *A primer of drug action: A comprehensive guide to the actions, uses, and side effects of psychoactive drugs* (12th ed.). New York: Worth Publishers.

Karp, J. F., Weiner, D. K., Dew, M. A., Begley, A., Miller, M. D., & Reynolds, C. F. III. (2010). Duloxetine and care management treatment of older adults with comorbid major depressive disorder and chronic low back pain: Results of an open-label pilot study. *International Journal of Geriatric Psychiatry, 25*(6), 633–642.

Katzman, M. A. (2011). Aripiprazole: A clinical review of its use for the treatment of anxiety disorders as a comorbidity in mental illness. *Journal of Affective Disorders, 128* (suppl. 1), S11–S20.

Kodish, I., Rockhill, C., Ryan, S. & Varley, C. (2011). Pharmacotherapy for anxiety disorders in children and adolescents. *Pediatric Clinics of North America, 58*(1), 55–72.

Kohen, I., Lester, P. E., & Lam, S. (2010). Antipsychotic treatments for the elderly: Efficacy and safety of aripiprazole. *Neuropsychiatric Disease and Treatment, 6*, 47–58.

Kornum, J. B., Nielsen, R. B., Pedersen, L., Mortensen, P. B., & Norgaard, M. (2010). Use of selective serotonin-reuptake inhibitors during pregnancy and risk of congenital malformations: Updated analysis. *Clinical Epidemiology, 2*, 29–36.

Krystal, J. H., Rosenheck, R. A., Cramer, J. A., Vessicchio, J. C., Jones, K. M., Vertrees, J. E., et al. (2011). Adjunctive risperidone treatment for antidepressant-resistant symptoms of chronic military service–related PTSD: A randomized trial. *JAMA: Journal of the American Medical Association, 306*(5), 493–502.

Laredo, L., Vargas, E., Blasco, A. J., Aguilar, M. D., Moreno, A., & Portoles, A. (2011). Risk of cerebrovascular accident associated with use of antipsychotics: Population-based case-control study. *Journal of the American Geriatric Society, 59*(7), 1182–1187.

Lenze, E.J., Mantella, R. C., Shi, P., Goate, A. M., Nowotny, P., Butters, M. A., et al. (2011). Elevated cortisol in older adults with generalized anxiety disorder is reduced by treatment: A placebo-controlled evaluation of escitalopram. *International Journal of Geriatric Psychiatry, 19*(5), 482–490.

Lewis, G., Rice, F., Harold, G. T., Collishaw, S., & Thapar, A. (2011). Investigating environmental links between parent depression and child depressive/anxiety symptoms using an assisted conception design. *Journal of the American Academy of Child and Adolescent Psychiatry, 50*(5), 451–459.

Luby, J. L. (2009). Early childhood depression. *American Journal of Psychiatry, 166*(9), 974–979.

Luby, J. L. (2010). Preschool depression: The importance of identification of depression early in development. *Current Directions in Psychological Sciences, 19*(2), 91–95.

Luby, J. L., Si, X., Belden, A. C., Tandon, M., & Spitznagel, E. (2009). Preschool depression: Homotypic continuity and course over 24 months. *Archives of General Psychiatry, 66*(8), 897–905.

Madhusoodanan, S., & Shah, P. (2008). Management of psychosis in patients with Alzheimer's disease: Focus on aripiprazole. *Clinical Interventions in Aging, 3*(3), 491–501.

Maher, A. R., Maglione, M., Bagley, S., Suttorp, M., Hu, J. H., Ewing, B., et al. (2011). Efficacy and comparative effectiveness of atypical antipsychotic medications for off-label uses in adults: A systematic review and meta-analysis. *JAMA: Journal of the American Medical Association, 306*(12), 1359–1369.

Manthey, L., van Veen, T., Giltay, E. J., Stoop, J. E., Neven, A. K., Penninx, B. W., & Zitman, F. G. (2011). Correlates of (inappropriate) benzodiazepine use: The Netherlands Study of Depression and Anxiety (NESDA). *International Journal of Clinical Pharmacology, 71*(2), 263–272.

Masi, G., Pfanner, C., Millepiedi, S., & Berloffa, S. (2010). Aripiprazole augmentation in 39 adolescents with medication-resistant obsessive-compulsive disorder. *Journal of Clinical Psychopharmacology, 30*(6), 688–693.

Mehta, S., Chen, H., Johnson, M., & Aparasu, R. R. (2011). Risk of serious cardiac events in older adults using antipsychotic agents. *International Journal of Geriatric Pharmacotherapy, 9*(2), 120–132.

Mohr, N., Vythilingum, B., Emsley, R. A., & Stein, D. J. (2002. Quetiapine augmentation of serotonin reuptake inhibitors in obsessive-compulsive disorder. *International Clinical Psychopharmacology, 17*(1), 37–40.

Pediatric OCD Treatment Study (POTS) Team. (2004). Cognitive-behavior therapy, sertraline, and their combination for children and adolescents with obsessive-compulsive disorder: The Pediatric OCD Treatment Study (POTS) randomized controlled trial. *JAMA: Journal of the American Medical Association, 292*(16), 1969–1976.

Ramsawh, H. J., Chavira, D. A., & Stein, M. B. (2010). The burden of anxiety disorders in pediatric medical settings: Prevalence, phenomenology, and a research agenda. *Archives of Pediatric and Adolescent Medicine, 164*(10), 965–972.

Rao, S., & Zisook, S. (2009). Anxious depression: Clinical features and treatment. *Current Psychiatric Reports, 11*(6), 429–436.

Rao, U., Chen, L. A., Bidesi, A. S., Shad, M. U., Thomas, M. A., & Hammen, C. L. (2010). Hippocampal changes associated with early-life adversity and vulnerability to depression. *Biological Psychiatry, 67*(4), 357–364.

Robb, A. S., Cueva, J. E., Sporn, J., Yang, R., & Vanderburg, D. G. (2010). Sertraline treatment of children and adolescents with posttraumatic stress disorder: A double-blind, placebo-controlled trial. *Journal of Child and Adolescent Psychopharmacology, 20*(6), 463–471.

Rynn, M., Puliafico, A., Heleniak, C., Rikhi, P., Ghalib, K., & Vidair, H. (2011). Advances in pharmacotherapy for pediatric anxiety disorders. *Depression and Anxiety, 28*(1), 76–87.

Sansone, R. A., & Sansone, L. A. (2011). SNSIs pharmacological alternatives for the treatment of obsessive compulsive disorder? *Innovations in Clinical Neuroscience, 8*(6), 10–14.

Sepić-Grahovac, D., Grahovac, T., Ružić-Baršić, A., & Dadić-Hero, E. (2011). Lamotrigine treatment of a patient affected by epilepsy and anxiety disorder. *Psychiatria Danubina, 23*(1), 111–113.

Serafini, G., Pompili, M., Del Casale, A., Mancini, M., Innamorati, M., Lester, D., et al. (2010). Duloxetine versus venlafaxine in the treatment of unipolar and bipolar depression. *Clinica Terapeutica, 161*(4), 321–327.

Serretti, A., Chiesa, A., Calati, R., Perna, G., Bellodi, L., & De Ronchi, D. (2011). Novel antidepressants and panic disorder: Evidence beyond current guidelines. *Neuropsychobiology, 63*(1), 1–7.

Strawn, J. R., Keeshin, B. R., DelBello, M. P., Geracioti, T. D. Jr., & Putnam, F. W. (2010). Psychopharmacological treatment of posttraumatic stress disorder in children and adolescents: A review. *Journal of Clinical Psychiatry, 71*(7), 932–941.

Tennant, F. (2010, May). Making practical sense of cytochrome P450. *Practical Pain Management*, pp. 12–18.

Vulink, N. C., Figee, M., & Denys, D. (2011). Review of atypical antipsychotics in anxiety. *European Neuropsychopharmacology, 21*(6), 429–449.

Walkup, J. T., Albano, A. M., Piacentini, J., Birmaher, B., Compton, S. N., Sherrill, J. T., et al. (2008). Cognitive-behavioral therapy, sertraline, or a combination in childhood anxiety. *New England Journal of Medicine, 359*(26), 2753–2766.

Psychosocial Treatment of Anxiety Disorders Across the Lifespan

Michael Sweeney, Jessica Levitt, Robert Westerholm, Clare Gaskins, and Christina Lipinski

This chapter provides a review of psychosocial interventions for the treatment of anxiety, with a particular emphasis on how the interventions are applied differently at various developmental stages. Provided in this introduction is an overview of the nature of anxiety and the interrelationship between anxiety and development as they pertain to psychosocial interventions. The subsequent sections will discuss the psychosocial interventions across all stages of development: with young children (ages 2 through 7), school-aged children (ages 8 through 12), adolescence (ages 13 through young adulthood), and, lastly, adulthood. A conclusion section will complete the chapter with general recommendations for the application of psychosocial interventions at different developmental stages.

THE NATURE OF ANXIETY

Understanding the nature of anxiety in relation to psychosocial interventions requires an appreciation of several factors: (1) Anxiety is a complicated condition resulting from a dynamic interplay of many internal and external factors. (2) Psychosocial treatments flow directly from one's understanding of anxiety. (3) The distinction between causal and maintaining factors is important for developing effective treatments. (4) Evidence-based interventions for anxiety focus on altering cognitions and behavior as a means of reducing avoidance of the feared situation. Each of these factors will be discussed in turn.

Anxiety Is Complicated

Many factors contribute to the development and maintenance of anxiety. Extensive research has documented the contribution of genetic, physiological, neuroanatomical, developmental, attachment, cognitive, perceptual, behavioral, and learning among other factors in the etiology of anxiety (Kinsella &

Monk, 2009; Monk, Leight, & Fang, 2008; Norrholm & Ressler, 2009; O'Connor, Heron, Golding, & Glover, 2003; Yehuda, Halligan, & Bierer, 2001). Further complicating matters, anxiety has various presentations. Anxiety can present as a cognitive (anxious thoughts), affective (a feeling of fear), behavioral (an avoidance of situations), or physiological (headaches, stomachaches) event. Lastly, the focus of one's anxiety and the symptom presentation changes across the developmental spectrum. Young children, for whom the greatest developmental challenge is independence, are more likely to fear separation. Older children, who have become aware of the judgments of others, are more likely to have social or performance anxieties. For any given anxious individual, the causal pathway to their current state is best understood as a dynamic and fluid interplay of all of the above-listed factors.

What One Believes About Anxiety and What One Does to Treat It are Intertwined

Psychosocial interventions evolve from one's assumptions about the nature of the condition. If one believes pathological anxiety results from childhood experiences, one develops a treatment that focuses on early life. With inaccurate, anxiety-laden beliefs as the cause, one constructs a treatment focused on challenging the anxious person's beliefs. If one believes that avoidance of feared situations is a paramount factor, the implication is that one should develop a smart way to expose the anxious person to feared situations. The interrelationship between one's beliefs about the nature of anxiety and the nuts and bolts of what one does to help the anxious individual makes it especially important that the clinician have an understanding of the nature of anxiety and the implications for psychosocial intervention (Wells, 2005).

Understanding the Distinction between Causal and Maintaining Factors is Important

The factors that led to development of an anxiety disorder (causal) may not be the same as the factors that are perpetuating the anxiety (maintaining). In broad terms, factors such as genetics and temperament are seen as causal. Factors such as cognition, learning, behavior, social pressures, and avoidance may serve a causal role but garner the greatest attention for their function as maintaining factors. A treatment focused on altering the maintaining factors is thought to be the quickest route to change. Several examples illustrate this point. A young child fears sleeping alone and goes to the parent's bed. The causal factor of this fear of sleeping alone may well be an anxious temperament. The maintaining variable may be a parent who provides an easy opportunity for avoidance, thus unintentionally discouraging independent sleeping. The focus of this treatment might be cognitive (changing the mother's attitudes and expectations about the need to foster independence in this situation) and behavioral (having a reasonable plan for keeping the child in his or her room at night). An example from a later developmental stage would be the socially phobic young adult who avoids dating. Causal factors for the current social anxiety might include bad social experiences from high school. In contrast, the maintaining factors might include current beliefs about his or her social desirability and the avoidance of social setting that creates the possibility of positive feedback. The focus of the treatment would not be a review of the experiences of high school (causal). A focus would be challenging the person's current cognitions about social desirability and a plan for what social settings to engage in and how to engage in those settings (Hoffman, 2007).

Evidence-Based Interventions Focus on Altering Cognitions and Behavior

The focus on altering cognitions and behavior is in service of reducing the avoidance of feared situations—the treatment's ultimate endpoint. Concerning cognition, one can employ methods such as thinking differently, holding more accurate and realistic expectations, keeping reassuring thoughts in mind, and anticipating the successful navigation of the anxious event. Cognitive interventions have many benefits; however, the interventions are premised on the individual's ability to think about what they are thinking (metacognition). Consequently, the interventions are most appropriately applied to individuals who have reached a formal operational stage of thinking, typically adolescence and older (see the following section on development). Concerning behavior, one can learn how to act differently, prepare for a situation, practice different skills, etc. Behavioral interventions are very practical and have proven very effective. Importantly, behavioral interventions can be used with individuals at every stage of the developmental process. Consequently, behavioral interventions are the first line of treatment in younger and school-aged children. The most important outcome is typically behavioral; the individual no longer avoids the feared situation(s) (Wells, 1999).

DEVELOPMENT IS A DYNAMIC PROCESS COMPRISING SEVERAL STAGES

Each developmental stage is marked by a new set of challenges, a new set of skills, and a new set of corresponding concerns. These challenges, skills, and concerns evolve in a dynamic interplay known as a stage. At each stage the interplay between challenge, skill, and concern is intricately interwoven in a rich and detailed manner into every aspect of one's daily experience. The focus, expression, and treatment of anxiety are different at each stage. The interchange between challenge, skill, and anxiety for four distinct developmental stages is illustrated in what follows.

EARLY CHILDHOOD

This section will review the prevalence, clinical presentation and psychosocial treatment of anxiety disorders in early childhood (ages 2–7).

Anxiety is common in early childhood

A normative stage of separation anxiety exists for all children and is developmentally appropriate. This normative stage ranges from 8 to 24 months, peaking between 14 and 18 months of age, and decreases in severity and frequency during the preschool years. When concerns about separating from caregivers persist later into childhood, a separation anxiety disorder may emerge (Kagan, Reznick, & Snidman, 1988; Kagan & Snidman, 1999). For most children the early childhood anxiety is transient, but for others it presages a lifelong struggle.

The tendency toward anxiety is part of a child's temperament

Kagan (1989) conducted seminal research on the influence of temperament. His research followed a large sample of children from age 4 months through middle childhood. Children were categorized as high- or low-reactive on the basis of their response to novel stimuli; high-reactive children would move vigorously, fret, and cry when presented with novel stimuli. The children who were high-reactive infants were more likely to be classified as shy and demonstrated fewer spontaneous comments and smiles at age 4. At age 7, anxiety symptoms such as nightmares and fear of the dark, thunder, lightning, etc. were present in 45% of the children who were high-reactive as infants but only 15% of children who were low-reactive as infants. Kagan's research demonstrates that a proclivity to anxiety can be identified in early childhood, and that early-childhood high reactivity predicts a significantly higher rate of anxiety problems in later childhood.

Parents play a central role in the treatment of anxiety in early childhood

There is growing, albeit limited, empirical support for behavioral and cognitive-behavioral interventions for young children with anxiety (Comer et al., 2012; Hirshfeld-Becker et al., 2010; Pincus, Santucci, Ehrenreich, & Eyberg, 2008). Central to all these treatments is the involvement of parents, because parents are the most influential agents in the life of a young child. The parents of an anxious child need to do several things. First, they must recognize that the anxiety is a problem that is limiting the child's life. Childhood anxiety is often easily minimized, or rationalized as a passing stage. A minimized view of the problem provides insufficient motivation for the parent to push back against the child's anxiety. Second, they must be thoughtful about any inadvertent ways they may be encouraging the anxiety. Examples include providing unnecessary warnings, allowing the child's anxious mood to be a mechanism by which he or she gains greater parental attention, and not holding the child to age-appropriate standards. Third, they can focus on and express pride in the occasions where the child acts in opposition to the fears. Fourth, they must help the child practice a plan for the occasions when they will be worried. Fifth, they can set out some system of rewards for the child for "brave" behavior.

Separation Anxiety Disorder in Early Childhood

Epidemiology

SEPARATION ANXIETY IS THE MOST COMMON ANXIETY DISORDER IN YOUNG CHILDREN

The prevalence of separation anxiety disorder (SAD) among children in early childhood (ages 2–5) is estimated to be 2.4% (Egger & Angold, 2006), occurring at higher rates in this stage than among any other age group. Notably, when prevalence rates are estimated strictly on *DSM–V–R* criteria, which specify that a child must have three or more SAD symptoms that cause distress *or* impairment (as opposed to impairment alone), prevalence rates are as high as 8.6% (Egger & Angold, 2006) for preschool-aged children.

SEPARATION ANXIETY DISORDER IS ESPECIALLY SENSITIVE TO FAMILY FACTORS

Separation anxiety occurs in the context of a family, and that family context will make itself known in the treatment in very practical ways. As it is a disorder of early childhood, treatment is undertaken by typically newer, less-experienced parents. The treatment requires parents to be firm on occasions when the child is anxious. The need to be firm will expose the difference between parents in their belief in the need to be and in their ability to be firm. SAD youth often have young siblings. Homes with several young children can be very busy places at bedtime; children need to complete evening routines and be put to bed, children of different ages have differing bedtimes, etc. The additional busyness of having several children complicates being calm, being prepared, and having the time to deal with the exceptional needs of the SAD youth.

Clinical Vignette: Sally, a typically developing 5-year-old with separation anxiety

Sally's behavior at the first meeting reflected her anxiety over separation. She sat curled up beside her mother on the couch and would hide her face in her mother's side when asked a question. Attempts to engage Sally were unsuccessful. The ordinary process of spending some time alone with the child had to be skipped as it was clear that Sally would refuse to be without her mother at her side. Sally refused to meet one-on-one with the clinician. Engaging Sally would be a trying process and much of the treatment would proceed by including the mother as a type of co-therapist. During the first parent meeting, Sally's mother admitted that she was uncertain about how to handle Sally's behavior when she refused to cooperate, and would often give in when Sally became distressed, as she hated to see her daughter so upset.

Most of the treatment was delivered by using the parent as co-therapist. First, one ensures the mother has the right orientation to treatment. A brief discussion about the mother's family of origin revealed an important fact: the mother experienced her parents as unpleasantly autocratic and had sworn to take a more egalitarian approach in raising her children. It was explained to the parent that parenting in reaction to one's own childhood is not the best strategy; a better method was responding to the facts of the current situation in a thoughtful and planned-out manner. It was also evident that the mother was more comfortable with a consensus-building interpersonal style; she had difficulty asserting her authority. It was explained to the mother that raising children includes leading them, and Sally was far too young to be part of every decision-making process. One must also make sure the mother is sufficiently motivated for what will be at times difficult. Second, one provides the mother with an education about anxiety. Genetics and temperament are important. Life circumstances encourage or discourage the experience of anxiety in one's life. Parents must be careful not to amplify fears by overly attending to them, providing the child with too many fear-based communications, or enabling by allowing the child to avoid fearful situations. Third, one provides the parents with specific plans for high- and low-anxious times. Low-anxious times offer the greatest opportunity to make therapeutic gains. One can talk to a child during low-anxious times: teach them something about anxiety, encourage them to be brave, and agree on a plan to prepare for coming high-anxiety times. Lastly, the therapist makes sure to provide the mother with emotional support for the arduous job of shepherding their child through a difficult educational process.

Sally's mother needed guidance on how to effectively respond to her daughter's anxious behavior. The clinician explained to Sally's mother that her tendency to pay particular attention to Sally when she was distressed and to remain home when Sally protested helped reinforce Sally's inclination to become unraveled and avoid separations. Together, the clinician and Sally's mother role-played ways to attend to and praise Sally's brave and independent behavior and to provide brief coaching statements when she appeared distressed or non-compliant.

Given Sally's non-compliance, her mother needed to implement clearer rules and expectations at home. The clinician worked with the parent to script clear, simple, and effective commands. In addition, the clinician developed a behavior management program in which Sally could earn stickers and small rewards for complying with parental requests (e.g., to clean up toys). Compliance is the ability to feel one way but act another. One wants to keep playing but is able to make oneself stop and clean up. The ability to push back against emotions in any one setting is practice for pushing back against emotions in another setting.

Sally and her mother must work as a team to practice brave behavior. In parent–child sessions, the family began to work on progressively challenging exposures in session (e.g., Sally sitting on couch and Mom on a chair across the room; Sally spending a portion of the session with the therapist with Mom outside the room; Mom leaving the clinic while Sally was in session; Mom arriving late to pick up Sally) so she could practice independent behavior. The clinician continued to coach Sally's mother on ways to attend to, praise, and reward brave behavior and ignore avoidant and anxious behavior. The family extended this work to challenges at home (e.g., playing in a different room for 30 minutes without calling or checking on Mom, staying with a relative while Mom runs a quick errand; remaining with babysitter while Mom goes out for progressively longer periods of time; falling asleep without Mom in the room; going to a play-date without Mom).

MIDDLE CHILDHOOD

This section will review the prevalence, clinical presentation, and psychosocial treatment of anxiety disorders in middle childhood (ages 8–12).

Anxiety can interfere with developing a sense of mastery

According to Piaget (1971), it is during middle childhood that youth develop a sense of industry and mastery in their work at school and in their interactions with peers and family. For anxious children who are fearful or withdrawn in one or more settings, it is often all the more challenging to develop confidence. Anxious children have been found to differ from non-anxious children in their levels of self-esteem, quality of peer relations, attention, social behavior and school performance (Strauss, Frame, & Forehand, 1987). Comparatively, childhood anxiety has even stronger associations with problematic family processes such as parent–child discord (Ezpeleta, Keeler, Alaatin, Costello, & Angold, 2001).

Co-occurring disorders are the rule, not the exception

Children who present with anxiety disorder often present with other difficulties. Estimates suggest that 40–60% of anxious children meet criteria for more than one anxiety disorder (Benjamin, Costello, & Warren, 1990). Childhood anxiety also places youth at much greater risk for depression (Angold, Costello, & Erkanli, 1999). It is particularly troubling, at a time when school plays such a central role in a child's identity, that many anxious youth meet criteria for a learning or language disorder (Gregory et al., 2007).

CBT treatments have a solid empirical foundation

Cognitive-behavioral treatment for anxious youth have been extensively investigated and found to be efficacious (Silverman, Pina, & Viswesvaran, 2008) when delivered in individual (Kendall, 1994; Kendall et al., 1997, Walkup et al., 2008), family (Kendall, Hudson, Gosch, Flannery-Schroeder, & Suveg, 2008), and group modalities (Hudson et al., 2009). Cognitive-behavioral treatment for school-aged youth typically covers relaxation, cognitive restructuring, problem solving, social skills, and *in vivo* exposure.

Specific Phobia in Middle Childhood

Epidemiology

SPECIFIC FEARS ARE COMMON AMONG CHILDREN

Among the most common fears in childhood are fears of animals, fear of natural environments, and fear of the dark. The prevalence of specific phobia among youth in community samples is thought to range from 5% to 10% (Kessler et al., 2005). Retrospective studies of adults suggest that specific phobias commonly first emerge in early to middle childhood, with lifetime prevalence rates of 12.5% (Kessler et al., 2005).

SPECIFIC PHOBIAS ARE LINKED TO MOOD AND ANXIETY PROBLEMS IN ADULTHOOD

A prospective follow-back investigation found that specific phobias in adulthood were often preceded by phobias in childhood but not by other anxiety or mood problems (Gregory et al., 2007). Additionally, adulthood mood and anxiety disorders in this sample were preceded by childhood phobias more than any other childhood anxiety or mood problem.

Clinical Vignette: Mark, a typically developing 11-year-old boy presenting with a fear of the dark

Mark's fear of the dark interfered with his independence at home as well as his ability to engage in age-appropriate activities with his peers.

Simplified cognitive strategies are effectively integrated into treatment with children. After explaining the link between anxious thoughts, feelings, and behaviors, the clinician worked with Mark to identify the worried thoughts he had about being in the dark. ("Bad things happen in the dark. Scary creatures hide in the dark. If I can't see, then I can't protect myself.") The clinician helped him to develop brave talk and cheerleading statements, including "I am safe. Just because it is dark doesn't mean something bad is going to happen. Even if there were monsters hiding in the dark, they've never hurt me."

Children respond to challenges that replace fearful associations with fun or pleasant feelings and build a sense of mastery. Homework challenges were designed to promote new, positive associations with the dark (e.g., going on scavenger hunts in the house with a flashlight, playing with a glow-in-the-dark soccer ball in the basement) and to help Mark gain confidence and independence in completing normal activities (e.g., running an errand for Mom upstairs; bringing clothes to the laundry room first in the daylight and then in the evening).

Fear associated with concerns about being alone often manifests in difficulties with independent sleep in childhood. As Mark developed greater confidence during the day and evening hours, the clinician worked with the family to eliminate safety behaviors (e.g., running between rooms, turning on lights). Independence at bedtime continued to be a challenge as Mark's imagination had a tendency to run wild when lying in bed. In session, Mark practiced a guided imagery exercise in which he imagined himself running down the field and scoring a soccer goal. He was encouraged to practice this exercise at bedtime. His parents were also coached to change their involvement in the bedtime routine. After they had read one story together, his mother wished him goodnight, turned off the light, moved from the bed to the hallway, and finally transitioned to her own room. Each step toward independence brought Mark closer to a final reward of hosting a sleepover with his closest friends.

ADOLESCENCE

This section will first discuss how the presentation and treatment of anxiety is influenced by developmental changes that occur during adolescence, and the epidemiology, presentation, and treatment of social anxiety disorder in adolescence will be reviewed.

Adolescence is an especially eventful period of development

If one is inclined to worry, perhaps no other developmental stage will offer such a rapid-fire succession of potential foci of worry. Anxious concerns that are especially prevalent in adolescence can be divided into two categories: personal worries, and worries that turn on the evaluation of others. Personal worries include the onset of puberty, the development of romantic attraction, concern with appearance, and increased autonomy. Evaluation worries include a widening social circle and a greater focus on popularity, dating ability, academic competence, and athletic performance. The clinician anticipates these worries in this age group precisely because they are the developmental concerns specific to the age. For an unlucky subset of adolescents, these ordinary concerns intermingle with their inclination for excessive worry, forming the basis of a potential social anxiety or generalized anxiety disorder.

Cognitive developments greatly enhance the variety and sophistication of anxiety management strategies

Cognitive developments in adolescence include an increased capacity for planning, focusing attention, social perspective taking, metacognition, and persistence in adhering to a plan. Therapists can build upon these emerging skills to help individuals cope with anxious feelings. For example, anxious individuals tend to perceive events in distorted and overly pessimistic ways. Planning is a useful mood-management tool. One can plan a stress-relieving event to follow a long day of exams. One can plan to bring a friend or plan what to say at a social event. The allocation of one's attention is important for mood management. The hypochondriac who feels compelled toward internet illness searches can intentionally divert his or her attention to a more adaptive topic. The development of metacognition is the capacity to think about one's own thinking. The capacity to identify when one's thinking has become distorted creates the opportunity for the adolescent to challenge his or her own thoughts about themselves, others, and the future and to then develop a more helpful and realistic perspective. Therapists can teach adolescents how to mobilize these novel abilities in order to better cope with anxiety-provoking experiences. The last skill is an increased ability to persist; changing something about oneself is hard, and persistence is essential.

Parents still matter

Much attention is rightly paid to adolescents' individuation from the family of origin; however, parents remain a primary influence. The therapist must carefully consider the role of the parent(s) in the treatment of the anxious adolescent. Parents contribute in ways good and bad. Many parents too suffer from anxiety. A parent's personal struggle with anxiety can be a bridge to understanding the experience of their anxious child. Anxious parents can also be overly sympathetic, finding it hard to push the anxious adolescent to face fears. Parents have to be mindful about the amount of reassurance they provide. Parents can provide too much reassurance, unintentionally facilitating a dependent child who has inadequate practice at reassuring themselves. Parents are most practically thought of as co-therapists. Parents can join with the therapist to clarify expectations, share personal experiences, and push for compliance with exposure to feared situations. The trajectory of adolescence is to evolve from being largely reliant upon one's parents toward more independent mood management. Becoming successful at independently managing one's anxiety is contingent upon a few factors, including the acquisition of skills, a bit of a push toward independence by parents, and the draw of the attractive elements of an independent life.

Social Phobia in Adolescence

Epidemiology

SOCIAL PHOBIA IN ADOLESCENCE IS COMMON, PERSISTENT, AND IMPAIRING

Social phobia (social anxiety disorder, SAD) is an enduring fear of embarrassment or negative feedback in a social or performance situation that results in significant limitation in social and school functioning (American Psychiatric Association, 1994). Lifetime prevalence rates of social anxiety disorder in adolescence range from 2% to 9% (Essau, Conradt, & Petermann, 1999; Fehm, Pelissolo, Furmark, & Wittchen, 2005) and social anxiety symptoms tend to be stable across the four years of high school (Hayward et al., 2008). Socially phobic adolescents lag behind peers in achieving developmental tasks such as the development of identity, independence from family, dating, or seeking employment (Albano, Chorpita, & Barlow, 2003). These youth typically have poor self-esteem, high self-critique, hypersensitivity to rejection and criticism, and often underachieve academically owing to infrequent classroom participation, poor test performance, or school refusal (Albano & DiBartolo, 2007; Kearney, 2001).

SOCIAL EVALUATION FEARS INCREASE IN ADOLESCENCE

Social evaluation fears increase in adolescence in lockstep with the development of perspective-taking and attending to one's internal dialogue (Alfano, Beidel, & Turner, 2002; Westenberg, Gullone, Bokhorst, Heyne, & King, 2007). Socially phobic adolescents have an internal dialogue fraught with apprehension and self-doubt, e.g., "I will forget what I am supposed to say," "Everyone will know I'm nervous," "The whole class will laugh at me if I make a mistake." The anxiogenic internal voice leads to increased anxiety as well as a greater likelihood of perceived or actual poor performance. As already described, it is the adolescent's very ability to identify and attend to internal dialogue that forms the cornerstone of cognitive intervention and makes it possible for them to engage in cognitive restructuring of maladaptive cognitions.

Cognitive-behavioral Therapy

There is considerable research documenting the efficacy of individual and group CBT for social phobia in adolescents (e.g., Crawley, Beidas, Benjamin, Martin, & Kendall, 2008; Garcia-Lopez et al., 2006; Hayward et al., 2000; Kashdan & Herbert, 2001). CBT for social anxiety includes education about anxiety, practice in identifying and challenging one's anxiogenic cognitions, social skills training, and practice socializing with others. Parents are often utilized as "co-therapists" to facilitate skill development. Treatment begins by providing the adolescent with education about social phobia and constructing a hierarchy of anxiety-provoking social situations ordered from least to most anxiety-provoking. The cognitive component details the reciprocal interaction of anxious thoughts, anxious physiological feelings, and anxious behaviors, the nature of maladaptive automatic thoughts (e.g., overestimation of the severity and likelihood of negative social interactions), and cognitive restructuring. Cognitive restructuring is the CBT term for becoming thoughtful about one's thinking—noticing anxiogenic thoughts and replacing them with more rational and encouraging thoughts. The skills training component focuses on teaching the adolescent the necessary social skills and behavioral relaxation techniques to engage in successful social interactions via didactics and role-play/modeling. Finally, and often most important, the exposure component entails graduated exposure to both simulated and *in vivo* anxiety-provoking social situations while the adolescent utilizes their cognitive and behavioral skills to successfully cope with their anxiety and engage in adaptive social interaction.

Clinical Vignette: Christopher, a high school freshman with social anxiety

Christopher's anxious expectations and concordant social avoidance were a target of intervention. Turning on the adolescent ability to think abstractly and take the perspective of another, the therapist engaged Christopher in a collaborative investigation of the origin and influence of his anxiogenic thoughts. Christopher began to track anxiety-provoking social situations, his automatic thoughts, and the impact of the thoughts on his anxiety and avoidant behavior. The therapist assisted Christopher in examining the evidence for and against his automatic thoughts and calling attention to maladaptive beliefs that lacked credibility. Christopher and the therapist collaboratively challenged and restructured those beliefs in order to generate more accurate and adaptive explanations of the social situations. For example, when a classmate to whom Christopher was talking in the hall stated that they had to go, Christopher immediately thought, "They must be annoyed with me." However, through a process of collaborative empiricism Christopher was able to see that this assumption lacked evidence and that he had been overlooking meaningful details that suggested the peer had been enjoying the conversation but was late for an extracurricular activity. This discovery led to greater confidence that enabled Christopher to engage in similar and more frequent casual conversations rather than avoid these interactions altogether. As treatment progressed, Christopher became better able to examine the evidence, challenge his anxious and often inaccurate expectations, and engage in increasingly difficult social situations.

Christopher also needed training in social skills. While much of his social difficulty was fueled by inaccurate and maladaptive cognitions, deficits in his social skills also played a significant role. Social skills needed for a high school freshman are particular to the demands of the age and gender of the individual. Initially, the therapist and Christopher focused on basic skills such as maintaining eye contact (rather than averting his gaze), having good posture (as opposed to slouching), conversational skills (e.g., ways to keep a conversation going), and assertiveness training. However, it was also important to ensure Christopher had an adequate fund of knowledge for topics considered "cool" by peers his age. These included knowledge of current music, sports, popular TV shows, and contemporary clothing. Christopher developed conversation starters for the various groups with whom he could interact: sports questions for boys in gym class, TV topics for peers in study hall, and so on.

Christopher's parents were engaged in a co-therapist-like role. Despite his initial desire for complete autonomy and discomfort with parental involvement, Christopher's parents provided much-needed support, encouragement, and feedback to facilitate improved socialization. His parents were able to remind him of and reinforce cognitive and behavioral skills learned during treatment in the home environment, where much of Christopher's social planning took place. They were also able to provide the therapist with helpful information to understand why certain aspects of treatment might not be going as planned (e.g., Christopher's initial attempts at peer interaction entailed posting vague messages on Facebook). However, it was also important for the therapist to work with Christopher's parents (who were both anxious themselves) to normalize Christopher's individuation from his family and increased influence of peers. In this way, his parents were better able to participate in the treatment without its feeling intrusive or infantilizing to Christopher. At times, the parents were able to play a more active role in the treatment, such as when his father purchased three tickets to a football game and Christopher was allowed to bring a friend of his choice. In addition to setting the stage for an enjoyable social activity, the father used the opportunity to observe Christopher while he socialized and report helpful details to the therapist that were the focus of subsequent therapy sessions.

ADULTHOOD

This section will review the epidemiology, presentation, and cognitive-behavioral treatment of anxiety disorders in adulthood.

Adulthood encompasses many developmental challenges

Young adults must contend with living away from home, dating, marriage, employment, and career development. In middle adulthood, many focus on starting a family, parenting, balancing career and family life, caring for aging parents, and learning how to adjust to the physical changes of middle age. Among seniors, the developmental challenge involves shifting one's orientation to life away from planning for the future and toward a more retrospective direction that involves building a sense of satisfaction with one's life and accomplishments. Anxiety is common in each of these stages. The focus and treatment of anxiety, however, may differ.

Adulthood is the culmination of acquired skills learned through the course of development. As discussed earlier, the psychosocial treatment options for young children are circumscribed by their capacity to participate in treatment. Young children have limited ability to plan, have trouble thinking about what they are thinking, can only persist for so long, and so on. Similar limitations extend, albeit to a lesser extent, into adolescence. Among mature adults the psychosocial therapist may unleash the full palate of interventions. By adulthood, most individuals are able to learn and apply information in sophisticated ways to meet the demands of specific situations. They should be able learn specific skills, engage in abstract reasoning, and look at problems from multiple perspectives. Adults typically have the capacity for metacognition such that they can learn to notice and challenge the veracity of their anxiogenic thoughts. Adults are also capable of mindfulness, including the emotional maturity to acknowledge their feelings and push back against the impulse to judge or react.

Panic Disorder with and without Agoraphobia in an Adult

Epidemiology

PANIC DISORDER IS COMMON, PERSISTENT, AND SIGNIFICANTLY IMPAIRING

Panic disorder is diagnosed in 1–2% of adults annually, with 1.5–3.5% of adults being diagnosed with panic at some point during their lives (APA, 1994). Panic disorder is a chronic problem with low rates of remission and high rates of relapse (APA, 1994; Keller et al., 1994; Pollack et al., 1990). Furthermore, it is associated with increased rates of death, mostly from cardiovascular disease and suicide (Coryell, Noyes, & Clancy, 1982; Coryell, Noyes, & House, 1986).

PANIC IS A DISORDER OF ADOLESCENCE AND ADULTHOOD

Panic attacks are rarely seen in childhood. Panic has a bimodal distribution of onset: it peeks between ages 15 and 24 and again between ages 45 and 54 (Eaton, Kessler, Wittchen, & Magee, 1994). The median age of onset is estimated at 24 years (Burke, Burke, Regier, & Rae, 1990). Initial psychological or psychiatric treatment for panic disorder is usually sought around age 34 (Breier, Charney, & Heninger, 1986; Craske, Miller, Rotunda, & Barlow, 1990).

PANIC HAS MANY PHYSICAL SYMPTOMS, WHICH AFFECTS THE PATH TO TREATMENT

The physical symptoms that accompany a panic attack (dizziness, shortness of breath, chest pains) lead many panic suffers to seek medical evaluations. Individuals with panic often first present for treatment at primary, specialty care, or emergency-room settings (Markowitz, Weissman, Ouellette, Lish, & Klerman, 1989; Sartorius, Ustun, Lecrubier, & Witcchen, 1996; Spitzer et al., 1995). Because of the symptom cluster, they are frequently referred to neurologists, otolaryngologists, and cardiologists (Kennedy & Schwab, 1997; Roy-Byrne & Katon, 2000). Individuals presenting at medical settings with complaints of noncardiac chest pain, palpitations, unexplained faintness, irritable bowel syndrome, and vertigo and dizziness are highly likely meet criteria for panic disorder (Beitman et al., 1987; Katon et al., 1988; Roy-Byrne & Katon, 2000).

Clinical Vignette: Nicole, a 37-year-old wife and mother who has begun to experience panic attacks

Nicole has sought treatment because her panic attacks are interfering with her ability to do things on her own.

Panic attacks are not harmful. Because adults have developed the intellectual capacity to comprehend complex, abstract information and to use advanced reasoning skills to apply information to real-world phenomena, education about the nature of panic and anxiety is often an important intervention. Nicole was particularly receptive to psychoeducation as she had been a good student and was quick to take the information presented to her and apply it to her own situation. Nicole's therapist carefully explained that panic attacks are normal physical reactions to a feared event. These reactions serve to prepare the body to respond to the perceived danger. The preparations produce physical sensations that are meant to protect the individual from harm. When panic attacks occur in the absence of a real danger, they are merely false alarms that may feel uncomfortable but are harmless. From this information, Nicole came to understand that she had become afraid of the physical sensations themselves because she had believed that they truly signaled danger when in fact they did not. Armed with this new understanding, Nicole was ready to believe that the feared physical sensations were not likely to be as dangerous as she had previously thought and she was willing to learn how to tolerate them instead of avoid them.

Nicole learned coping skills to help her better respond to anxiety and its physical expression. Nicole was taught breathing and thinking skills to use when anxious thoughts, feelings, and physical sensations occurred. The therapist taught Nicole to use slow, diaphragmatic breathing when feeling anxious. The plan was for Nicole to be able to regulate her breathing so that the anxiety symptoms did not intensify. The breathing skills were also meant to help her face the anxiety-provoking sensations and situations as calmly as possible so that she could remain in them until the anxious feelings had dissipated rather than escaping while feeling highly anxious. Escape and avoidance only serve to strengthen anxiety. In order to overcome anxiety, Nicole would need to respond to the feared situation calmly and remain there until her fear went away. It is only through this kind of experience that she could learn that her fears were unrealistic and that it was possible to deal with the situation.

The development of metacognition enables the identification of thought patterns that are likely to trigger or exacerbate panic. Metacognition also allows individuals to reflect upon and challenge those patterns, and then to develop alternative ways of thinking that are ultimately more rational and helpful. Thinking skills such as cognitive restructuring are based on this ability. Nicole identified that she held a number of erroneous beliefs that led her to experience increased anxiety and could trigger the onset of a panic attack. In particular, she initially believed that a physical sensation such an increased heart rate was an indication of some kind of rare and serious heart problem or cancer that had yet to be diagnosed. The therapist helped Nicole to identify these anxiety-provoking thoughts and to challenge them when they occurred. Then, they worked together to develop alternative thoughts that would be more helpful in reducing anxiety. For example, instead of believing the she could be about to have a heart attack, Nicole learned to remind herself that increased heart rate could occur for a number of other reasons, such as anxiety, hyperventilation, caffeine, exercise, or excitement. Additionally, Nicole also trained herself to remember that the odds were very low that she would have a heart attack and die, go crazy, or lose control. She generated other thoughts that she could use in the moment such as: "It's normal for my heart rate to change sometimes. Maybe my heart isn't beating any faster than usual but I'm just paying too much attention to it. Even if my heart is beating quickly, it's not dangerous." Nicole further learned to tell herself that the less attention she paid to her increased heart rate, the sooner it would probably go away. She developed the ability to change her thoughts away from the possible negative consequences of panic symptoms and onto strategies for coping with panic attacks.

Nicole gradually confronted anxiety-provoking sensations and situations that she had associated with an increased risk of panic attacks. Nicole's drive toward autonomy and independence was being threatened by her fear of panic attacks. Nicole was extremely motivated to regain her confidence to go places and do things independently. Moreover, she wanted to feel comfortable being alone with her children, taking them to activities, and being fully involved in their lives. The therapist built upon this motivation by engaging Nicole in exposure exercises that allowed her to practice using her coping skills and learn that the feared negative consequences would not occur. They developed a fear hierarchy that included physical sensations as well as particular situations. They began by having Nicole do interoceptive exposures in the office. For example, Nicole raised her heart rate by jogging in place and doing jumping jacks. Then she practiced using her breathing and thinking skills to cope until the anxious feelings subsided. They did this exercise in the office many times until Nicole felt confident that she could tolerate the sensations and her anxiety levels stayed low throughout the entire exercise. Next, Nicole began to practice doing exposures outside the office. Initially, she began in the privacy of her apartment, where she felt most safe. She replicated the office exposure by jogging in place to raise her heart rate and then used her coping skills while her anxiety level came down. After getting comfortable with this, she moved up her hierarchy and went jogging with her husband. As she became more comfortable, she continued to move up her hierarchy. Eventually she went to places that she had been avoiding. Using her coping skills, she was able to make it through an entire dinner with friends at a big, popular restaurant, and on another occasion she was able to see an entire movie at the local movie theater. Finally, she went food shopping alone and spent an entire day caring for her children by herself.

Mindfulness training can help to prevent relapse. Through treatment, Nicole became more confident in her ability to tolerate her physical sensations and control her worries about panic attacks, and with this new confidence she was able to regain her independence and her prior level of functioning. To prevent relapse, the therapist integrated mindfulness-based strategies into the treatment. Nicole learned how to be more aware of her automatic reactions to any particular situation that she experienced and to pay attention to her thoughts and feelings on a moment-to-moment basis without judging or reacting to them. She learned to accept her thoughts and feelings even when they were unpleasant, and to attend to them with an open and curious attitude. This allowed her to have a greater perspective on her experience and to better recognize how to help herself feel better and address her concerns in healthy ways. In this way, the therapist trained Nicole to be her own therapist, so that she could maintain her gains even after the formal therapy had ended.

CONCLUSION

The psychosocial treatment of anxiety requires an appreciation of the complexity of the illness, the known evidence-based treatments, and the developmentally sensitive delivery of those treatments. Anxiety is a complicated illness. It originates from factors as wide-ranging as physiology, cognition, attachment, and learning. Anxiety has cognitive, affective, and physiological expressions. Anxiety disorders coalesce with the challenges particular to one's developmental stage; young children often have fears related to demands for autonomy, while fears of social evaluation and performance have an onset later in life.

There are well-documented evidence-based treatments for anxiety. These comprise different interventions, including psychoeducation, relaxation training, diaphragmatic breathing, systematic desensitization, positive self-talk, cognitive restructuring, and mindfulness, among others. Different interventions are indicated for different anxiety disorders. The end goal of all the interventions is the same: to lessen phobic avoidance.

Developmental considerations enter into the selection and delivery of interventions. People exist in a developmental context. Young children are dependent upon their parents. Consequently, the treatment of young children must address the anxiety of the parents and include the parents as co-therapists. Older children, adolescents, etc. should become more independent in managing their emotions. Consequently, in these cases parents are encouraged to play a less prominent role.

Each of the interventions requires a different developmental skill of the patient. For example, cognitive restructuring requires the person have the intellectual sophistication to think about what they are thinking. Mindfulness requires both an intellectual sophistication and a level of emotional maturity to attend but not respond. The successful psychosocial treatment of anxiety requires the clinician to juggle all of the above concerns.

Clinical Points to Remember

1. Empathy is an essential ingredient in treatment. The anxious patient is in a difficult position. At any given moment it is easier to give in to the anxiety and stay with the well-worn habits of avoidance. To push back against your fears requires that you summon your courage and push aside feelings of shame, inadequacy, hopelessness, and depression. The situation is even more difficult for a child, who must confront all of these issues without the benefit of intellectual and emotional maturity, which are ordinarily the province of adulthood.

2. Anxiety is complicated. Many factors contribute to the development and maintenance of anxiety: genetic, physiological, neuroanatomical, developmental, attachment, cognitive, perceptual, behavioral, learning, etc. Additionally, anxiety presents with affective, cognitive, behavioral, and somatic features. A good assessment is mindful of the combined impact of all of these factors.

3. Anxiety is influenced by developmental factors. Anxiety disorders exist throughout the lifespan from early childhood through the end of life. The experience, presentation, and treatment of anxiety change as one develops. The clinician must be sensitive to the role of development to appropriately assess and treat anxiety.

4. There are well-established psychosocial treatments for anxiety disorders. No longer must a clinician grope through the empirical wilderness of just a generation ago; today, known evidence-based treatments exist. Clinical trial data now provide the clinician with a road map of proven interventions.

5. Psychosocial treatments are based on skill acquisition. The premise of psychosocial treatments is to teach the individual skills to better manage anxiety. The clinician must select a skill that is sensitive to the developmental status of the patient. Intellectually and emotionally sophisticated individuals can make good use of the most sophisticated skills, while younger patients must utilize simpler skills. For the youngest of patients, skills are often taught to the parents, who act as co-therapists.

6. Avoidance is anxiety's best friend. Avoiding feared situations permits the anxiety to further develop and become more fully integrated into one's life. The skills taught in psychosocial treatments are in service of facilitating the individual's engagement of the feared situation in order to neutralize and extinguish the fear.

REFERENCES

Albano, A. M., Chorpita, B. F., & Barlow, D. H. (2003). Anxiety disorders. In E. J. Mash & R. A. Barkley (Eds.), *Child psychopathology* (2nd ed., pp. 196–241). New York: Guilford Press.

Albano, A. M., & DiBartolo, P. M. (2007). *Cognitive-behavioral therapy for social phobia in adolescents: Stand up, speak out (therapist guide).* New York: Oxford University Press.

Alfano, C. A., Beidel, D. C., & Turner, S. M. (2002). Cognition in childhood anxiety: Conceptual, methodological, and developmental issues. *Clinical Psychology Review, 22*, 1209–1238.

American Psychiatric Association (APA). (1994). *Diagnostic and statistical manual of mental disorders* (4th ed.). Washington, DC: APA.

Angold, A., Costello, E. J., & Erkanli, A. (1999). Comorbidity. *Journal of Child Psychology and Psychiatry, 40*, 57–87.

Beitman, B. D., Lamberti, J. W., Mukerji, V., DeRosear, L., Basha, I., & Schmid, L. (1987). Panic disorder in cardiology patients with atypical or non-anginal chest pain: A pilot study. *Journal of Anxiety Disorders, 1*, 277–282.

Benjamin, R. S., Costello, E. J., & Warren, M. (1990). Anxiety disorders in a pediatric sample. *Journal of Anxiety Disorders, 4*, 293–316.

Breier, A., Charney, D., & Heninger, G. R. (1986). Agoraphobia with panic attacks. *Archives of General Psychiatry, 43*, 1029–1036.

Burke, K. C., Burke, J. D. Jr., Regier, D. A., & Rae, D. S. (1990). Age at onset of selected mental disorders in five community populations. *Archives of General Psychiatry, 47*, 511–518.

Comer, J. S., Puliafico, A. C., Aschenbrand, S. G., McKnight, K., Robin, J. A., Goldfine, M. E., & Albano, A. M. (2012). A pilot feasibility evaluation of the CALM Program for anxiety disorders in early childhood. *Journal of Anxiety Disorders, 26*, 40–49. doi:10.1016/j.janxdis.2011.08.011

Coryell, W., Noyes, R., & Clancy, J. (1982). Excess mortality in panic disorder: A comparison with unipolar depression. *Archives of General Psychiatry, 39*, 701–703.

Coryell, W., Noyes, R., & House, J. D. (1986). Mortality among outpatients with anxiety disorders. *American Journal of Psychiatry, 143*, 508–510.

Craske, M. G., Miller, P. P., Rotunda, R., & Barlow, D. H. (1990). A descriptive report of features of initial unexpected panic attacks in minimal and extensive avoiders. *Behaviour Research and Therapy, 28*, 395–400.

Crawley, S., Beidas, R., Benjamin, C., Martin, E., & Kendall, P. C. (2008). Treating socially phobic youth with CBT: Differential outcomes and treatment considerations. *Behavioural and Cognitive Psychotherapy, 36*, 379–389.

Eaton, W. W., Kessler, R. C., Wittchen, H. U., & Magee, W. J. (1994). Panic and panic disorder in the United States. *American Journal of Psychiatry, 151*, 413–420.

Egger, H. L., & Angold, A. (2006). Common emotional and behavioral disorders in preschool children: presentation, nosology, and epidemiology. *Journal of Child Psychology and Psychiatry, 47*, 313–337.

Essau, C. A., Conradt, J., & Petermann, F. (1999). Frequency and comorbidity of social phobia and social fears in adolescents. *Behaviour Research and Therapy, 37*, 831–843.

Ezpeleta, L., Keeler, G., Alaatin, E., Costello, E. J., & Angold, A. (2001). Epidemiology of psychiatric disability in childhood and adolescence. *Journal of Child Psychology and Psychiatry, 42*, 901–914.

Fehm, L., Pelissolo, A., Furmark, T., & Wittchen, H.-U. (2005). Size and burden of social phobia in Europe. *European Neuropharmacology, 15*, 453–462.

Garcia-Lopez, L. J., Olivares, J., Beidel, D. C., Albano, A. M., Turner, S. M., & Rosa, A. I. (2006). Efficacy of three treatment protocols for adolescents with social anxiety disorder: A five-year follow up assessment. *Journal of Anxiety Disorders, 20*, 175–191.

Gregory, A. M., Caspi, A., Moffitt, T. E., Koenen, K., Eley, T. C., & Poulton, R. (2007). Juvenile mental health histories of adults with anxiety disorders. *American Journal of Psychiatry, 164*, 301–308.

Hayward, C., Varady, S., Albano, A. M., Thieneman, M., Henderson, L., & Schatzberg, A. F. (2000). Cognitive behavioral group therapy for female socially phobic adolescents: Results of a pilot study. *Journal of the American Academy of Child and Adolescent Psychiatry, 39*, 721–726.

Hayward, C., Wilson, K. A., Lagle, K., Kraemer, H. C., Killen, J. D., & Taylor, C. B. (2008). The developmental psychopathology of social anxiety in adolescents. *Depression and Anxiety, 25*, 200–206.

Hirshfeld-Becker, D. R., Masek, B., Henin, A., Blakely, L. R., Pollock-Wurman, R. A., McQuade, J., et al. (2010). Cognitive behavioral therapy for 4- to 7-year-old children with anxiety disorders: A randomized clinical trial. *Journal of Consulting and Clinical Psychology, 78*, 498–510.

Hoffman, S. G. (2007). Cognitive factors that maintain social anxiety disorder: a comprehensive model and its treatment implications. *Cognitive Behaviour Therapy, 36*(4), 193–209.

Hudson, J. L., Rapee, R. M., Deveney, C., Schniering, C. A., Lyneham, H. J., & Bovopoulous, N. (2009). Cognitive-behavioral treatment versus an active control for children and adolescents with anxiety disorders: A randomized trial. *Journal of the American Academy of Child and Adolescent Psychiatry, 48*, 533–544.

Kagan, J. (1989). Temperamental contributions to social behavior. *American Psychologist, 44,* 668–674.

Kagan, J., Reznick, J. S., & Snidman, N. (1988). Biological bases of childhood shyness. *Science, 240,* 167–171.

Kagan, J., & Snidman, N. (1999). Early predictors of adult anxiety disorders. *Biological Psychiatry, 46,* 1536–1541.

Kashdan, T. B., & Herbert, J. D. (2001). Social anxiety disorder in childhood and adolescence: Current status and future directions. *Clinical Child and Family Psychology Review, 4,* 37–61.

Katon, W., Hall, M., Russo, J., Cormier, L., Hollifield, M., Vitaliano, P., & Beitman, B. (1988). Chest pain: Relationship of psychiatric illness to coronary arteriographic results. *American Journal of Medicine, 84,* 1–9.

Kearney, C. A. (2001). *School refusal behavior.* Washington, DC: American Psychological Association.

Keller, M. B., Yonkers, K. A., Warshaw, M. G., Pratt, L. A., Golan, J., Mathews, A. O., et al. (1994). Remission and relapse in subjects with panic disorder and agoraphobia: A prospective short interval naturalistic follow-up. *Journal of Nervous and Mental Disorders, 182,* 290–296.

Kendall, P. C. (1994). Treating anxiety disorders in children: Results of a randomized clinical trial. *Journal of Consulting and Clinical Psychology, 62,* 100–110.

Kendall, P. C., Flannery-Schroeder, E., Panichelli-Mindel, S. M., Southam-Gerow, M., Henin, A., & Warman, M. (1997). Therapy for youths with anxiety disorders: A second randomized trial. *Journal of Consulting and Clinical Psychology, 65,* 366–380.

Kendall, P. C., Hudson, J. L., Gosch, E., Flannery-Schroeder, E., & Suveg, C. (2008). Cognitive-behavioral therapy for anxiety disordered youth: A randomized clinical trial evaluating child and family modalities. *Journal of Consulting and Clinical Psychology, 76,* 282–297.

Kennedy, B., & Schwab, J. (1997). Utilization of medical specialists by anxiety disorder patients. *Psychosomatics, 38,* 109–112.

Kessler, R. C., Berglund, P., Demler, O., Jin, R., Merikangas, K. R., & Walters, E. E. (2005). Lifetime prevalence and age-of-onset distribution of DSM-IV disorders in the National Comorbidity Survey Replication. *Archives of General Psychiatry, 62,* 593–602.

Kinsella, M. T. & Monk, C. (2009). Impact of maternal stress, depression and anxiety on fetal neurobehavioral development. *Clinical Obstetrics and Gynecology, 52(3),* 425–440.

Markowitz, J. S., Weissman, M. M., Ouellette, R., Lish, J. D., & Klerman, G. L. (1989). Quality of life in panic disorder. *Archives of General Psychiatry, 46,* 984–992.

Monk, C., Leight, K. L., & Fang, Y. (2008). The relationship between women's attachment style and perinatal mood disturbance: implications for screening and treatment. *Archives of Women's Mental Health, 11,* 117–129.

Norrholm, S. D., & Ressler, K. J. (2009). Genetics of anxiety and trauma-related disorders. *Neuroscience, 164,* 272–287.

O'Connor, T. G., Heron, J., Golding, J., Glover, V., & the ALSPAC Study Team. (2003). Maternal antenatal anxiety and behavioural/emotional problems in children: A test of a programming hypothesis. *Journal of Child Psychology and Psychiatry, 44(7),* 1025–1036.

Piaget, J. (1971). *The theory of stages in cognitive development: Measurement and Piaget.* New York: McGraw-Hill Green.

Pincus, D., Santucci, L. C., Ehrenreich, J. T., & Eyberg, S. M. (2008). The implementation of modified Parent–Child Interaction Therapy for Youth with separation anxiety disorder. *Cognitive and Behavioral Practice, 15,* 118–125.

Pollack, M. H., Otto, M. W., Rosenbaum, J. F., Sachs, G., O'Neil, C., Asher, R., & Meltzer-Brody, S. (1990). Longitudinal course of panic disorder: Findings from the Massachusetts General Hospital naturalistic study. *Journal of Clinical Psychiatry, 51,* 12–16.

Roy-Byrne, P. P., & Katon, W. (2000). Anxiety management in the medical setting: Rationale, barriers to diagnosis and treatment, and proposed solutions. In D. I. Mostofsky & D. H. Barlow (Eds.), *The management of stress and anxiety in medical disorders* (pp. 1–14). Boston: Allyn & Bacon.

Sartorius, N., Ustun, T., Lecrubier, Y., & Witcchen, H. U. (1996). Depression comorbid with anxiety: Results from the WHO Study on Psychological Disorders in Primary Health Care. *British Journal of Psychiatry, 168* (Suppl. 30), 38–43.

Silverman, W. K., Pina, A. A., & Viswesvaran, C. (2008). Evidence-based psychosocial treatments for phobic and anxiety disorders in children and adolescents. *Journal of Clinical Child and Adolescent Psychology, 37,* 105–130.

Spitzer, R. L., Kroenke, K., Linzer, M., Hahn, S. R., Williams, J. B. W., deGruy, F V. III, et al. (1995). Health related quality of life in primary care patients with mental disorders: Results from the PRIME MD 1000 Study. *JAMA: Journal of the American Medical Association, 274*(19), 1511–1517.

Strauss, C. C., Frame, C. L., & Forehand, R. (1987). Psychosocial impairment associated with anxiety in children. *Journal of Clinical Child Psychology, 16,* 235–239.

Walkup, J. T., Albano, A. M., Piacentini, J., Birmaher, B., Compton, S. N., Sherrill, J. T., & Kendall, P. C. (2008). Cognitive behavioral therapy, sertraline, or a combination in childhood anxiety. *New England Journal of Medicine, 359,* 2753–2766.

Wells, A. (1999). A metacognitive model and therapy for generalized anxiety disorder. *Clinical Psychology and Psychotherapy, 6,* 86–95.

Wells, A. (2005). Generalized anxiety disorder. In A. Freeman et al. (Eds.), *Encyclopedia of cognitive behavior therapy* (pp. 195–198). New York: Springer. doi:10.1007/0-306-48581-8_56

Westenberg, P. M., Gullone, E., Bokhorst, C. L., Heyne, D. A., & King, N. J. (2007). Social evaluation fear in childhood and adolescence: Normative developmental course and continuity of individual differences. *British Journal of Developmental Psychology, 25,* 471–483.

Yehuda, R., Halligan, S. L., & Bierer, L. M. (2001) Relationship of parental trauma exposure and PTSD to PTSD, depressive and anxiety disorders in offspring. *Journal of Psychiatric Research, 35,* 261–270.

Part II

Treatment

CHAPTER 5

Generalized Anxiety Disorder

Joseph E. Comaty and Claire Advokat

INTRODUCTION

Generalized anxiety disorder (GAD) is a relatively recent independent diagnosis, first appearing in the 1980 *DSM–III* (Gorman, 2002; Tyrer & Baldwin, 2006). Before then, it was to be found in the category of "general neurotic syndrome" (Allgulander, 2010) "or anxiety neurosis." Freud first placed it in the category "unattached fearfulness," but this included the symptom of panic, which Klein determined to be a separate illness (Tyrer & Baldwin, 2006). Therefore, the aspect of anxiety neurosis that did not include panic became known as generalized anxiety disorder.

DSM Criteria

Although a recent diagnostic entity, "[n]o diagnostic category has changed over the past 25 years as much as GAD" (Davidson et al., 2010, p. 5). In the *DSM–III* the requirement was persistent anxiety for at least 1 month, in the absence of other anxiety or psychiatric disorders. The symptoms had to come from three of the four categories of (1) motor tension, (2) autonomic hyperactivity, (3) apprehensive expectation, and (4) being at least 18 years old.

The description changed in the *DSM–III–R* to "unrealistic or excessive worry about 2 or more circumstances" present for more days than not, over 6 months. This version required six symptoms from three categories (motor tension, autonomic hyperactivity, and vigilance/scanning). The disorder could not occur exclusively during the course of a mood disorder, and it could be diagnosed in children. In the *DSM–IV* (1994) and *DSM–IV–TR* (2000) the "excessive worry" was required to be "difficult to control," and to cause significant distress or impairment. The number of symptom categories was again increased to six, of which three or more had to be present: (1) muscle tension, (2) feeling restless, keyed up or on edge, (3) being easily fatigued, (4) having difficulty concentrating, (5) irritability, and (6) sleep disturbance.

The symptoms have always included a combination of psychological and somatic complaints. The latter are more prominent in the WHO's International Statistical Classification of Diseases and Related Health Problems, 10th Revision (ICD–10), which requires at least one symptom of autonomic arousal, indicated by such responses as palpitations, sweating, trembling, dry mouth, difficulty breathing, chest pain, nausea, dizziness, irritable bowel syndrome, difficulty swallowing, aches and pains, and other somatic reactions (Katzman, 2009; Tyrer & Baldwin, 2006).

GAD criteria are still controversial. Current debate concerns the duration and number of symptoms, the requirement of "excessive worry," and the relationship between GAD and major depressive disorder (MDD) (M. B. Stein, 2009; Tyrer & Baldwin, 2006; Weisberg, 2009). Not surprisingly, the prevalence of GAD increases as the duration requirement decreases. It is also unclear whether or not three symptoms are optimal; arguments have been made to *increase* the number to four and to *decrease* the number to two. Defining "excessive" worry has also been problematic, and this criterion was associated with the lowest interrater agreement. There is also a large and bidirectional overlap between anxiety and depression: almost three-quarters of people with GAD will have depression in their lifetime. Usually, anxiety precedes depression, but they are both likely to occur in the same year, and the evidence suggests they are linked in some way (M. B. Stein, 2009; Weisberg, 2009).

For the next version of the *DSM* (expected in 2013), major changes include a reduction in the duration of excessive anxiety and worry from 6 to 3 months and a reduction in the number of symptoms from six to one. A new addition to the *DSM–V* is a requirement for at least one of four behaviors that represent attempts to avoid situations that induce anxiety, result in increased time preparing for situations in which negative outcomes could occur, procrastination in decision making due to worries, or repeatedly seeking reassurance due to worries. This was included to be consistent with criteria in other anxiety disorders (www.dsm5.org/Pages/Default.aspx).

In addition to MDD, GAD has a high rate (over 90%; Katzman, 2009) of comorbidity with other psychiatric disorders, including bipolar disorder, substance use disorders and other anxiety disorders (Simon, 2009). "The high prevalence of concurrent psychiatric disorders is the most damaging criticism of the diagnosis of generalized anxiety disorder" (Tyrer & Baldwin, 2006, p. 2158).

Prevalence

In spite of the diagnostic difficulties, it is often stated that GAD is the most common anxiety disorder in primary care, where the prevalence may be as high as 8.3% (Katzman, 2009), and that anxiety symptoms are also common in the community (Baldwin, Ajel, & Garner, 2010; Baldwin, Waldman, &

Allgulander, 2011; Garner, Möhler, Stein, Mueggler, & Baldwin, 2009; Samuel, Zimovetz, Gabriel, & Beard, 2011). Estimates of 12-month and lifetime prevalence in the United States are 3.1% and 5.7%, respectively, with women affected more than men in a 2:1 ratio (Katzman, 2009; Pollack, 2009; Weisberg, 2009). Worldwide lifetime and 12-month prevalence ranges are reported to be 2.8–6.6% and 0.9–3.6%, respectively. While GAD may occur at any point in a person's lifetime, it is relatively uncommon before the age of 20 years, and the median age of onset in the United States is estimated at 31 years (Katzman, 2009; Weisberg, 2009). The highest rates are reported in the 45- to 55-year age group, and it is the most common anxiety disorder among individuals aged 55 to 85 years (Baldwin et al., 2011), with estimates in the elderly being as high as 10.2% (Davidson et al., 2010).

Prognosis

GAD is a chronic disorder with a waxing and waning course, and it is not unusual for patients to have experienced active symptoms for more than 10 years before they seek treatment. Although spontaneous remission can occur, rates over 5 years are less than 40% and most patients are still symptomatic 6–12 years after diagnosis (Davidson et al., 2010; Tyrer & Baldwin, 2006). Continued treatment is often necessary; 25% of patients may relapse within a month (Pollack, 2009). In the large Harvard/Brown Anxiety Research Project, recovery over the 12-year naturalistic follow-up period was only achieved by 58% of GAD patients, which was a lower percentage than for panic disorder (82%) or MDD (73%). Of those who did recover, nearly one-half eventually had a recurrence (Bruce et al., 2005). However, some epidemiological data suggest a more optimistic long-term prognosis. In a 40-year follow-up study of 59 GAD patients, only about 17% were still diagnosed with GAD (Rubio & López-Ibor, 2007). In a non-patient cohort of community participants, the course of the GAD spectrum over 20 years was similar: only 16% (12) of the 75 individuals were rediagnosed as having GAD (Angst, Gamma, Baldwin, Ajdacic-Gross, & Rössler, 2009).

The human and economic costs of GAD are substantial. Functional impairment of pure GAD is comparable in magnitude to that of pure MDD (Pollack, 2009), and in the range of chronic medical conditions (D. L. Hoffman, Dukes, & Wittchen, 2008). Medical disorders associated with anxiety often involve the adrenal system, which mediates the various physiological effects of stress on the body. Consequences may include pain conditions, such as arthritis, migraine, and back pain; gastrointestinal illness, ulcers; cardiovascular conditions, such as coronary heart disease; endocrine disorders such as diabetes; and respiratory conditions such as asthma and chronic obstructive pulmonary disease (Culpepper, 2009). GAD patients use primary care and gastroenterology services significantly more often than those without the disorder, and are twice as likely to consult gastroenterologists as to consult psychiatrists. As a result of lost work productivity and high medical resource use, GAD is associated with considerable economic costs, and the per-patient cost of GAD is reported to be higher than that of any of the other anxiety disorders studied (D. L. Hoffman et al., 2008).

SOLITARY TREATMENT APPROACHES

Pharmacological Treatment

Treatment efficacy for GAD has been established in randomized, placebo-controlled clinical trials for drugs from several classes, including benzodiazepines (BZDs), azapirones (buspirone), selective serotonin reuptake inhibitors (SSRIs), serotonin–norepinephrine reuptake inhibitors (SNRIs), atypical antipsychotics, antihistamines, and anticonvulsants. Other agents that are not officially indicated for this condition may also be effective (Davidson, 2009). Because benzodiazepines and azapirones have essentially been superseded by the antidepressants and newer agents, their clinical application will be summarized first.

Benzodiazepines

Benzodiazepines (BZDs) have been available since the 1960s and used therapeutically not only for the treatment of anxiety but also for their hypnotic, anticonvulsant, and muscle-relaxant properties. These actions are mediated by binding to the γ-aminobutyric acid receptor (GABA) complex, specifically the $GABA_A$ subtype, which potentiates the effect of GABA on chloride ion channels, hyperpolarizing neurons and reducing neurotransmission. Unlike barbiturates, BZDs cannot activate the chloride channel directly, independently of GABA, and this is believed to be the reason they are very safe in overdose. The agents have similar anxiolytic efficacy, and clinical use is primarily determined by their duration—that is, whether they are short-, intermediate- or long-acting (because of variables like lipid solubility and active metabolites) (Gorman, 2002).

BZDs have the advantage of a short latency to response, usually within 15–60 minutes (Tyrer & Baldwin, 2006), and can be used on an as-needed basis for situational anxiety as well as for continued therapy and for augmentation if other agents are insufficient (Pollack, 2009). Some of them (lorazepam, oxazepam, and temazepam) have no active metabolites, which means they are less likely to produce problems from drug–drug interactions. On the other hand, a few antidepressants (such as fluoxetine and fluvoxamine) inhibit the enzyme that metabolizes some of the BZDs, which might require a dose reduction (Carlat, 2011).

Although BZDs, particularly diazepam, alprazolam, and lorazepam, have been used for decades as effective treatments for GAD (Martin et al., 2007; Mitte, Noack, Steil, & Hautzinger, 2005), therapeutic guidelines for these medications have undergone major changes. Twenty years ago they were considered first-line treatment for many anxiety disorders, but now they are considered second-line options because of their abuse potential (Feltner & Haig, 2011) and the difficulty of discontinuation, and are not recommended for more than 2–4 weeks (Cloos, 2010).

The benefit of these medications is primarily in the relief of somatic symptoms rather than the psychological aspects of "worry." And BZDs do not reduce symptoms of depression, which is a disadvantage, considering the high comorbidity of the two disorders. It has been proposed that BZDs are most useful in two types of situations: for brief reactions in response to stress, or where somatic symptoms are more prominent than psychic symptoms. BZDs are not recommended when GAD presents with significant hostility, impatience, irritability, and impulsivity, as these behaviors may be worsened by BZDs (Davidson et al., 2010).

BZDs also have several undesirable side effects, such as sedation, motor impairment, and cognitive disturbances, which may be synergistic with alcohol. These drugs have been particularly associated with automobile accidents and increased falls in the elderly (Gorman, 2002).

Although tolerance develops to many effects of these drugs within weeks, patients taking BZDs for long periods of time generally do not increase their dose, and, except for individuals with preexisting substance abuse, BZD abuse is rare (Cloos, 2010; Gorman, 2002; Pollack, 2009). Nevertheless, as little as 2 weeks of chronic use can produce physical dependence and withdrawal effects upon discontinuing the medication. These include rebound anxiety, agitation, insomnia, and other reactions, which are more severe after longer administration, high doses, and abrupt termination. BZDs should always be tapered slowly when discontinued, even as gradually as 5% every two days (Carlat, 2011). To avoid physiological dependence, it is common to prescribe "as-needed" use. However, intermittent use results in fluctuating blood levels, which may worsen anxiety, reduce efficacy, and impair cognition. These effects may be especially detrimental in regard to psychological treatment, as the chronic continued use of BZDs may interfere with the efficacy of cognitive-behavioral treatment. For these reasons, a regular time-fixed dosing schedule may be preferred for preventing anxiety symptoms, rather than reducing them after they occur (Cloos, 2010).

In brief, the recommended approach is to use BZDs for short-term treatment (until an alternative medication, such as an antidepressant, begins to work, and to protect against occasional worsening of anxiety at the start of alternate treatment), and in patients who have not responded to at least two previous treatments (Baldwin et al., 2009; Davidson et al., 2010). Once patients are stabilized on another treatment, the goal would be to taper the BZD (Ravindran & Stein, 2010). Nevertheless, "clinical reality" does not always match the guidelines, and BZDs are still commonly prescribed for acute and chronic anxiety disorders (Carlat, 2011; Cloos, 2010).

Azapirones: buspirone

Buspirone is a partial $5HT1_a$ (serotonin) agonist that has short-term efficacy for GAD; it is the only azapirone approved for anxiety treatment, and the first non-BZD to demonstrate efficacy in controlled trials (Rickels, Downing, Schweizer, & Hassman, 1993). It acts by reducing the firing of serotonergic neurons at presynaptic serotonin autoreceptors (Gorman, 2002). Mitte et al. (2005) describe results from 10 studies of buspirone, of which eight showed an acceptable effect relative to placebo. A Cochrane systematic review (Chessick et al., 2006) summarized results from six studies of buspirone compared to placebo, 12 studies compared to BZDs, and one study compared to the antidepressant venlafaxine, and found buspirone superior to placebo and similar to the BZDs. While buspirone may be beneficial for initial GAD treatment, particularly in patients who have not been exposed to BZDs, its slow onset of action (2–3 weeks) and modest efficacy have reduced its use as monotherapy. It may be helpful for augmenting other anxiolytics, in comorbid depression treatment, or in patients with antidepressant-induced sexual dysfunction. Because it is not addictive, it is thought to be useful in patients with alcohol dependence, but there is little evidence in this regard (Davidson et al., 2010; Pollack, 2009; Tyrer & Baldwin, 2006). In contrast to BZDs, buspirone primarily improves psychic symptoms. It does not interact with other central nervous system depressants, does not impair cognition or motor function, and does not produce significant negative somatic effects upon discontinuation. Buspirone's adverse effects are mild, mostly dizziness, headache, and nausea, but this may reflect its short plasma half-life, which often requires three daily doses. This characteristic reduces compliance and may contribute to its low efficacy. The fact that it lacks antidepressant benefit is also a drawback (Gorman, 2002; Ravindran & Stein, 2010).

Antidepressants

As early as 1962, antidepressants were reported to have anxiolytic efficacy, mostly in conjunction with the treatment of panic attacks and phobias. The tricyclic antidepressant (TCA) imipramine was more effective than placebo or the BZD chlordiazepoxide in a patient population with "anxiety neurosis," and comparable to alprazolam in reducing both psychic and somatic symptoms (Hoehn-Saric, McLeod, & Zimmerli 1988; McLeod, Hoehn-Saric, Porges, &

Zimmerli, 1992; Rickels et al., 1993). These positive outcomes prompted a double-blind, placebo-controlled trial of imipramine and trazodone, compared with diazepam, in patients who met the *DSM–III* criteria for GAD without major depression or panic disorder.

In what has since become typical of these studies, participants were predominantly white females, aged 35 and older, who had had their first episode 5–10 years earlier. The baseline Hamilton Anxiety Scale (HAM-A) score was at least 18, with the group average in the mid 20s. The trial lasted 8 weeks, with mean maximum daily doses of imipramine (143 mg), trazodone (255 mg), and diazepam (26 mg). During the first 2 weeks, diazepam produced significantly more improvement than imipramine and trazodone, with greater effect on somatic than on psychic symptoms. By week 3, all three active drugs produced comparable improvement, but by week 8 only imipramine had sustained a statistically significant improvement compared with placebo. The overall completion rate was 65%, with no difference in attrition among the four treatments. With the exception of drowsiness, both antidepressants caused more side effects than diazepam. While sedative side effects waned, the antidepressant-induced anticholinergic responses did not. As assessed by the patients, global improvement was statistically significant for all three medications, compared with placebo: 73% for imipramine, 67% for trazodone, 66% for diazepam, and 39% for placebo (Rickels et al., 1993).

In a subsequent study, Rickels et al. (2000) compared imipramine and buspirone in the management of BZD discontinuation in GAD patients who had been taking BZDs for an average of 8.5 years. There were several phases: a BZD stabilization phase, 4 weeks of imipramine (180 mg/day), buspirone (38 mg/day) or placebo with BZD maintenance, a 4- to 6-week BZD taper, and a 5-week post-taper phase with imipramine, buspirone, and placebo treatment continued for another 3 weeks, followed by 2 weeks of placebo. Of the 107 patients who entered the study, 32 did not complete the pre-taper phase. During that period, patients taking imipramine reported more adverse reactions than patients in the other two groups. During the actual taper phase, neither buspirone nor imipramine reduced the severity of the BZD discontinuation effects, and the patients receiving imipramine even reported significantly more severe symptoms. But at the 3-month follow-up, patients receiving imipramine had a significantly higher success rate of taper (82.6%) than those given placebo (37.5%), while the difference between these treatments and buspirone (67.9%) did not reach statistical significance. At 12 months, 80% of the patients BZD-free at 3 months were still free (32 out of 40). For 57 patients who provided data at 12 months, 39 (68.4%) were BZD-free and 18 (31.6%) were still taking BZDs. Most importantly, BZD-free patients reported significantly lower levels of anxiety and depression than those still taking the drugs.

Selective serotonin reuptake inhibitors (SSRIs)

PAROXETINE

The poor side-effect profile of TCAs, particularly the potential for lethal over-dose, limited their use. Subsequently, the SSRI antidepressants were also found effective for GAD, as well as other anxiety disorders. Paroxetine was one of the earliest to be evaluated, in an open comparison with imipramine and 2'-chlord-esmethyldiazepam, and the first SSRI to be approved for the treatment of GAD. As before, all three drugs produced significant improvement, with diazepam initially more efficacious than the two antidepressants, and somatic symptoms showing the best response. But by the 4th week, paroxetine and imipramine were more effective than diazepam, with greater benefit for psychic symptoms (Rocca, Fonzo, Scotta, Zanalda, & Ravizza, 1997). These results were replicated in several double-blind, placebo-controlled studies in outpatients (Pollack et al., 2001; Rickels et al., 2003; Stocchi et al., 2003). Response and remission rates for paroxetine were 62–68% and 30–36%, respectively, with 46% and 20% respec-tively for the placebo groups. Significantly, more paroxetine than placebo patients reported adverse side effects, notably sexual dysfunction but also asthe-nia, constipation, and nausea, similar to those occurring during treatment for depression. In a continuation phase, responders were randomly assigned to double-blind treatment with paroxetine or placebo for another 24 weeks. Sig-nificantly fewer paroxetine patients relapsed (10.9%) than placebo patients (39.9%) (Sheehan & Mao, 2003; Stocchi et al., 2003).

SERTRALINE

Given that sertraline had demonstrated efficacy for panic disorder, obsessive-compulsive disorder, posttraumatic stress disorder, and social anxiety, it should not be surprising that studies demonstrated its effectiveness for GAD as well (Allgulander et al., 2004). In the first, 12-week, double-blind, placebo-controlled trial, sertraline (50–150 mg/day) showed significantly greater efficacy, relative to placebo, on all measures by the 4th week, which was maintained for all 12 weeks. Improvement was shown for both psychic and somatic factors (Dahl et al., 2005). This was in spite of the fact that some of the side effects of sertraline itself, as well as paroxetine (such as nausea, diarrhea and sweating), are similar to the somatic symptoms of anxiety. The response rate at endpoint was 56% for sertraline and 29% for placebo, and the respective remission rates were 31% and 18%. Adverse events that were greater for sertraline than placebo included nausea, insomnia, sweating, decreased libido in males and females, and diarrhea. Nevertheless, 80% of 147 participants given sertraline completed the study, as did 74% of placebo patients. In a second, 10-week trial, results again showed a statistically greater reduction in HAM-A scores with sertraline (average dose 149 mg/day) compared with placebo, although the difference in absolute scores was very small. In contrast to the previous findings, the psychic subscale ratings were better for the sertraline group—but not the somatic sub-scale ratings. On the other hand, the only adverse reactions reported significantly more by patients given sertraline were sexual side effects. In this study, there was an exceptionally high placebo response rate of 48.2% compared with 59.2% in the sertraline group (Brawman-Mintzer, Knapp, Rynn, Carter, & Rickels, 2006).

ESCITALOPRAM

Escitalopram, the enantiomer of citalopram, is currently the most selective serotonin reuptake inhibitor available. The efficacy, safety, and tolerability of this drug in the treatment of GAD were determined in three randomized double-blind placebo-controlled 8-week studies (Davidson, Bose, Korotzer, & Zheng, 2004; Goodman, Bose, & Wang, 2005). In each case, escitalopram reduced HAM-A total scores and both the psychic and the somatic anxiety sub-scales significantly more than placebo. Escitalopram produced significantly more responders (47.5% vs. 28.6%) and remitters (26.4% vs. 14.1%) than placebo. The dropout rate was relatively low, and 78% of both groups completed the 8-week trials. As might be expected, the primary adverse events for escitalopram compared with placebo were in regard to sexual dysfunction, as well as insomnia and fatigue.

Serotonin–norepinephrine reuptake inhibitors (SNRIs)

VENLAFAXINE

Extended release venlafaxine was the first antidepressant medication to receive U.S. Food and Drug Administration (FDA) approval for GAD. In the first trial, 75–150 mg/day was effective in an acute, 8-week study, producing a greater, though not statistically significant, reduction in HAM-A scores than placebo or buspirone (Davidson, DuPont, Hedges, & Haskins, 1999). Statistical significance required an additional dose of 225 mg/day (Rickels, Pollack, Sheehan, & Haskins, 2000). In particular, psychic symptoms were better relieved than somatic symptoms. Across five placebo-controlled studies, the difference between placebo and venlafaxine on the mean HAM-A score ranged from 1.6 to 4.2 (Gorman, 2002), which represents a clinically meaningful effect. Long-term treatment for 6 months with 75, 150, or 225 mg/day showed significantly greater response rates in venlafaxine patients (69% or higher beginning at week 6) than in placebo patients (42–46%). But the dropout rate was very high, with many placebo dropouts due to lack of response, and most venlafaxine dropouts from adverse reactions, particularly nausea, somnolence, dry mouth, and, in males, sexual dysfunction (Gelenberg et al., 2000).

A subsequent 24-week trial resulted in a better overall outcome, with lower doses (Allgulander, Hackett, & Salinas, 2001). In this case both 75 and 150 mg/day doses showed significant improvement relative to placebo on all of the primary efficacy variables. Venlafaxine was associated with more side effects than placebo even at the lowest dose, and the highest dose greatly increased the proportion of patients reporting nausea, vomiting, loss of appetite, tinnitus, dizziness, and light-headedness. Yet Montgomery, Mahé, Haudiquet, and Hackett (2002) found venlafaxine to be well tolerated, with adverse events not different from placebo. Meoni, Hackett, and Lader (2004) provide a meta-analysis of these results. For patients who responded to a 6-month trial and continued to take venlafaxine after an extended period of time (6–12 months), relapse rates were 9.8%, which was significantly better than the 53.7% of patients who relapsed on placebo (Rickels et al., 2010).

DULOXETINE

Duloxetine was approved in 2007 for GAD treatment on the basis of trial outcomes showing efficacy, safety, and relapse prevention. In a 10-week double-blind, progressive-titration, flexible-dose trial, adult outpatients with a *DSM–IV*-defined GAD diagnosis were randomized to duloxetine or placebo treatment. Duloxetine decreased HAM-A total scores statistically more (8.12, a 36% decline) than placebo group (5.89, a 25% decline) at a mean daily dose of 102 mg/day. The response rate of the drug group was 40%, compared with 32% for placebo, which was a statistical difference. But only 28% of drug-treated patients met remission criteria, compared with 23% for the placebo condition, which was not significant. Duloxetine elicited significantly more reports of nausea, dizziness, and tremor than placebo, although not sexual dysfunction, and the drug was associated with significant increases in heart rate and blood pressure (Rynn et al., 2008). In another comparison, venlafaxine produced more side effects during the tapering period, although both drugs were equally effective (Hartford et al., 2007). In a continuation phase of this trial, treatment responders in the 10-week phase of the study were randomly assigned to receive duloxetine or placebo for another 26 weeks. Relapse was defined as a ≥2-point increase in illness severity ratings, or dropout due to lack of efficacy. The relapse rate of placebo patients, 41.8%, was significantly greater than that of duloxetine patients, 13.7% (Davidson et al., 2008). A subsequent analysis of relapse variables in responders found that the strongest predictors of relapse were the magnitude of anxious mood and severity of pain (Bodkin et al., 2011).

Direct comparisons among the antidepressant drugs show minimal differences. In a head-to-head randomized, placebo-controlled trial of the two SNRIs, duloxetine (20 mg or 60–120 mg a day) and extended-release venlafaxine (75–225 mg/day), both drugs produced a significantly greater improvement on the HAM-A total score than placebo. Venlafaxine and the two higher doses of duloxetine also significantly improved both the psychic and the somatic symptom scores relative to placebo. However, duloxetine produced significantly more adverse events (especially nausea) than venlafaxine or placebo, especially at doses between 60 and 120 mg (Nicolini et al., 2009). In an 8-week double-blind comparison between the two SSRIs, paroxetine (mean dose 28.4 mg/day) and sertraline (mean dose 78.5 mg/day), both agents significantly and comparably reduced HAM-A scores. The percentage of treatment responders was 68% for paroxetine and 61% for sertraline; respective remission rates were 40% and 46%, and 20% of paroxetine and 18% of sertraline patients withdrew. The two drugs equally reduced the psychic symptoms more than the somatic symptoms (Ball, Kuhn, Wall, Shekhar, & Goddard, 2005). This study did not include a placebo arm, so it is not possible to know whether either medication was better than placebo. In a more recent comparison of the SSRI escitalopram (10–20 mg/day) and the SNRI venlafaxine extended release (75–225 mg/day), only venlafaxine (Bose, Korotzer, Gommoll, & Dayong, 2008) produced a greater decrease in HAM-A scores relative to placebo. However, neither drug had significantly more responders or remitters than placebo (for escitalopram, 52.8% and 31.2%; venlafaxine, 52.0% and 31.2%; placebo, 42.2% and 23.7%), and both drugs had more adverse reactions than placebo, particularly in regard to sexual dysfunction.

One new approach is the drug agomelatine, an agonist at melatonergic (MT_1, MT_2) receptors and an antagonist at $5HT_{2C}$ serotonergic receptors. It has no effect on monoamine uptake and no affinity for adrenergic, histaminergic, cholinergic, dopaminergic, BZD receptors, or other serotonergic receptors. During clinical trials in which it was tested for antidepressant efficacy, it showed some anxiolytic action and was assessed for GAD (at 25–50 mg/day) in a randomized, placebo-controlled 12-week study (D. J. Stein, Ahokas, & de Bodinat, 2008). Agomelatine decreased the HAM-A total score significantly more than placebo. Although both psychic and somatic scores declined, only the latter decline reached statistical significance relative to placebo. Significantly more patients responded to the drug than to placebo (66.7% vs. 46.6%, respectively), and significantly more remitted under the drug (41.3% vs. 22.4%). Very few patients withdrew from the study (three out of 55 from placebo and five out of 63 from agomelatine), and adverse events were minimal (mainly dizziness, 7.9% vs. 3.4%, and nausea, 4.8% vs. 1.7%, for agomelatine compared to placebo). Considering the high baseline HAM-A score of ≥22, the outcome indicates that agomelatine may have anxiolytic benefit.

Anticonvulsants

PREGABALIN

Pregabalin is an anticonvulsant used for neuropathic pain and as adjunct therapy for partial seizures. In 2007 it was approved for GAD in the European Union (Mula, Pini, & Cassano, 2007). Pregabalin inhibits the release of several neurotransmitters, including glutamate, noradrenaline, and substance P. The mechanism is believed to be due to potent binding to the $\alpha_2\delta$ subunit of the voltage-gated calcium channel, which reduces calcium influx in nerve terminals, thereby preventing transmitter release.

Several dose-finding placebo-controlled trials (4–6 weeks' duration) have been conducted, and have also compared pregabalin to lorazepam (6 mg/day) (Feltner et al., 2003; Pande et al., 2003; Pohl, Feltner, Fieve, & Pande, 2005), alprazolam (1.5 mg/day) (Rickels et al., 2005) and venlafaxine (75 mg/day) (Montgomery, Tobias, Zornberg, Kasper, & Pande, 2006). Pregabalin doses across these studies ranged from 150, 300, 400, 450, 600, 800, to 1350 mg/day. In each case, the active drugs were significantly more effective than placebo at reducing HAM-A scores. Data pooled from these trials found that at 450 mg/day, pregabalin produced a peak reduction in anxiety symptoms; psychic symptoms peaked at 400 mg/day, while somatic anxiety symptoms continued to improve up to the maximum dose of 600 mg/day (Boschen, 2012). Side effects of pregabalin, across studies, included somnolence, dizziness, incoordination, dry mouth, euphoria, blurred vision, ataxia, and asthenia. Weight gain was also more prominent with pregabalin, especially at high doses. Dropout rates from pregabalin ranged from 10.1% to 29%.

Continuation treatment with pregabalin was assessed in a multiple-phase trial in which patients who responded to 450 mg/day in an 8-week open-hase period were maintained for a 24-week double-blind phase (Feltner et al., 2008). By the end of the 6-month period, 42.3% of the pregabalin- and 65.3% of the placebo-treated patients had relapsed. Interestingly, a 16.7% incidence of euphoria to pregabalin was seen during the open-phase period, which lasted for a mean of 4 days, although pregabalin is not considered to have abuse potential and no additional pill taking was seen in this study. Attrition was high in the pregabalin group (36%) compared to the placebo group (22%), although most patients in both groups had met the response criterion at the time of premature discontinuation. A thorough review of pregabalin can be found in Boschen (2011).

OTHER ANTICONVULSANTS

Given the positive results reported for pregabalin, it is not surprising that other anticonvulsants have been assessed for GAD. Tiagabine inhibits the reuptake of the inhibitory transmitter GABA, and was initially evaluated in GAD patients in a 10-week randomized open-label trial with paroxetine as a positive control (Rosenthal, 2003). At a mean final dose of 10 mg/day for tiagabine, or 27 mg/day for paroxetine, the two drugs significantly, and equally, reduced HAM-A total scores as well as the psychic and somatic subscales. The percentage of responders and remitters was 40% and 20% for tiagabine and 60% and 20% for paroxetine, respectively. Tiagabine produced a higher rate of adverse effects, including headache, nausea, anorexia, dizziness, somnolence, diarrhea, increased appetite, vasodilation, and vomiting, while paroxetine produced more insomnia and sexual dysfunction. However, a subsequent 8-week trial comparing tiagabine with placebo found no difference between the two treatments on the primary HAM-A endpoint (Pollack et al., 2005).

A more successful outcome was reported for another gabaergic agent, valproate. Valproic acid increases GABA concentration in the brain by increasing its synthesis or inhibiting its metabolism. It may also decrease excitatory neurotransmission. In a 6-week double-blind, randomized, placebo-controlled trial, drug-treated patients (500 mg of valproate, three times a day) were significantly more likely to respond than placebo patients (72.2% vs. 15.8%) and their scores on the HAM-A scale were reduced significantly more. The primary adverse effects of valproate were dizziness and nausea. Although this drug is generally well tolerated, and metabolic interactions with other psychotropic agents are minor, it produces weight gain and alopecia. Moreover, like other anticonvulsants, it is teratogenic, and can elevate liver enzymes, causing rare but fatal hepatotoxicity (Aliyev & Aliyev, 2008).

Zonisamide is a novel anticonvulsant approved for the adjunctive treatment of partial seizures in adults with epilepsy. It reduces neuronal firing by blocking voltage-sensitive ion channels and reducing glutamatergic excitation. One small open-label study assessed the efficacy of adjunctive zonisamide in 10 patients with any anxiety disorder who were refractory to anxiolytic therapy. At the endpoint, mean of 9.2 weeks, 60% of the patients had responded, at a mean dose of 160 mg/day (Kinrys, Vasconcelos e Sa, & Nery, 2007).

The glutamate presynaptic release modulator riluzole was evaluated in an 8-week open-label, fixed-dose study (100 mg/day) in 18 GAD patients. By 8 weeks, eight patients were in remission. The most common side effects were insomnia, nausea, and sedation (Mathew et al., 2005). These encouraging results may warrant further investigation.

Atypical antipsychotics

In contrast to the modest but promising support for anticonvulsant efficacy in the treatment of GAD, the results of several second-generation antipsychotic (SGA) studies are more equivocal. Several recent reviews of the evidence describe the outcomes of randomized, double-blind, parallel-group studies of SGA augmentation versus placebo, or SGA monotherapy versus placebo and an active comparator, while additional studies were open label without comparison groups (Gao, Sheehan, & Calabrese, 2009; Huh, Goebert, Takeshita, Lu, & Kang, 2011; LaLonde & Van Lieshout, 2011; Lorenz, Jackson, & Saitz, 2010; Samuel et al., 2011).

In one augmentation study, risperidone (0.5–1.5 mg/day), added to other anxiolytics in a 4-week double-blind trial, reduced the HAM-A total and psychic factor scores significantly more than placebo treatment. However, other outcome variables, including response rates, were not significantly different (Brawman-Mintzer, Knapp, & Nietert, 2005). In a subsequent study, risperidone augmentation in a group of anxious patients, of whom 16 out of 30 had GAD, led to a statistically significant but clinically small decrease in the HAM-A (Simon et al., 2006). Adjunctive risperidone was ineffective, relative to placebo, in another group of patients with residual GAD symptoms (Pandina, Canuso, Turkoz, Kujawa, & Mahmoud, 2007).

A similar unsatisfactory outcome was found when olanzapine (mean dose 8.7 mg) was combined with fluoxetine or placebo in GAD patients who had insufficient response to the antidepressant after 6 weeks. The decrease in symptoms with olanzapine was not significantly greater than with placebo, although the number of olanzapine responders was barely, although statistically, greater. As might be expected, olanzapine produced significant weight gain (Pollack et al., 2006). In a 12-week open-label, flexible-dose study of quetiapine augmentation (mean dose 386 mg/day) of "traditional medication," HAM-A scores were substantially reduced, and the remission rate was 72.1% (Katzman et al., 2008). However, in a follow-up trial that compared quetiapine augmentation with placebo in GAD patients receiving paroxetine, there was no significant benefit from the antipsychotic (Simon et al., 2008). In a small study of GAD patients who were partial responders to SSRI treatment, a low (50 mg/day) dose of quetiapine improved outcomes on the HAM-A, and increased the number of responders and remitters, but not to a statistically significant degree (Altamura, Serati, Buoli, & Dell'Osso, 2011).

In a very small open-label augmentation pilot trial, aripiprazole (mean dose 13.9 mg/day) produced a response in five out of nine patients, and remission in one. However, three out of the nine developed akathisia within the first week, as well as other side effects, including weight gain (Menza, Dobkin, & Marin, 2007). In an 8-week flexible-dose, open-label augmentation trial, aripiprazole was added to failed treatments of antidepressants or BZDs in 13 patients with GAD, or GAD with panic disorder (Hoge et al., 2008). Both anxiety groups had a significant reduction in their symptoms. An open-label pilot study of ziprasidone (20–80 mg/day) in 13 treatment-resistant GAD patients showed significant reductions from baseline in all measures, with 54% and 38% of subjects meeting criteria for response and remission, respectively. However, no placebo or active control was included (Snyderman, Rynn, & Rickels, 2005). In a follow-up 8-week randomized, double-blind, placebo-controlled, flexible-dose trial, 62 GAD patients received either placebo or ziprasidone, either as an augmentation of continued medications or as monotherapy. There was no difference between the ziprasidone groups and placebo, although the data indicated a better outcome for those patients receiving ziprasidone alone compared with those taking the antipsychotic in conjunction with other medications. Out of 41 ziprasidone patients, 13 dropped out, compared with two of 21 placebo patients (Lohoff, Etemad, Mando, Gallop, & Rickels, 2010).

Currently, the only randomized placebo-controlled clinical trials with SGA monotherapy have been conducted with quetiapine. The first randomized controlled trial (RCT) consisted of a 1- to 4-week enrollment/washout period, 8 weeks of active treatment, and 2 weeks of post-treatment drug discontinuation (Bandelow et al., 2010). Quetiapine extended release (50 or 150 mg) was compared with paroxetine (20 mg) or placebo. At week 8, all active agents had significantly reduced HAM-A total and psychic subscale scores relative to placebo; only 150 mg quetiapine reduced the somatic subscale scores. Quetiapine, but not paroxetine, scores separated significantly from placebo by day 4. Remission rates at week 8 were significantly higher for quetiapine extended release 150 mg (42.6%) and paroxetine (38.8%) versus placebo (27.2%). While fewer patients reported sexual dysfunction with quetiapine, both drugs produced significantly more side effects "potentially related to extrapyramidal symptoms." Across four studies, participants randomized to receive quetiapine (150 mg) were more likely to reach a clinical response or remission, and a greater decrease in the HAM-A rating scores than placebo patients. However, quetiapine also increased all-cause dropouts, from adverse events, sedation, or extrapyramidal side effects, and produced notable weight gain (Depping, Komossa, Kissling, & Leucht, 2010; LaLonde & Van Lieshout, 2011). In the most recent trial (Khan et al., 2011), quetiapine again showed a statistically significant, albeit quantitatively modest, improvement compared to placebo.

As discussed by Gao et al. (2009), the atypical antipsychotics raise different concerns relative to antidepressants and BZDs. In short-term studies the metabolic changes were modest, but until long-term safety data are available, all GAD patients treated with SGAs should be monitored closely, as recommended by the American Diabetes Association, the American Psychiatric Association, the American Association of Clinical Endocrinologists, and the North American Association for the Study of Obesity. This requires the monitoring of weight (BMI), waist circumference, blood pressure, fasting plasma glucose, and fasting lipid profile at baseline and then from every 4 weeks for weight gain to every 5 years for fasting lipid profile, depending on the changes in those parameters.

HYDROXYZINE

In their Cochrane Review, Guaiana, Barbui, and Cipriani (2010) describe the results of five randomized controlled studies that compared this antihistamine to either placebo or another anxiolytic. Hydroxyzine was comparable to BZDs and buspirone in terms of efficacy, acceptability, and tolerability, although it was associated with more sleepiness or drowsiness. In one study, for example (Boerner, Garziella, & Achenbach, 2007), a total of 299 patients with GAD were administered an average of 45 mg/day for 4 weeks in an open ambulant study. The HAM-A score dropped significantly from 25.5 to 10.4. After 1 month, 61.5% of the patients had responded, and 42.2% reached remission. It was stated that even other types of anxiety symptoms were also reduced, such as phobic and panic attacks, and that even some depressive symptoms were improved.

Nutritional and herbal supplements

Lack of efficacy (especially for long-term remission) and undesirable side effects of approved medications for GAD continue to be a problem. As a result, there has been increased interest in the use of complementary and alternative medicines (CAM). Although there are few controlled studies, several reviews have summarized current evidence for the most commonly used substances.

KAVA KAVA

Kava kava is a beverage traditionally prepared from the rhizome of the kava plant, *Piper methysticum*, among Pacific Island cultures. It has become popular in the West because of its anxiolytic and sedative properties. The mechanism(s) of action is/are believed to be $GABA_A$ receptor binding and blockade of sodium and calcium voltage-gated ion channels, perhaps monoamine reuptake inhibition, and reversible monoamine inhibition. At least 10 randomized placebo-controlled trials and one observational study have been conducted with kava in patients diagnosed with anxiety. In seven of these studies, kava monotherapy was effective; four other reports showed that kava alone or in combination with St. John's Wort was not different from placebo. Moreover, kava has been implicated in liver failure, and this risk led the FDA to issue a consumer advisory warning about the potential for severe liver damage from kava in March 2002. However, in 2008 it was noted that kava was not considered to be very toxic until 1998, when the first report of liver hepatotoxicity occurred, and that this may be a rare side effect due to contaminants, overdose, prolonged exposure, and other drugs. It has been reported that kava inhibits P450 metabolic enzymes, which may alter the potency of other medications. Short-term use of up to 24 weeks may provide some anxiolytic benefit (Saeed, Bloch, & Antonacci, 2007) but kava's minimal efficacy and potential toxicity do not support maintained use (Kinrys, Coleman, & Rothstein, 2009; Lake, 2007; Lakhan & Vieira, 2010).

ST. JOHN'S WORT

Hypericum perforatum is derived from the flowering tops of a perennial shrub native to Europe, West Asia, and North America. It was recognized by the Greeks and Romans for its medicinal value, and is licensed in Germany for anxiety, depression, and sleep disorders. There is a substantial literature on its mechanism of action, and there may be numerous biochemical effects exerted by different plant components (Lakhan & Vieira, 2010). A few case studies of patients with GAD report successful treatment at doses of 900–1800 mg/day (Kinrys et al., 2009). However, much stronger evidence is needed before St. John's wort is considered a viable option for anxiety treatment (Saeed, Bloch, & Antonacci, 2007).

PASSIONFLOWER

Passionflower (*Passiflora incarnata Linn*) is indigenous to the southeastern United States, Argentina, and Brazil and has a long history of use as an anxiolytic in folklore. One double-blind, placebo-controlled study compared passionflower with the BZD oxazepam in 36 GAD patients. The results showed no difference between the two agents, with oxazepam producing more rapid onset of action but more impairment of job performance than passiflora (Miyasaka, Atallah, & Soares, 2007). Anxiolytic effects were also reported in patients given passionflower monotherapy before undergoing surgery, and individuals diagnosed with adjustment disorder treated with passionflower in combination with a variety of other substances (Kinrys, Coleman, & Rothstein, 2009; Lakhan & Vieira, 2010).

A variety of other non-standard substances have been used in the treatment of the anxiety disorders. L-Theanine (γ-ethylamino-L-glutamic acid) is an amino acid constituent of green tea, which has traditionally been used in Chinese medicine. According to anecdotal clinical experience, 50–200 mg once or twice daily produces a calming effect within 30–40 minutes that lasts 8–10 hours. Also, it was stated that L-theanine, unlike BZDs, does not increase drowsiness, slow reflexes, impair concentration, or produce tolerance, dependence, or serious adverse reactions (Lake, 2007). At least one randomized controlled trial of valerian root has been conducted in patients diagnosed with GAD. Results showed no difference between valerian and either placebo- or diazepam-treated groups on the HAM-A total scores, and no difference from placebo on the somatic or psychic factor scores (Miyasaka, Atallah & Soares, 2006). A 6-week controlled study evaluated the efficacy of silexan, a new oral lavender oil capsule preparation, in comparison with the BZD lorazepam. The HAM-A total, psychic, and somatic scores decreased significantly, and equally, in both drug groups (Woelk & Schläfke, 2010).

Clinical Vignette: Good outcome with pharmacotherapy

John is a 36-year-old married man who has worked at the same job for the past 10 years. About 1 year ago he began having overwhelming worries and anxiety for no apparent reason and unrelated to any events or situations. He would often be late for work and had difficulty concentrating. At home, he was often irritable and had trouble sleeping. He was receiving poor work performance ratings and his family was upset with his behavior and tended to avoid him when he was in one of his "moods." After a comprehensive assessment that included a physical exam and labs to rule out any physiological cause, he was diagnosed with GAD. Since John had never been exposed to medications, the prescriber decided to use buspirone. But, because buspirone requires at least 2–4 weeks to reach full effect and John was hesitant to take medications, the prescriber also started John on a low dose of a long-acting benzodiazepine to improve adherence. Within a few days, John began to feel much better. He was less irritable at home, was sleeping better, and his work performance improved. After 4 weeks the prescriber and John felt that he was doing very well and almost back to his baseline. Concerned about tolerance and dependence, the prescriber began slowly reducing the BZD, and over the next few weeks of tapering it was discontinued. John continued to do well on the buspirone, had no side effects or need for dose increase, and was referred to a skilled therapist who worked with him using cognitive-behavior therapy. John continued to do well and needed no further interventions other than routine monitoring

Clinical Vignette: Poor outcome with pharmacotherapy

Mark is a 21-year-old single college student. He was having trouble in class and his grades were suffering. He complained to his girlfriend that he was constantly worried about passing his courses and graduating from college in time to take advantage of a job offer. He was not sleeping, feeling restless all the time, and frequently tense and "uptight." Mark had always had an unusual degree of unrealistic worries, but over the past couple of years the anxiety had gotten worse. He attempted to reduce his anxiety by having a few drinks after classes. This worked temporarily and over time he began to drink more heavily and experimented with various drugs to help him sleep and feel calmer. Although he felt less anxious, his school performance was not improving, because of the adverse effects of the alcohol and drugs on his concentration and memory. His girlfriend persuaded Mark to go the university counseling center, where he was diagnosed with GAD; but Mark minimized his use of drugs and alcohol to the point that he was not identified as having a co-occurring substance use disorder. The prescriber started Mark on a short-acting benzodiazepine, which helped with his anxiety. However, because of its short half-life, Mark's anxiety returned before his next dose was due to be taken. He continued to use alcohol and drugs to mute the intermittent anxiety and also increased the BZD dose. He was doing no better in school and was in danger of not graduating. Owing to his continued drug use, Mark's relationship with his girlfriend was on the verge of breakup. When his current prescriber became concerned about his escalating BZD dosage and tried to wean him off it, Mark terminated and went to another prescriber to get a new prescription for benzodiazepines. This pattern continued, with Mark seeking multiple scripts from different prescribers. He shortly afterward left school without graduating and broke up with his girlfriend.

Psychosocial Treatment

In spite of the numerous pharmacological options for GAD, it is clear that current medications leave a lot to be desired. Short-term clinical trials routinely show limited efficacy (rarely above a 70% response rate), high placebo response rates, modest remission rates, high dropout rates, and high relapse rates. Many drug classes produce the same adverse effects of somnolence, insomnia, nausea, and gastrointestinal distress. Each drug class has additional characteristic side effects: abuse potential and dependence with BZDs; delayed onset, sexual dysfunction, suicidality, birth defects, and high blood pressure with antidepressants; delayed onset and birth defects with anticonvulsants; delayed onset and serious metabolic effects with antipsychotics—to name a few. These limitations make drug treatment less appealing and support the case for non-pharmacological approaches to GAD treatment.

Psychotherapy has several advantages over medication alone. Patients often prefer behavioral therapies to drug treatments, supported by lower dropout rates. There are fewer concerns with side effects and overdose. When effective, behavioral treatment reduces both psychic and somatic symptoms of anxiety, and may also reduce symptoms of other psychiatric disorders (Borkovec & Ruscio, 2001). Behavioral treatment may produce improvement as fast as medications, and evidence shows maintenance of recovery (Otto, Smits, & Reese, 2004) and no "withdrawal" syndrome.

The necessity for scheduling and attending multiple therapy sessions is one disadvantage of behavioral treatment. Cost has also been cited, but although psychotherapy may be more expensive in the short term, long-term successful treatment may be cost-effective (Otto et al., 2004). The cost–benefit ratio may also be improved by some technological advantages of CBT. A recent review of internet and computer-based delivery of CBT found that this format provided effective and acceptable treatment for both anxiety and depressive disorders compared to the (waitlist) control group (Andrews, Cuijpers, Craske, McEvoy, & Titov, 2010). Across the 22 studies included in the review, adherence to computerized CBT was good: 80% of those who began the programs completed all stages. Patients noted the advantages of convenience (working on the program when they had the time), ability to progress at their own pace, low cost, and privacy.

For patients who do not respond to pharmacotherapy, psychotherapy is an obvious alternative, but it is also beneficial for patients who choose to discontinue their medications or who are attempting to bolster treatment effectiveness (Otto et al., 2004).

What are the methods of psychotherapy for generalized anxiety disorder?

Early behavioral approaches to anxiety treatment involved relaxation training, such as muscular relaxation, biofeedback, and meditation. After GAD was independently categorized in the *DSM–III*, more research was conducted to increase and improve available techniques. Trials of psychotherapy for GAD are also relatively recent because of the difficulty of applying the techniques to noncircumscribed, "free-floating" stimuli, unlike exposure methods, which could be applied to other anxiety disorders.

Cognitive-behavioral treatment (CBT) is the approach for which there is the most information. This involves a variety of techniques. First, information in the form of *psychoeducation* can help patients realize that they are not alone in suffering with this condition; it can destigmatize the diagnosis, and motivate clients by explaining the reasons for the treatment approach and what to expect (Lang, 2004). Second, in *self-monitoring*, clients are trained to detect stimuli that elicit anxiety and to apply coping skills. Third, *relaxation training* provides exercises in breathing, relaxing imagery, meditation, and progressive muscle relaxation. These techniques are rehearsed in therapy sessions and practiced in daily life. Fourth, *cognitive restructuring* addresses ways of rethinking situations that elicit anxiety. What are they? How can they be prevented? What is the worst that could happen? How bad is that? How likely is that to occur? These techniques reduce immediate discomfort and help the client gain a sense of control (Borkovec & Ruscio, 2001; Lang, 2004).

In their review, Borkovec and Ruscio (2001) described the results of 13 high-quality psychotherapy studies of GAD, including the classic study of Borkovec and Costello (1993). Most patients in these studies were women in their late 30s who had had the disorder for an average of 7 years. Six of the studies included clients taking medication. On average, therapy required 11 sessions, with an average duration of about 70 minutes. All studies used CBT as the "active" treatment, with some including additional behavioral therapy (usually relaxation), with a variety of control conditions, such as supportive listening, pill placebo, and "waiting list no treatment."

Results showed CBT to be superior to "no treatment" in every case; to non-specific or alternative treatment in 82% of comparisons immediately after therapy, in 78% at follow-up; and to behavioral or cognitive components (separately) at post-therapy and follow-up. CBT always showed long-term maintenance or even an increase in outcome. HAM-A scores for CBT at pre-therapy, post-therapy, and follow-up were 21.5, 8.5, and 8.6, respectively. CBT was better than individual components (of behavior or cognitive therapy), than placebo treatment, and no treatment. The effect of CBT even increased from post-therapy to follow-up on both anxiety and depression measures relative to the single-component treatment. Furthermore, a subsequent analysis by Smits and Hofmann (2009) showed that even the control conditions used in psychotherapy treatment (such as therapist contact, support, and education) are modestly effective, producing a response rate of 25% with attrition of only 14.2%.

In an update, Lang (2004) described factors that were associated with poor treatment response: concurrent use of psychotropic medicine, comorbid diagnoses, chronic social stressors, and negative expectations about therapy. That review concluded that the clinical benefit of CBT for GAD was modest. In fact, a recent meta-analysis by Hofmann and Smits (2008) argued that CBT was no better than placebo for GAD. However, that outcome was based on only two studies: one that found a significant CBT effect, and a second paper, which reported no benefit of CBT in older adults. But, as noted by Lang (2004), GAD presents differently in older adults, in that, for example, more emphasis is placed on somatic symptoms. He argues that outcome to CBT in older adults may be improved with memory-enhancing techniques (video- or audiotapes), visual imagery, planning ahead to reduce physical impairments or fatigue, transportation support, large print, etc.

Lang (2004) described several other ways to improve efficacy. One modification was to focus on reducing erroneous beliefs about worry. Another intervention was designed to address overriding beliefs about worry in general. Additional approaches include methods of improving interpersonal interactions; training in emotion regulation; incorporation of mindfulness (to increase relaxation); and acceptance strategies (acknowledging that some situations are out of our control).

Subsequent studies have confirmed the effectiveness of CBT compared with people who received treatment as usual or who were on a waiting list. Results show that the number of dropouts is greater among older patients (confirming that CBT is less successful in this population) and those who received group therapy. On the other hand, these studies did not assess the long-term effectiveness of CBT. There are also few studies comparing CBT to other psychological treatments; in fact, several reports on supportive therapy found differing results (Hunot, Churchill, Teixeira, & Silva de Lima, 2007).

However, the first randomized controlled trial comparing CBT with psychodynamic therapy was recently conducted. Each therapy was administered according to the respective procedures described in treatment manuals, and included up to 30 (50-minute) sessions. CBT used the standard techniques: relaxation, problem-solving, planning, etc. Psychodynamic treatment used supportive-expressive therapy, which "focuses on the core conflictual relationship theme associated with the symptoms of generalized anxiety disorder" (Leichsenring et al., 2009, p. 68) in which the emphasis is placed on a "positive therapeutic alliance" (p. 69). Both treatments significantly reduced all outcome measures, which were maintained at the 6-month follow-up. CBT treatment was superior in some measures.

Recent studies have also assessed various "formulations" of CBT. Metacognitive therapy (MCT) was compared with applied relaxation (AR) in a pilot trial in 20 outpatients with GAD. At the end of the 8–12 weekly sessions, and at 6- and 12-month follow-up, MCT was superior to AR, and there were no dropouts with MCT (Wells et al., 2010). In contrast, the first randomized controlled trial to directly compare CBT alone with an augmentation strategy "targeting interpersonal problems and emotional processing" did not show a benefit of this additional component. Both treatments significantly, but comparably, reduced GAD symptoms for up to 2 years post-therapy (Newman et al., 2011).

Clinical Vignette: Good outcome with psychotherapy

Samantha is a 36-year-old married woman who has been successfully treated for anxiety with psychotropic medications for nearly 10 years. Initially, she responded well to paroxetine, but the sexual side effects of this drug eventually became a problem. Fortunately, the sexual dysfunction remitted, while effectiveness was retained, when she was switched to the anticonvulsant drug pregabalin. However, now she and her husband would like to start a family, and she is concerned about the lack of information about this drug in regard to congenital defects. Fortunately, she discussed this issue with her practitioner in sufficient time to start tapering the pregabalin before she tried to become pregnant, while, at the same time, she initiated cognitive-behavioral therapy. Samantha gradually discontinued her pregabalin during several months of CBT sessions, and subsequently became pregnant. Before her baby was due, she arranged to continue her CBT therapy at home, via the internet, so that she would not need to travel to her therapist's office during the first months after the baby was born.

Clinical Vignette: Poor outcome with psychotherapy

Nancy is a 65-year-old woman who recently lost her husband of 35 years. She has been grieving for several months, and, rather than getting better, she is becoming more nervous. She is not used to managing the finances and is concerned about having enough money to live on. She has developed insomnia, lost her appetite, and is losing weight. She complains of aches and pains. Her physician recognizes her symptoms and diagnoses her anxiety and developing depression. He suggests some medication for acute relief of the anxiety—specifically, benzodiazepines. But Nancy worries about the side effects, especially the cognitive impairment and risk of falling. She prefers not to take pills. Her doctor arranges for CBT sessions. Although Nancy makes all her appointments, she is not responding well to the behavioral treatment. She has trouble concentrating on the "homework" and finds the effort very fatiguing. For her, CBT is not effective. Eventually, Nancy agrees to try medication. Because she is generally healthy and has no cardiac risk factors, he starts her on venlafaxine. Within a few weeks Nancy feels much better, she has more energy, and finds that she is able to handle her personal affairs more easily than before.

COMBINED THERAPY

Most patients initiating behavioral therapy for anxiety are already taking anxiolytic medication, and the majority state that they prefer a combined approach. In one of the few studies involving GAD patients, Power, Simpson, Swanson, and Wallace (1990) compared the effect of CBT and diazepam (DZ), alone and in combination. There were five groups: CBT, diazepam, placebo, CBT + diazepam and CBT + placebo, over a 10-week trial. HAM-A scores declined in all five groups, but the DZ + CBT group had the largest percentage of patients showing "clinically significant change" on all the rating scales. Patients in the CBT, CBT + placebo, and CBT + DZ groups were also less likely to receive further psychological therapy or medication during the 6-month poststudy period. In this study, CBT was a viable method of anxiety reduction. The poor outcome of diazepam alone was somewhat surprising, but partly attributed to the fixed low-dose regimen.

The usefulness of CBT in facilitating BZD discontinuation was demonstrated in a study by Gosselin, Ladouceur, Morin, Dugas, and Baillargeon (2006), which was the first study in GAD patients to compare CBT with a non-specific intervention control (NST). In weekly standardized exercises of 20–25 minutes, patients practiced applying CBT techniques, including psychoeducation procedures, cognitive restructuring, problem-solving training, cognitive exposure to worries, situational exposure, and relapse prevention training, including ways of dealing with tapering. Drug tapering consisted of decreasing the daily dose by 25% at intervals of 2–3 weeks over a 12-week trial. In addition to BZD intake, and urine analyses, measures included several rating scales, such as the Penn State Worry Questionnaire and the Worry and Anxiety Questionnaire, the Intolerance of Uncertainty Scale, the Negative Problem Orientation Questionnaire, the Cognitive Avoidance Questionnaire, and the Credibility and Expectancy Scale.

At the end of the 12-week study, 74.2% of the CBT patients and 36.7% of the NST group had stopped taking BZDs. At 12 months the values were 64.5% and 30.0%, respectively, with the CBT group statistically better in each comparison. At 3 and 12 months, significantly more CBT than NST patients did not have GAD symptoms. Withdrawal symptoms were few and weak, and the CBT group had a significantly lower tendency to worry, and less cognitive avoidance. On the other hand, there was no difference between the groups in insomnia and depression. And, although there was a significant decline in BZD dose, this decrease was equal in the two groups, and among those patients that were still using BZDs, there was no difference in the amount of drug at either 3 or 12 months post-treatment.

Because CBT techniques are non-specific, and because there is much comorbidity among anxiety disorders, a flexible psychotherapeutic treatment delivery model, Coordinated Anxiety Learning and Management (CALM), has been developed as an intervention applicable to more than one anxiety disorder. This approach is intended for the treatment of panic disorder, social anxiety disorder, and posttraumatic stress disorder, in addition to GAD, even when they occur with depression. CALM optimizes treatment by allowing patients to choose their treatment modality—pharmacotherapy, CBT, or both—as well as additional treatment when necessary.

Roy-Byrne et al. (2010) recently conducted a clinical trial of CALM compared with usual care (UC). The intervention was administered to 1004 primary care patients across 17 clinics over 10–12 weeks. The CALM protocol consisted of a web-based monitoring system with a computer-assisted CBT program of motivational interviewing, a medication algorithm for anxiety, and outreach strategies for minority groups. The CBT program included several modules that were applicable for all conditions (education, self-monitoring, hierarchy development, breathing training, and relapse prevention), and some that were specific to the four disorders (cognitive restructuring, and exposure to internal and external stimuli). Personnel (Anxiety Clinical Specialists) were trained in the application of the treatment, administered over 6–8 weeks in conjunction with medication.

The goal of CALM treatment was either clinical remission, sufficient improvement such that the patient did not want further treatment, or improvement with residual symptoms warranting a different therapeutic treatment. Clinical remission was defined as a score of 8 on a symptom scale (the Overall Anxiety Severity and Impairment Scale) of 0 to 20. If necessary, patients could receive additional treatment of the same or the alternative modality. At the end of the study, patients were maintained with continued care in the form of monthly follow-up phone calls.

The patients consisted of 71% women, 44% non-white, with a broad age range. They were fairly ill: more than half had at least two chronic medical conditions and at least two anxiety disorders, and two-thirds had comorbid depression. At 6, 12, and 18 months, significantly more CALM patients than UC patients responded and remitted. By 18 months, response rate was 64.6% versus 51.5% and remission rates were 51.6% versus 36.8%, respectively. While the outcomes supported the effectiveness of the CALM intervention model, it was acknowledged that the program is expensive and the necessary reimbursement mechanisms for broad implementation are not available. In addition, the approach is not feasible for small or rurally located practices.

Effective psychotherapeutic methods continue to be refined and improved. One modification that has received much recent attention is cognitive bias modification (CBM) (see reviews by Bar-Haim, 2010; Beard, 2011; Browning, Holmes, & Harmer, 2010; Hakamata et al., 2010). This approach is derived from research showing that anxious individuals are likely to attend preferentially to threat-relevant stimuli in their environment. The model has been tested experimentally by recording the reaction time for recognizing threatening words compared with neutral words. Anxious people have faster responses relative to non-anxious people, a phenomenon termed cognitive bias modification of attention (CBM-A), or sometimes attention bias modification (ABM). A similar paradigm has shown that anxious individuals are also more likely to respond faster when negative words rather than positive words are used to clarify ambiguous phrases. This phenomenon is termed interpretation bias—that is, cognitive bias modification for interpretation (CBM-I). These models propose that attention and interpretation biases serve as cognitive indices of anxious behavior, and that manipulations of these behaviors can be used to treat excessive anxiety. This approach differs from standard CBT therapy, which attempts to help anxious patients learn to explicitly divert their attention away from anxiety-provoking thoughts. In contrast, ABM is directed at shifting early, implicit, automatic, and presumably unconscious attentional biases away from threatening stimuli (Bar-Haim, 2010).

An example of the CBM-A paradigm is provided by the one randomized controlled trial that has been conducted to date in individuals diagnosed with GAD. In this study (Amir, Beard, Burns, & Bomyea, 2009), GAD patients were randomly allocated to an attentional training condition or an attentional control condition. In each condition, pairs of words were presented for 500 milliseconds on a computer screen. Some trials included one neutral word ("dishwasher") and one threat word ("humiliated"), while in other trials both words were neutral. After the word pairs had been presented, a "probe" stimulus appeared on the computer screen, either the letter "E" or "F." The probe could appear in the same spot where either the neutral or the threat word had been located. Participants had to indicate which probe had appeared.

Both groups were presented with pairs of neutral or threat words. For the experimental group the probe *always* followed the neutral word. In other words, although there was no specific instruction to direct attention away from the threat word, the position of the neutral word predicted the subsequent position of the probe. In the control condition the presentation of stimulus word pairs was the same, but the probe appeared equally often in the position of the neutral or threat word. The idea is that participants learn to direct attention toward the type of stimuli that predict the probe location. Therefore, when the probe replaces the neutral stimulus, participants are learning to avoid threat.

After eight training sessions over 4 weeks, the experimental group had a significant decrease in their HAM-A scores, but those in the control group did not. There were also significant reductions in a variety of self-report measures, and a "significantly larger proportion of the AMP participants (50%) compared with the ACC group (13%) no longer met diagnostic criteria for GAD" (Amir et al., 2009, p. 31). Although the long-term maintenance of this result remains to be seen, this preliminary outcome is encouraging. A large component of this technology is automated, and the training methods are well established. The equipment is portable, and the system is cost-effective for administration to underserved, e.g. rural, populations.

Mindfulness-based therapy, derived from Buddhist practice, is another psychotherapeutic intervention that has been integrated into CBT for treating various psychiatric disorders, including anxiety. Classical mindfulness has characteristics that may directly target specific diagnostic features of GAD. In their excellent review, Rapgay, Bystritsky, Dafter, and Spearman (2011) provide a brief summary of CBT treatment of GAD and a discussion of how to incorporate the processes associated with mindfulness practice. In their comprehensive review of clinical trials for GAD treatment, Gale and Millichamp (2011) provide summary tables and conclusions for most of these pharmacological and behavioral therapies.

Clinical Vignette: Combined treatment

Julia is a divorced woman in her mid 30s, living with her elderly father. Her mother passed away many years ago. Her father is becoming senile and is often irritable and emotionally abusive. Julia finds herself constantly on edge as she tries to take care of the household and her father in addition to working full-time as an elementary school teacher. She has difficulty concentrating, and has insomnia. When, one day, she takes her father to his doctor's appointments, the physician becomes aware of Julia's growing anxiety. The physician cannot spend much time with Julia, who is not her patient, but manages to discuss the situation with Julia enough to feel comfortable writing a prescription for sertraline to help the anxiety. Julia obtains some benefit from the SSRI, but even after several months is still nervous and tense when she spends too much time interacting with her father. A friend mentions a colleague who has had a good experience with psychotherapy, particularly a treatment that incorporates a cognitive approach that provides some training in coping with everyday frustrations and anxiety-provoking interpersonal situations. Julia decides to explore this option and initiates a behavioral treatment that includes training in problem solving and planning, and cognitive restructuring of her environment. After several sessions, Julia finds that she is better able to prepare for interactions with her father, and to plan alternative ways of reacting to and interpreting stressful situations. Eventually she finds that the combination of cognitive therapy and the SSRI has relieved her anxiety and allowed her to relax and develop new interpersonal skills.

FUTURE DIRECTIONS

Although current pharmacological and behavioral GAD treatments leave much room for improvement, efforts to address therapeutic limitations continue. One study reported positive results on the HAM-A, and an excellent safety profile, with an experimental drug, ocinaplon, that is a positive allosteric modulator of the $GABA_A$ receptor (Czobor, Skolnick, Beer, & Lippa, 2010).

A reexamination of opioids in the neurobiology of anxiety has recently been proposed (Colasanti, Rabiner, Lingford-Hughes, & Nutt, 2011). Similarly, a recent neurobiological analysis of fear extinction discusses the relevance of this behavioral paradigm to the anxiety disorders (Graham & Milad, 2011). Clearly, the need for more effective methods of treating generalized anxiety disorder is recognized and new developments are in progress.

Clinical Points to Remember

1. It is important to carry out a comprehensive assessment to differentiate GAD from related disorders, especially co-occurring depression and substance use disorders.
2. It is important to consider age, gender, pregnancy status, and other factors when choosing medications to treat GAD. For example, some SSRIs might actually worsen anxiety symptoms initially. Avoid benzodiazepines in the elderly, because of cognitive problems and the risk of falls; Use of anti-epileptic medications in women who may become or who are pregnant requires consideration of effects of medications on the developing fetus.
3. Since GAD is by definition a chronic disorder, there is a need to determine how long to treat with medications. It is important to periodically reassess the need for continued treatment. For example, use of benzodiazepines leads to tolerance, dependency, and withdrawal upon termination.
4. Psychodynamic or cognitive psychotherapy should always be considered as part of the treatment package. These therapies are cost-effective, more effective in the long run, and allow for medication reduction and termination.
5. Some of the medications used to treat GAS are difficult to stop, owing to dependency and rebound anxiety. Prepare the patient for eventual discontinuation from the beginning of treatment, and when the decision to discontinue is made, taper gradually and monitor closely for increased anxiety.

REFERENCES

Aliyev, N. A., & Aliyev, Z. N. (2008). Valproate (depakine-chrono) in the acute treatment of outpatients with generalized anxiety disorder without psychiatric comorbidity: Randomized, double-blind placebo-controlled study. *European Psychiatry*, *23*, 109–114.

Allgulander, C. (2010). Novel approaches to treatment of generalized anxiety disorder. *Current Opinion in Psychiatry, 23*, 37–42.

Allgulander, C., Dahl, A. A., Austin, C., Morris, P. L. P., Sogaard, J. A., Fayyad, R., et al. (2004). Efficacy of sertraline in a 12-week trial. *American Journal of Psychiatry, 161*, 1642–1649.

Allgulander, C., Hackett, D., & Salinas, E. (2001). Venlafaxine extended release (ER) in the treatment of generalized anxiety disorder. *British Journal of Psychiatry, 179*, 15–22.

Altamura, A. C., Serati, M., Buoli, M., & Dell'Osso, B. (2011). Augmentative quetiapine in partial/nonresponders with generalized anxiety disorder: A randomized, placebo-controlled study. *International Clinical Psychopharmacology, 26*, 201–205.

Amir, N., Beard, C., Burns, M., & Bomyea, J. (2009). Attention modification program in individuals with generalized anxiety disorder. *Journal of Abnormal Psychology, 118*, 28–33.

Andrews, G., Cuijpers, P., Craske, M. G., McEvoy, P., & Titov, N. (2010). Computer therapy for the anxiety and depressive disorders is effective, acceptable and practical health care: A meta-analysis. *PLoS ONE, 5*, e13196, 1–6.

Angst, J., Gamma, A., Baldwin, D. S., Ajdacic-Gross, V., & Rössler, W. (2009). The generalized anxiety spectrum: Prevalence, onset, course and outcome. *European Archives of Psychiatry and Clinical Neuroscience, 259*, 37–45.

Baldwin, D. S., Ajel, K. I., & Garner, M. (2010). Pharmacological treatment of generalized anxiety disorder. *Current Topics in Behavioral Neurosciences, 2*, 453–467.

Baldwin, D. S., Waldman, S., & Allgulander, C. (2011). Evidence-based pharmacological treatment of generalized anxiety disorder. *International Journal of Neuropsychopharmacology, 14*, 697–710.

Ball, S. G., Kuhn, A., Wall, D., Shekhar, A., & Goddard, A. W. (2005). Selective serotonin reuptake inhibitor treatment for generalized anxiety disorder: A double-blind, prospective comparison between paroxetine and sertraline. *Journal of Clinical Psychiatry, 66*, 94–99.

Bandelow, B., Chouinard, G., Bobes, J., Ahokas, A., Eggens, I., Liu, S., & Eriksson, H. (2010). Extended-release quetiapine fumarate (quetiapine XR): A once-daily monotherapy effective in generalized anxiety disorder: Data from a randomized, double-blind, placebo- and active-controlled study. *International Journal of Neuropsychopharmacology, 13*, 305–320.

Bar-Haim, Y. (2010). Research review: Attention bias modification (ABM): A novel treatment for anxiety disorders. *Journal of Child Psychology and Psychiatry, 51*, 859–870.

Beard, C. (2011). Cognitive bias modification for anxiety: Current evidence and future directions. *Expert Review in Neurotherapy, 11*, 299–311.

Bodkin, J. A., Allgulander, C., Llorca, P. M., Spann, M. E., Walker, D. J., Russell, J. M., & Ball, S. G. (2011). Predictors of relapse in a study of duloxetine treatment for patients with generalized anxiety disorder. *Human Psychopharmacology: Clinical and Experimental, 26*, 258–266.

Boerner, R. J., Garziella, M., & Achenbach, U. (2007). Efficacy and tolerance of hydroxyzine in the treatment of patients with generalized anxiety disturbance (GAD): Results of an open ambulant study. *Psychopharmakotherapie, 14*, 23–30.

Borkovec, T. D., & Costello, E. (1993). Efficacy of applied relaxation and cognitive-behavioral therapy in the treatment of generalized anxiety disorder. *Journal of Consulting and Clinical Psychology, 61*, 611–619.

Borkovec, T. D., & Ruscio, A. M. (2001). Psychotherapy for generalized anxiety disorder. *Journal of Clinical Psychiatry, 62* (Suppl. 11), 37–42.

Boschen, M. J. (2011). Generalized anxiety disorder in adults: Focus on pregabalin. *Clinical Medicine Insights: Psychiatry, 4,* 17–35.

Boschen, M. J. (2012). Pregabalin: Dose–response relationship in generalized anxiety disorder. *Pharmacopsychiatry, 45,* 51–56.

Bose, A., Korotzer, A., Gommoll, C., & Dayong, L. (2008). Randomized, placebo-controlled trial of escitalopram and venlafaxine XR in the treatment of generalized anxiety disorder. *Depression and Anxiety, 25,* 854–861.

Brawman-Mintzer, O., Knapp, R. G., & Nietert, P. J. (2005). Adjunctive risperidone in generalized anxiety disorder: A double-blind, placebo-controlled study. *Journal of Clinical Psychiatry, 66,* 1321–1325.

Brawman-Mintzer, O., Knapp, R. G., Rynn, M., Carter, R. E., & Rickels, K. (2006). Sertraline treatment for generalized anxiety disorder: A randomized, double-blind, placebo-controlled study. *Journal of Clinical Psychiatry, 67,* 874–881.

Browning, M., Holmes, E. A., & Harmer, C. J. (2010). The modification of attentional bias to emotional information: A review of the techniques, mechanisms, and relevance to emotional disorders. *Cognitive, Affective, and Behavioral Neuroscience, 10,* 8–20.

Bruce, S. E., Yonkers, K. A., Otto, M. W., Eisen, J. L., Weisberg, R. B., Pagano, M., et al. (2005). Influence of psychiatric comorbidity on recovery and recurrence in generalized anxiety disorder, social phobia, and panic disorder: A 12-year prospective study. *American Journal of Psychiatry, 162,* 1179–1187.

Carlat, D. (2011). Benzodiazepines: A guide to safe prescribing. *Carlat Psychiatry Report, 9,* 1–4.

Chessick, C. A., Allen, M. H., Thase, M. E., Batista Miralha da Cunha, A. A. B. C., Kapczinski, F. F. K., Silva de Lima, M., & dos Santos Souza, J. J. S. S. (2006). Azapirones for generalized anxiety disorder. *Cochrane Database of Systematic Reviews, 3,* Art. No.: CD006115.

Cloos, J.-M. (2010, July). Benzodiazepines and addiction: Myths and realities (Part 1). *Psychiatric Times,* pp. 26–29.

Colasanti, A., Rabiner, E. A., Lingford-Hughes, A., & Nutt, D. J. (2011). Opioids and anxiety. *Journal of Psychopharmacology, 25,* 1415–1433.

Culpepper, L. (2009). Generalized anxiety disorder and medical illness. *Journal of Clinical Psychiatry, 70* (Suppl. 2), 20–24.

Czobor, P., Skolnick, P., Beer, B., & Lippa, A. (2010). A multicenter, placebo-controlled, double-blind, randomized study of efficacy and safety of ocinaplon (DOV 273,547) in generalized anxiety disorder. *CNS Neuroscience and Therapeutics, 16,* 63–75.

Dahl, A. A., Ravindran, A., Allgulander, C., Kutcher, S. P., Austin, C., & Burt, T. (2005). Sertraline in generalized anxiety disorder: Efficacy in treating the psychic and somatic anxiety factors. *Acta Psychiatrica Scandinavica, 111,* 429–435.

Davidson, J. R. T. (2009). First-line pharmacotherapy approaches for generalized anxiety disorder. *Journal of Clinical Psychiatry, 70* (Suppl. 2), 25–31.

Davidson, J. R. T., Bose, A., Korotzer, A., & Zheng, H. (2004). Escitalopram in the treatment of generalized anxiety disorder: Double-blind, placebo controlled, flexible-dose study. *Depression and Anxiety, 19,* 234–240.

Davidson, J. R. T., DuPont, R. L., Hedges, D., & Haskins, J. T. (1999). Efficacy, safety, and tolerability of venlafaxine extended release and buspirone in outpatients with generalized anxiety disorder. *Journal of Clinical Psychiatry, 60*, 528–535.

Davidson, J. R. T., Wittchen, H.-U., Llorca, P.-M., Erickson, J., Detke, M., Ball, S. G., & Russell, J. M. (2008). Duloxetine treatment for relapse prevention in adults with generalized anxiety disorder: A double-blind placebo-controlled trial. *European Neuropsychopharmcology, 18*, 673–681.

Davidson, J. R., Zhang, W., Conner, K. M., Ji, J., Jobson, K., Lecrubier, Y., et al. (2010). A psychopharmacological treatment algorithm for generalized anxiety disorder (GAD). *Journal of Psychopharmacology, 24*, 3–26.

Depping, A. M., Komossa, K., Kissling, W., & Leucht, S. (2010). Second-generation antipsychotics for anxiety disorders. *Cochrane Database of Systematic Reviews, 12*, Art. No.: CD008120. doi:10.1002/14651858.CD008120.pub2

Feltner, D. E., Crockatt, J. G., Dubovsky, S. J., Cohn, C. K., Shrivastava, R. K., Targum, S. D., et al. (2003). A randomized, double-blind, placebo-controlled, fixed-dose, multicenter study of pregabalin in patients with generalized anxiety disorder. *Journal of Clinical Psychopharmacology, 23*, 240–249.

Feltner, D. E., & Haig, G. (2011). Evaluation of the subjective and reinforcing effects of diphenhydramine, levetiracetam, and valproic acid. *Journal of Psychopharmacology, 25*, 763–773.

Feltner, D. E., Wittchen, H. U., Kavoussi, R., Brock, J., Baldinetti, F., & Pande, A. C. (2008). Long-term efficacy of pregabalin in generalized anxiety disorder. *International Clinical Psychopharmacology, 23*, 18–28.

Gale, C. K., & Millichamp, J. (2011). Generalized anxiety disorder. *Clinical Evidence, 10*, 1–73.

Gao, K., Sheehan, D. V., & Calabrese, J. R. (2009). *Expert Review of Neurotherapeutics, 9*, 1147–1158.

Garner, M., Möhler, H., Stein, D. J., Mueggler, T., & Baldwin, D. S. (2009). Research in anxiety disorders: From the bench to the bedside. *European Neuropsychopharmacology, 19*, 381–390.

Gelenberg, A. J., Lydiard, R. B., Rudolph, R. L., Aguiar, L., Haskins, J. T., & Salinas, E. (2000). Efficacy of venlafaxine extended-release capsules in nondepressed outpatients with generalized anxiety disorder. *JAMA: Journal of the American Medical Association, 283*, 3082–3088.

Goodman, W. K., Bose, A., & Wang, Q. (2005). Treatment of generalized anxiety disorder with escitalopram: Pooled results from double-blind, placebo-controlled trials. *Journal of Affective Disorders, 87*, 161–167.

Gorman, J. M. (2002). Treatment of generalized anxiety disorder. *Journal of Clinical Psychiatry, 63* (Suppl. 8), 17–23.

Gosselin, P., Ladouceur, R., Morin, C. M., Dugas, M. J., & Baillargeon, L. (2006). Benzodiazepine discontinuation among adults with GAD: A randomized trial of cognitive-behavioral therapy. *Journal of Consulting and Clinical Psychology, 74*, 908–919.

Graham, B. M., & Milad, M. R. (2011). The study of fear extinction: Implications for anxiety disorders. *American Journal of Psychiatry, 168*, 1255–1265.

Guaiana, G., Barbui, C., & Cipriani, A. (2010). Hydroxyzine for generalized anxiety disorder. *Cochrane Database of Systematic Reviews, 12*, Art. No.: CD006815. doi:10.1002/14651858.CD006815.pub2.

Hakamata, Y., Lissek, S., Bar-Haim, Y., Britton, J. C., Fox, N. A., Leibenluft, E., et al. (2010). Attention bias modification treatment: A meta-analysis toward the establishment of novel treatment of anxiety. *Biological Psychiatry, 68*, 982–990.

Hartford, J., Kornstein, S., Liebowitz, M., Pigott, T., Russell, J., Detke, M., et al. (2007). Duloxetine as an SNRI treatment for generalized anxiety disorder: Results from a placebo and active-controlled trial. *International Clinical Psychopharmacology, 22*, 167–174.

Hoehn-Saric, R., McLeod, D. R., & Zimmerli, W. D. (1988). Differential effects of alprazolam and imipramine in generalized anxiety disorder: Somatic versus psychic symptoms. *Journal of Clinical Psychiatry, 49*, 293–301.

Hoffman, D. L., Dukes, E. M., & Wittchen, H.-U. (2008). Human and economic burden of generalized anxiety disorder. *Depression and Anxiety, 25*, 72–90.

Hofmann, S. G., & Smits, J. A. J. (2008). Cognitive-behavioral therapy for adult anxiety disorders: A meta-analysis of randomized placebo-controlled trials. *Journal of Clinical Psychiatry, 69*, 621–632.

Hoge, E. A., Worthington, J. J. III, Kaufman, R. E., Delong, H. R., Pollack, M. H., & Simon, N. M. (2008). Aripiprazole as augmentation treatment of refractory generalized anxiety disorder and panic disorder. *CNS Spectrum, 13*, 522–527.

Huh, J., Goebert, D., Takeshita, J., Lu, B. Y., & Kang, M. (2011). Treatment of generalized anxiety disorder: A comprehensive review of the literature for psychopharmacologic alternatives to newer antidepressants and benzodiazepines. *Primary Care Companion for CNS Disorders, 13*, PCC.08r00709. doi:10.4088/PCC.08r00709blu

Hunot, V., Churchill, R., Teixeira, V., & Silva de Lima, M. (2007). Psychological therapies for generalized anxiety disorder. *Cochrane Database of Systematic Reviews, 1*, Art. No.: CD001848. doi:10.1002/14651858.CD001848.pub4

Katzman, M. A. (2009). Current considerations in the treatment of generalized anxiety disorder. *CNS Drugs, 23*, 103–120.

Katzman, M. A., Vermani, M., Jacobs, L., Marcus, M., Kong, B., Lessard, S., et al. (2008). Quetiapine as an adjunctive pharmacotherapy for the treatment of nonremitting generalized anxiety disorder: A flexible-dose, open-label pilot trial. *Journal of Anxiety Disorders, 22*, 1480–1486.

Khan, A., Joyce, M., Atkinson, S., Eggens, I., Baldytcheva, I., & Eriksson, H. (2011). A randomized, double-blind study of once-daily extended release quetiapine fumarate (quetiapine XR) monotherapy in patients with generalized anxiety disorder. *Journal of Clinical Psychopharmacology, 31*, 418–428.

Kinrys, G., Coleman, E., & Rothstein, E. (2009). Natural remedies for anxiety disorders: potential use and clinical applications. *Depression and Anxiety, 26*, 259–265.

Kinrys, G., Vasconcelos e Sa, D., & Nery, F. (2007). Adjunctive zonisamide for treatment refractory anxiety. *International Journal of Clinical Practice, 61*, 1050–1053.

Lake, J. (2007). Integrative management of anxiety, Part 1. *Psychiatric Times, 24*, 1–9.

Lakhan, S. E., & Vieira, K. F. (2010). Nutritional and herbal supplements for anxiety and anxiety-related disorders: Systematic review. *Nutrition Journal, 9*, 1–14.

LaLonde, C. D., & Van Lieshout, R. J. (2011). Treating generalized anxiety disorder with second generation antipsychotics. *Journal of Clinical Psychopharmacology, 31*, 326–333.

Lang, A. J. (2004). Treating generalized anxiety disorder with cognitive behavioral therapy. *Journal of Clinical Psychiatry, 65* (Suppl. 13), 14–19.

Leichsenring, F., Salzer, S., Jaeger, U., Kächele, H., Kreische, R., Leweke, F., et al. (2009). Short-term psychodynamic psychotherapy and cognitive-behavioral therapy in generalized anxiety disorder: A randomized, controlled trial. *American Journal of Psychiatry, 166,* 875–881.

Lohoff, F. W., Etemad, B., Mandos, L.A., Gallop, R., & Rickels, K. (2010). Ziprasidone treatment of refractory generalized anxiety disorder. *Journal of Clinical Psychopharmacology, 30,* 185–189.

Lorenz, R. A., Jackson, C. W., & Saitz, M. (2010). Use of atypical antipsychotics for treatment-resistant generalized anxiety disorder. *Pharmacotherapy, 30,* 942–951.

Martin, J. L. R., Sainz-Pardo, M., Furukawa, T. A., Martín-Sánchez, E., Seoane, T., & Galán, C. (2007). Benzodiazepines in generalized anxiety disorder: Heterogeneity of outcomes based on a systematic review and meta-analysis of clinical trials. *Journal of Psychopharmacology, 21,* 774–782.

Mathew, S. J., Amiel, J. M., Coplan, J. D., Fitterling, H. A., Sackeim, H. A., & Gorman, J. M. (2005). Open-label trial of riluzole in generalized anxiety disorder. *American Journal of Psychiatry, 162,* 2379–2381.

McLeod, D. R., Hoehn-Saric, R., Porges, S. W., & Zimmerli, W. D. (1992). Effects of alprazolam and imipramine on parasympathetic cardiac control in patients with generalized anxiety disorder. *Psychopharmacology, 107,* 535–540.

Menza, M. A., Dobkin, R. D., & Marin, H. (2007). An open-label trial of aripiprazole augmentation for treatment-resistant generalized anxiety disorder. *Journal of Clinical Psychopharmacology, 22,* 207–210.

Meoni, P., Hackett, D., & Lader, M. (2004). Pooled analysis of venlafaxine XR efficacy on somatic and psychic symptoms of anxiety in patients with generalized anxiety disorder. *Depression and Anxiety, 19,* 127–132.

Mitte, K., Noack, P., Steil, R., & Hautzinger, M. (2005). A meta-analytic review of the efficacy of drug treatment in generalized anxiety disorder. *Journal of Clinical Psychopharmacology, 25,* 141–150.

Miyasaka, L. S., Atallah, A. N., & Soares, B. G. (2006). Valerian for anxiety disorders. *Cochrane Database of Systematic Reviews, 4,* Art. No.: CD004515.

Miyasaka, L. S., Atallah, A.N., & Soares, B. G. (2007). Passiflora for anxiety disorder. *Cochrane Database of Systematic Reviews, 1,* Art. No.: CD004518.

Montgomery, S. A., Mahé, H., Haudiquet, V., & Hackett, D. (2002). Effectiveness of venlafaxine extended release formulation, in the short-term and long-term treatment of generalized anxiety disorder: Results of a survival analysis. *Journal of Clinical Psychopharmacology, 22,* 561–567.

Montgomery, S. A., Tobias, K., Zornberg, G. L., Kasper, S., & Pande, A. C. (2006). Efficacy and safety of pregabalin in the treatment of generalized anxiety disorder: A 6-week, multicenter, randomized, double-blind, placebo-controlled comparison of pregabalin and venlafaxine. *Journal of Clinical Psychiatry, 67,* 771–782.

Mula, M., Pini, S., & Cassano, G. B. (2007). The role of anticonvulsant drugs in anxiety disorders: A critical review of the evidence. *Journal of Clinical Psychopharmacology, 27,* 263–272.

Newman, M. G., Castonguay, L. G., Borkovec, T. D., Fisher, A. J., Boswell, J. F., Szkodny, L. E., & Nordberg, S. S. (2011). A randomized controlled trial of cognitive-behavioral therapy for generalized anxiety disorder with integrated techniques from emotion-focused and interpersonal therapies. *Journal of Consulting and Clinical Psychology, 79,* 171–181.

Nicolini, H., Bakish, D., Duenas, H., Spann, M., Erickson, J., Hallberg, C., et al. (2009). Improvement of psychic and somatic symptoms in adult patients with generalized anxiety disorder: Examination from a duloxetine, venlafaxine extended-release and placebo-controlled trial. *Psychological Medicine, 39*, 267–276.

Otto, M. W., Smits, J. A. J., & Reese, H. E. (2004). Cognitive-behavioral therapy for the treatment of anxiety disorders. *Journal of Clinical Psychiatry, 65* (Suppl. 5), 43–41.

Pande, A. C., Crockatt, J. G., Feltner, D. E., Janney, C. A., Smith, W. T., Weisler, R., et al. (2003). Pregabalin in generalized anxiety disorder: A placebo-controlled trial. *American Journal of Psychiatry, 160*, 533–540.

Pandina, G. J., Canuso, C. M., Turkoz, I., Kujawa, M., & Mahmoud, R. A. (2007). Adjunctive risperidone in the treatment of generalized anxiety disorder: A double-blind, prospective, placebo-controlled, randomized trial. *Psychopharmacology Bulletin, 40*, 41–57.

Pohl, R. B., Feltner, D. E., Fieve, R. R., & Pande, A. C. (2005). Efficacy of pregabalin in the treatment of generalized anxiety disorder. *Journal of Clinical Psychopharmacology, 25*, 151–158.

Pollack, M. H. (2009). Refractory generalized anxiety disorder. *Journal of Clinical Psychiatry, 70* (Suppl. 2), 453–467.

Pollack, M. H., Roy-Byrne, P. P., Van Ameringen, M., Snyder, H., Brown, C., Ondrasik, J., & Rickels, K. (2005). The selective GABA reuptake inhibitor tiagabine for the treatment of generalized anxiety disorder: Results of a placebo-controlled study. *Journal of Clinical Psychiatry, 66*, 1401–1408.

Pollack, M. H., Simon, N. M., Zalta, A. K., Worthington, J. J., Hoge, E. A., Mick, E., et al. (2006). Olanzapine augmentation of fluoxetine for refractory generalized anxiety disorder: A placebo-controlled study. *Biological Psychiatry, 59*, 211–215.

Pollack, M. H., Zaninelli, R., Goddard, A., McCafferty, J. P., Bellew, K. M., Burnham, D. B., & Iyengar, M. K. (2001). Paroxetine in the treatment of generalized anxiety disorder: Results of a placebo-controlled, flexible-dosage trial. *Journal of Clinical Psychiatry, 62*, 350–357.

Power, K. G., Simpson, R. J., Swanson, V., & Wallace, L. A. (1990). A controlled comparison of cognitive behavior therapy, diazepam and placebo, alone and in combination for the treatment of generalized anxiety disorder. *Journal of Anxiety Disorders, 4*, 267–297.

Rapgay, L., Bystritsky, A., Dafter, R. E., & Spearman, M. (2011). New strategies for combining mindfulness with integrative cognitive behavioral therapy for the treatment of generalized anxiety disorder. *Journal of Rational-Emotive and Cognitive Behavior Therapy, 29*, 92–119.

Ravindran, L. N., & Stein, M. B. (2010). The pharmacologic treatment of anxiety disorders: A review of progress. *Journal of Clinical Psychiatry, 71*, 839–854.

Rickels, K., DeMartinis, N., García-España, F., Greenblatt, D. J., Mandos, L. A., & Rynn, M. (2000). Imipramine and buspirone in treatment of patients with generalized anxiety disorder who are discontinuing long-term benzodiazepine therapy. *American Journal of Psychiatry, 157*, 1973–1979.

Rickels, K., Downing, R., Schweizer, E., & Hassman, H. (1993). Antidepressants for the treatment of generalized anxiety disorder. *Archives of General Psychiatry, 50*, 884–895.

Rickels, K., Etemad, B., Khalid-Khan, S., Lohoff, F. W., Rynn, M. A., & Gallop, R. J. (2010). Time to relapse after 6 and 12 months' treatment of generalized anxiety disorder with venlafaxine extended release. *Archives of General Psychiatry, 67,* 1274–1281.

Rickels, K., Pollack, M. H., Feltner, D. E., Lydiard, R. B., Zimbroff, D. L., Bielski, R. J., et al. (2005). Pregabalin for treatment of generalized anxiety disorder. *Archives of General Psychiatry, 62,* 1022–1030.

Rickels, K., Pollack, M. H., Sheehan, D. V., & Haskins, J. T. (2000). Efficacy of extended-release venlafaxine in nondepressed outpatients with generalized anxiety disorder. *American Journal of Psychiatry, 157,* 968–974.

Rickels, K., Zaninelli, R., McCafferty, J., Bellew, K., Iyengar, M., & Sheehan, D. (2003). Paroxetine treatment of generalized anxiety disorder: A double-blind, placebo-controlled study. *American Journal of Psychiatry, 160,* 749–756.

Rocca, P., Fonzo, V., Scotta, M., Zanalda, E., & Ravizza, L. (1997). Paroxetine efficacy in the treatment of generalized anxiety disorder. *Acta Psychiatrica Scandinavica, 95,* 444–450.

Rosenthal, M. (2003). Tiagabine for the treatment of generalized anxiety disorder: A randomized, open-label, clinical trial with paroxetine as a positive control. *Journal of Clinical Psychiatry, 64,* 1245–1249.

Roy-Byrne, P., Graske, M. G., Sullivan, G., Rose, R. D., Edlund, M. J., Lang, A. J., et al. (2010). Delivery of evidence-based treatment for multiple anxiety disorders in primary care. *Journal of the American Medical Association, 303,* 1921–1928.

Rubio, G., & López-Ibor, J. J. (2007). Generalized anxiety disorder: A 40-year follow-up study. *Acta Psychiatrica Scandinavica, 115,* 372–379.

Rynn, M., Russell, J., Erickson, J., Detke, M. J., Ball, S., Dinkel, J., et al. (2008). Efficacy and safety of duloxetine in the treatment of generalized anxiety disorder: A flexible-dose, progressive-titration, placebo-controlled trial. *Depression and Anxiety, 25,* 182–189.

Saeed, S. A., Bloch, R. M., & Antonacci, D. J. (2007). Herbal and dietary supplements for treatment of anxiety disorders. *American Family Physician, 76,* 549–556.

Samuel, M., Zimovetz, E. A., Gabriel, Z., & Beard, S. M. (2011). Efficacy and safety of treatments for refractory generalized anxiety disorder: A systematic review. *International Clinical Psychopharmacology, 26,* 63–68.

Sheehan, D. V., & Mao, C. G. (2003). Paroxetine treatment of generalized anxiety disorder. *Pharmacological Bulletin, 37* (Suppl. 1), 64–75.

Simon, N. M. (2009). Generalized anxiety disorder and psychiatric comorbidities such as depression, bipolar disorder, and substance abuse. *Journal of Clinical Psychiatry, 70* (Suppl. 2), 10–14.

Simon, N. M., Conner, K. M., LeBeau, R. T., Hoge, E. A., Worthington, J. J. III, Zhang, W., et al. (2008). Quetiapine augmentation of paroxetine CR for the treatment of refractory generalized anxiety disorder: Preliminary findings. *Psychopharmacology, 197,* 675–681.

Simon, N. M., Hoge, E. A., Fischmann, D. Worthington, J. J. III, Christian, K. M., Kinrys, G., & Pollack, M. H. (2006). An open-label trial of risperidone augmentation for refractory generalized anxiety disorders. *Journal of Clinical Psychiatry, 67,* 381–385.

Smits, J. A. J., & Hofmann, S. G. (2009). A meta-analytic review of the effects of psychotherapy control conditions for anxiety disorders. *Psychological Medicine, 39,* 229–239.

Snyderman, S. H., Rynn, M. A., & Rickels, K. (2005). Open-label pilot study of ziprasidone for refractory generalized anxiety disorder. *Journal of Clinical Psychopharmacology, 25,* 497–499.

Stein, D. J., Ahokas, A. A., & de Bodinat, C. (2008). Efficacy of agomelatine in generalized anxiety disorder: A randomized, double-blind, placebo-controlled study. *Journal of Clinical Psychopharmacology, 28,* 561–566.

Stein, M. B. (2009). Neurobiology of generalized anxiety disorder. *Journal of Clinical Psychology, 70* (Suppl. 2), 15–19.

Stocchi, F. S., Nordera, G., Jokinen, R. H., Lepola, U. M., Hewett, K., Bryson, H., & Iyengar, M. K. for the Paroxetine Generalized Anxiety Disorder Study Team. (2003). Efficacy and tolerability of paroxetine for the long-term treatment of generalized anxiety disorder. *Journal of Clinical Psychiatry, 64,* 250–258.

Tyrer, P., & Baldwin, D. (2006). Generalized anxiety disorder. *Lancet, 368,* 2156–2166.

Weisberg, R. B. (2009). Overview of generalized anxiety disorder: Epidemiology, presentation and course. *Journal of Clinical Psychiatry, 70* (Suppl. 2), 4–9.

Wells, A., Welford, M., King, P., Papageorgiou, C., Wisely, J., & Mendel, E. (2010). A pilot randomized trial of metacognitive therapy vs applied relaxation in the treatment of adults with generalized anxiety disorder. *Behaviour Research and Therapy, 48,* 429–434.

Woelk, H., & Schläfke, S. (2010). A multi-center, double-blind, randomized study of the lavender oil preparation Silexan in comparison to lorazepam for generalized anxiety disorder. *Phytomedicine, 17,* 94–99.

CHAPTER 6

Obsessive-Compulsive Disorder

Jonathan S. Abramowitz and Ryan J. Jacoby

INTRODUCTION

Obsessive-compulsive disorder (OCD) is an anxiety disorder involving obsessive thoughts and compulsive rituals (to be defined shortly) that occupy significant time, cause personal distress, or interfere with work or school, social relationships, and/or with activities of daily living (e.g., using the bathroom, leaving the house). Its psychopathology is among the most complex of the psychological disorders, as sufferers struggle against seemingly ubiquitous unwanted thoughts and urges that, while senseless, are also anxiety-provoking. The wide array and intricate associations between thoughts and behaviors can perplex even the most experienced of clinicians. Moreover, because OCD is under-recognized by sufferers and professionals alike, and because of its sometimes embarrassing symptoms, affected individuals might go for 10 years or more without receiving appropriate treatment. In this chapter we describe the nature of OCD before turning to a review and illustration of the most effective forms of pharmacological, psychological, and combined treatment approaches.

DSM Criteria

According to the *Diagnostic and Statistical Manual of Mental Disorders* (*DSM–IV–TR*; American Psychiatric Association, 2000), OCD is defined by *obsessions* or *compulsions* that produce significant distress and cause noticeable interference with various aspects of academic, occupational, social, leisure, and/or family functioning. *Obsessions* are defined as intrusive thoughts, ideas, images, impulses, or doubts that the person experiences as senseless and that evoke distress (i.e., anxiety, doubt). Common examples include unwanted sexual thoughts, ideas of harming loved ones, thoughts that one is contaminated with germs from the toilet, suspicions that one has behaved in an immoral or negligent way, and the feeling that objects are not arranged "just right." *Compulsions* are urges to perform observable (e.g., ordering, checking, cleaning) or mental rituals (e.g., repeating phrases, such as "God loves me") to counteract an obsessional doubt). Such rituals are performed in response to obsessions and according to self-imposed "rules." Abramowitz (2006) provides a more in-depth description of the nature of these symptoms.

Behavioral avoidance

Although not formally listed in the *DSM* criteria, avoidance behavior is present to some degree in most people with OCD, and is intended to prevent exposure to situations that would provoke obsessional thoughts and compulsive urges. For some patients, avoidance serves to prevent specific feared consequences, such as acting on unwanted thoughts; whereas in others it is focused on preventing obsessional thoughts from occurring in the first place. For example, one man avoided going to swimming pools because seeing children in bathing suits evoked unwanted thoughts of child molestation. Other patients engage in avoidance so that they do not have to carry out compulsive rituals. For instance, a woman with obsessional fears of accidentally hitting pedestrians avoided all driving in order to not have to perform elaborate and time-consuming rituals involving stopping the car to check the roadside for injured or dead bodies.

Subtypes and dimensions of OCD

The *DSM* presents OCD as a homogeneous disorder, yet research has identified reliable and valid *subtypes* or *dimensions* of OCD symptoms (Abramowitz et al., 2010; for a review, see McKay et al., 2004). These include (1) harming (aggressive obsessions and checking rituals), (2) contamination (contamination obsessions and decontamination rituals), (3) symmetry (obsessions about order or neatness and arranging rituals), (4) unacceptable immoral or violent thoughts with mental rituals and neutralization, and (5) hoarding symptoms. Most recently, however, research suggests that hoarding is not a symptom of OCD, but rather a separate psychological disorder (e.g., Abramowitz, Wheaton, & Storch, 2008).

Poor insight and overvalued ideation

Although the majority of people with OCD recognize at some point that their obsessions and compulsions are senseless and excessive, there exists a *continuum* of insight into the irrationality of these symptoms, with 4% of patients *convinced* that these symptoms are realistic (that is, they have poor insight; Foa & Kozak, 1995). The *DSM–IV* criteria for OCD include the specifier "with poor insight" to denote individuals who fall into this category. Poorer insight appears to be associated most strongly with the presence of religious obsessions, fears of mistakes, and aggressive obsessional impulses (Tolin, Abramowitz, Kozak, & Foa, 2001).

Prevalence of OCD

Once considered extremely rare, OCD is now considered one of the most common psychological disorders, with lifetime prevalence estimates as high as 2.9% (Kolada, Bland, & Newman, 1994; Kessler et al., 2005). The disorder typically begins by age 25, yet childhood or adolescence onset is common (Rasmussen & Tsuang, 1986). The mean age of onset is slightly earlier in males (about 21 years of age) than in females (22–24 years) (Rasmussen & Eisen, 1992). OCD has a low rate of spontaneous remission, and when left untreated tends to gradually worsen over time. Finally, periods of increased life stress are associated with increased symptom severity.

SOLITARY TREATMENT APPROACHES

There are two approaches to monotherapy for OCD that have received empirical support: pharmacotherapy primarily using serotonin reuptake inhibitor medication, and cognitive-behavioral therapy (CBT) using exposure and response prevention (ERP) procedures. These treatments have been evaluated in hundreds of studies and with thousands of patients worldwide. In this section we will focus on these two approaches, reviewing the conceptual foundation and most convincing outcome trials available for these treatments. Interpreting the results of OCD treatment studies is aided by the use of a common metric: the 10-item Yale–Brown Obsessive Compulsive Scale (Y–BOCS; Goodman et al., 1989a, 1989b), which is regarded as the "gold standard" measure of OCD severity and used as the primary outcome measure in most studies. This enables comparisons across studies and provides readers with a means of deriving clinically meaningful data from study results. The Y–BOCS yields a total score ranging from 0 (no symptoms) to 40 (extremely severe). Scores of 0–7 indicate subclinical symptoms, 8–15 indicate mild OCD, 16–25 represent moderate symptomatology, 26–30 represent severe symptoms, and 31–40 indicate profound or extreme symptoms.

Pharmacological Treatment

Conceptual foundation

Pharmacotherapy for OCD is based on a hypothesized dysregulation in the brain's serotonin neurotransmitter system. Specifically, OCD is thought to be associated with hypersensitivity of postsynaptic serotonin receptors (Gross, Sasson, Chopra, & Zohar, 1998). Dysfunctions in the serotonin transporter gene (5-HTT) and serotonin receptor gene (5HT2A) have also been hypothesized (Greenberg et al., 2000). Importantly, these hypothesized abnormalities have not been consistently identified (e.g., Saiz et al., 2008). It is also proposed that the glutamate and dopamine neurotransmitter systems are dysregulated in OCD (e.g., Greist, Jefferson, Kobak, Katzelnick, & Serlin, 1995; Chakrabarty, Bhattacharyya, Christopher, & Khanna, 2005), although findings are again inconsistent.

Review of randomized controlled trials (RCTs)

Despite the lack of consistent findings relating serotonin to OCD, pharmacotherapy using the serotonin reuptake inhibitors (SRIs) clomipramine (Anafranil), sertraline (Zoloft), fluoxetine (Prozac), fluvoxamine (Luvox), citalopram (Celexa), and paroxetine (Paxil) has been found effective for reducing OCD symptoms in over 30 double-blind, randomized, placebo-controlled trials (e.g., DeVeaugh-Geiss, Landau, & Katz, 1989; Montgomery et al., 1993; Price, Goodman, Charney, Rasmussen, & Heninger, 1987). A list of the medications evaluated in these RCTs appears in Table 6.1. Because of the large volume of studies, we turn to two meta-analyses that provide quantitative summaries of the RCT data. The first, by Greist et al. (1995), included several multicenter SRI trials of sertraline, fluoxetine, fluvoxamine, and clomipramine, revealing mean Y–BOCS reduction rates of about 20–40% (about 5–8 points from pre- to post-test) in comparison to placebo.

A more recent and comprehensive meta-analysis of 21 RCTs by Eddy, Dutra, Bradley, and Westen (2004) revealed a large effect size of 0.90 on the Y–BOCS, indicating that at post-test, SRI-treated patients were almost a full standard deviation better off than patients who had received placebo. The mean post-test Y–BOCS score, however, was 16.84 (SD =<th.1.83), suggesting that even following an adequate SRI trial, residual OCD symptoms of moderate severity are the norm. Clomipramine produced the strongest effects, followed by fluoxetine and sertraline.

TABLE 6.1
Medications Evaluated for Use with Obsessive-Compulsive Disorder

Brand Name	Generic Name	Effective Dose
Anafranil*	Clomipramine	Up to 250 mg/day
Luvox*	Fluvoxamine	Up to 300 mg/day
Paxil*	Paroxetine	40–60 mg/day
Prozac*	Fluoextine	40–80 mg/day
Zoloft*	Sertraline	Up to 200 mg/day
Effexor	Venlafaxine	75 mg/day
Celexa	Citalopram	Up to 60 mg/day

Note
*Approved by the U.S. Food and Drug Administration for the treatment of obsessive-compulsive disorder.

Review of other studies

Meta-analysis has also been used to determine the *relative* efficacy of various SRIs (e.g., Abramowitz, 1997; Eddy et al., 2004; Greist et al., 1995). The findings from these studies suggest that clomipramine (which is a tricyclic antidepressant with significant SRI properties) is superior to other SRIs (fluoxetine, fluvoxamine, and sertraline), and that the latter do not differ from one another in their efficacy. Despite clomipramine's efficacy, however, significant side effects (e.g., tachychardia, orthostatic hypotension, dry mouth, and constipation) and higher dropout rates have been reported (Eddy et al., 2004). As a result, SRIs other than clomipramine are often the first line of pharmacotherapy.

There has been very little research on the predictors of good and poor SRI outcome for OCD. In one study (Mataix-Cols, Rauch, Manzo, Jenike, & Baer, 1999), more severe pre-test OCD symptoms predicted more severe symptoms at post-test. In addition, patients with hoarding (then considered a symptom of OCD) fared worse than patients with other manifestations of OCD. In a second investigation (Ergovesi et al., 2001) a family history of OCD predicted good outcomes, while poor insight predicted poor outcomes.

Benefits and limitations of pharmacotherapy as the sole approach

Pharmacotherapy for the treatment of OCD has both pros and cons. Advantages include that it is beneficial for many patients and is relatively easy to administer, given that SRIs are safe and widely available. The medicine is usually taken orally and without the need for regular therapy sessions. On the other hand, a disadvantage of this approach is the relatively modest average improvement rate; even after adequate trials, many patients are left with clinically significant residual symptoms (in many studies, post-test Y–BOCS scores would still qualify for entry into the study). Moreover, selecting the most effective medication at the most effective clinical dose that also minimizes side effects is often a process of trial and error. Common SRI side effects are nausea, diarrhea, nervousness, jitteriness, insomnia, sexual dysfunction, and headaches. Finally, long-term improvement with SRIs is reliant on continuation of treatment since relapse typically occurs upon stoppage (e.g., Pato, Zohar-Kadouch, Zohar, & Murphy, 1988, Simpson et al., 2004).

Clinical Vignette: Good outcome with pharmacotherapy

Fred was 32 years old, yet he had suffered with OCD since his early 20s. His obsessions involved thoughts and unwanted impulses to look in the direction of people's genitals. As much as he tried, Fred could not get such thoughts out of his mind. His rituals involved repeating prayers and trying to reassure himself that he was not a "pervert." Fred had sought counseling from religious authorities but was never able to disclose the true nature of his obsessional thoughts for fear of embarrassment. At age 30, during a routine physical with his physician, Fred revealed that he was having problems with what he thought was OCD. Without being too specific, he described his obsessions and rituals, and was prescribed fluvoxamine at doses increasing to 300 mg/day over the course of a few weeks. After a few weeks, Fred noticed a reduction in his anxiety and the intrusive thoughts. His urges to seek assurance and pray had also decreased. Fred noticed mild side effects, such as a slightly reduced appetite and sex drive, but overall was pleased with his response to the medicine. Over the next two years, Fred remained on this dose, and although his symptoms waxed and waned, he was able to enjoy socializing without having to constantly battle the obsessional thoughts.

Clinical Vignette: Poor outcome with pharmacotherapy

Joanne, aged 40, had suffered with fears of contamination and washing rituals since the age of 18. While taking a college Abnormal Psychology class, she came to realize that her symptoms might be OCD, and after an evaluation with a psychiatrist on campus was prescribed clomipramine. Unfortunately, the side effects of this medicine were severe, and even after having her physician adjust the dose several times, Joanne was switched to fluoxetine. After a few months using this medicine, Joanne had not noticed any improvement—in fact, she was avoiding more and more situations and spending a greater amount of time with washing and showering rituals. Over the course of the next several years, Joanne tried several different SRI medications at various doses, sometimes augmented with other antidepresents, anxiolytics, and even antipsychotic agents in an attempt to quell her OCD symptoms; but none was effective, according to her own self-report, and most produced severe side effects.

Psychological Treatment

Exposure and response prevention (ERP) is based on a conceptualization of OCD as involving maladaptive thinking and behavior patterns (e.g., Kozak & Foa, 1997). The thinking patterns include exaggerating the importance of harmless unwanted intrusive thoughts; the behavior patterns include avoidance and compulsive rituals as a means of controlling the thoughts and anxiety. While these behaviors reduce anxiety in the short term, they also prevent the natural, long-term extinction of obsessional fears, thus maintaining the problem. Moreover, the behaviors are negatively reinforced by the short-term reduction in distress that they engender, leading to their habitual use.

Treatment using ERP aims to weaken the maladaptive thinking and behaving patterns by helping patients gradually confront obsession-provoking stimuli (i.e., *exposure*) in the form of actual encounters with the feared situations and imaginal confrontation with the feared consequences of doing so. Patients are encouraged to allow themselves to experience obsessional anxiety without performing rituals (*response prevention*) in order to learn that with time, the distress naturally subsides—a process known as *habituation*. With repeated exposure, habituation occurs more rapidly. A course of ERP begins with a thorough assessment of obsessions, rituals, avoidance behaviors, and feared consequences of confronting feared situations. This information is then used to plan the specific exposure exercises. ERP can be delivered over the course of 16–20 sessions (a full description can be found in Abramowitz, 2006).

Review of randomized controlled trials

Three RCTs have compared ERP with a credible psychotherapy control condition. The details and findings from these studies are summarized in Table 6.2. In the Fals-Stewart, Marks, and Schafer (1993) study, ERP patients were randomly assigned to 24 sessions of twice-weekly group or individual treatment over 12 weeks. Average improvement in the ERP groups was 41% on the Y–BOCS compared to only 9% in the relaxation control condition. In Lindsay, Crino, and Andrews's RCT (1997), ERP consisted of 15 daily sessions conducted over a three-week period. The anxiety management training (AMT) control intervention was delivered on a similar schedule and included breathing retraining, relaxation, and problem solving. The average pre- to post-test improvement with ERP was almost 62% on the Y–BOCS. In contrast, the AMT group showed no change in symptoms following treatment. Finally, Nakatani et al. (2005) in Japan compared ERP with a pill placebo to autogenic self-relaxation training and pill placebo for 12 weeks (a third group received fluvoxamine and autogenic training). Patients who received ERP had a greater than 50% reduction in Y–BOCS scores compared to a lack of improvement in the autogenic control group.

In all of these studies, post-test Y–BOCS scores among the ERP groups were significantly lower than with control treatments. This demonstrates a clear superiority of ERP over placebo therapies that control for non-specific factors such as expectancy, credibility, and attention from a therapist, indicating that improvement can be attributed to the specific ERP procedures themselves.

TABLE 6.2
Effects of Exposure and Response Prevention (ERP) in Randomized Controlled Trials with a Psychotherapeutic Control Condition

Study	Control Condition	Mean (SD) Y–BOCS Total Score					
		ERP Group			Control Group		
		n	Pre	Post	n	Pre	Post
Fals-Stewart, Marks, and Schafer (1993)[a]	Relaxation	31	20.2	12.1	32	19.9	18.1
Lindsay, Crino, and Andrews (1997)	Anxiety management	9	28.7 (4.6)	11.0 (3.8)	9	24.4 (7.0)	25.9 (5.8)
Nakatani et al. (2005)	Autogenic self-relaxation	10	29.9 (3.1)	12.9 (4.9)	8	30.5 (3.7)	28.4 (5.5)

Notes

Y–BOCS = Yale–Brown Obsessive Compulsive Scale.

a Standard deviation not reported in the study.

Moreover, post-test Y–BOCS scores following ERP are within the mild range of symptoms, indicating clinically significant improvement. Studies reporting follow-up data up to two years following treatment indicate that ERP produces durable treatment gains (e.g., Abramowitz, 1996); for example, across 16 uncontrolled studies, 76% of patients maintained at least 30% improvement (Foa & Kozak, 1996).

Review of other studies

Whereas RCTs substantiate the efficacy of ERP, such rigorously conducted studies may not generalize to routine clinical practice (e.g., Silberschatz in Persons & Silberschatz, 1998). RCT patient samples are not always representative of outpatients who present with multiple problems, and the extensive therapist training, supervision, and manualization of therapy are not typical of most outpatient settings. Accordingly, four studies have examined the effects of ERP as delivered outside of clinical studies. Franklin, Abramowitz, Foa, Kozak, and Levitt (2000) examined 110 consecutively referred outpatients with OCD, who received 15 daily sessions of ERP on a fee-for-service basis. No patients were excluded for reasons of comorbidity or previous treatment failure; half of the sample had comorbid Axis I or Axis II diagnoses, and many had failed previous trials of CBT (patients were only denied ERP if they were actively psychotic, abusing substances, or suicidal—all reasons not to begin ERP in any setting). These authors found that mean Y–BOCS scores improved from 26.8 to 11.8 (a 60% reduction in OCD symptoms). Moreover, only 10 patients dropped out of treatment prematurely. These findings closely parallel those of the RCTs described above.

A similarly designed study by Warren and Thomas (2001) included 26 patients treated with weekly ERP sessions (mean 16.4 hours of therapy) in a private practice setting. Thirty-two percent of these patients had comorbid conditions and 50% had previously received treatment for their OCD. Results were highly consistent with Franklin et al.'s (2000) study: Y–BOCS scores improved from 23.0 to 11.6 (a 48% reduction in OCD symptoms). Similarly, Houghton, Saxon, Bradburn, Ricketts, and Hardy (2010) reported results from 37 individuals with OCD, who received between one and 30 sessions of CBT (a combination of cognitive therapy and ERP). For the 27 patients who completed therapy, Y–BOCS scores improved from 23.2 to 13.0 (a 44% reduction in OCD symptoms).

Finally, Friedman and colleagues (2003) reported for a community sample of African American ($n = 15$), Caribbean American ($n = 11$), and Caucasian ($n = 36$) patients with OCD, who received a mean of 20 twice-weekly 45- to 90-minute sessions of ERP. While treatment was effective in reducing OCD and depressive symptoms, many patients reported significant residual symptoms after therapy: mean Y–BOCS scores for African American patients were 23.5 (pre-treatment) and 17.2 (post-treatment; a 27% reduction), and for Caucasians were 26.0 (pre) and 17.7 (post; a 23% reduction). There were no between-group dif-ferences in treatment outcome. The authors attributed the reduced effective-ness of ERP in this study to the use of less frequent treatment sessions (twice-weekly compared to daily), although the reader will note that Warren and Thomas (2001) obtained better results with a once-weekly ERP regimen.

Numerous studies have examined the relationship between outcome and the manner in which ERP is delivered (see Abramowitz, 1996, for a meta-analytic review). The results of this literature can be summarized as follows: ERP programs involving more in-session, therapist-supervised exposure pro-duced greater short- and long-term improvements than did programs in which all exposure was performed by the patient as homework assignments. Greater effectiveness is also achieved when treatment involves both exposure and response prevention (Foa, Steketee, Grayson, Turner, & Latimer, 1984). Not surprisingly, adherence with ERP instructions is associated with ERP outcome (Abramowitz, Franklin, Zoellner, & DiBernardo, 2002; Lax, Başoğlu, & Marks, 1992; O'Sullivan, Noshirvani, Marks, Monteiro, & Lelliott, 1991). Finally, whether ERP sessions are conducted in the therapist's office or in the patient's home (or other environment where OCD symptom are experienced) does not appear to make a difference in terms of outcome (Rowa et al., 2007).

Only two studies to date have compared group versus individual ERP or CBT (Anderson & Rees, 2007; Fals-Stewart et al., 1993). In concert, these stud-ies suggest that while individual treatment is associated with a more rapid treat-ment response, over time, group and individual exposure-based treatments are equally effective. This finding is encouraging, given that group treatments require significantly fewer therapist hours than individual therapy (Anderson & Rees, 2007; Fals-Stewart et al., 1993).

Lastly, the addition of cognitive therapy (CT), which aims to modify patients' misappraisal of their obsessional thoughts, has been examined as a possible adjunct to ERP. Vogel, Stiles, and Götestam (2004), for example, ran-domly assigned 35 patients to receive either ERP + CT ($n = 16$) or ERP plus relaxation ($n = 19$). Whereas both treatment programs were superior to wait list, ERP + CT was superior to ERP + relaxation at post-test (mean Y–BOCS scores were 11.3 and 16.4 respectively), a finding that disappeared at 1-year fol-low-up (Y–BOCS scores of 13.3 and 10.2 respectively). Importantly, the inclu-sion of CT was useful in reducing dropout. Thus, there are benefits to incorporating CT techniques along with ERP; perhaps CT techniques improve the acceptability of ERP.

Adding CT to ERP might be particularly helpful for individuals with severe obsessional thoughts and mental rituals. Freeston et al. (1997) treated 28 patients with this presentation of OCD, using ERP consisting of (1) education about the nature of intrusive thoughts, (2) loop-tape exposure to intrusive thoughts, (3) refraining from mental rituals and neutralizing behaviors, and (4) CT targeting exaggerated beliefs about the presence and meaning of obsessions. Y–BOCS scores improved from 23.9 to 9.8 after an average of 25.7 sessions over 19.2 weeks. Moreover, patients retained their gains at 6-month follow-up (the mean Y–BOCS score was 10.8).

A number of patient characteristics have been identified as predictors of response to ERP. These include the presence of poor insight (Foa, 1979; Foa, Abramowitz, Franklin, & Kozak, 1999), severe depression (Abramowitz & Foa, 2000; Abramowitz, Franklin, Street, Kozak, & Foa, 2000; Steketee, Chambless, & Tran, 2001), generalized anxiety disorder (Steketee et al., 2001), extreme emotional reactivity during exposure (Foa et al., 1983), and severe borderline personality traits (i.e., borderline; Steketee et al., 2001). The severity of OCD symptoms at pre-test has, with some inconsistency, also been found to predict more severe post-ERP symptoms (e.g., Foa et al., 1983; Franklin et al., 2000)

Benefits and limitations of psychological treatment as the sole approach

As with medications, there are pros and cons of ERP. The main advantage of this approach is its strong short- and long-term efficacy. CBT is also a relatively brief treatment in which skills are learned that the patient continues to use after formal therapy has ended. On the other hand, a downside is that ERP requires significant effort on the part of the patient (and therapist). Exposure therapy sessions typically provoke temporary anxiety and distress; thus, the patient must be willing to endure these feelings for the short term. The fact that relatively few treatment providers are adequately trained to deliver satisfactory ERP is also problematic; indeed, the most effective form of treatment for OCD is also the most difficult to find.

Clinical Vignette: Good outcome with psychotherapy

Hope, a 30-year-old woman with obsessions regarding bad luck from odd numbers, and rituals that involved counting and "evening" things out, sought treatment from our clinic. At intake her Y–BOCS score was 27, but she had good insight into the senselessness of her OCD symptoms. Following a description of ERP and discussion of its pros and cons, she agreed to begin our 16-session program. The first three sessions involved the therapist collecting information about Hope's obsessional triggers, avoidance behaviors, compulsive rituals, and feared consequences of exposure to fear triggers. The therapist also socialized Hope to the cognitive-behavioral model of OCD and made sure she understood the rationale behind ERP techniques. An exposure hierarchy was developed collaboratively that included gradually more fear-provoking stimuli. Hope began her first exposure during session 4 to writing down odd numbers. She was also helped how to resist her urges to count and "even count odd numbers." Other exposures included doing things an odd number of times, setting the alarm for an odd number on the clock, eating at odd times, and the like. For imaginal exposure, Hope practiced thinking about bad luck befalling her and her loved ones because of her ERP exercises. Hope was able to confront these situations and thoughts, and resist most of her ritualistic urges both in session and during her daily homework practice. Gradually, these tasks became easier when it became clear that her fears of bad luck were unfounded. After 16 treatment sessions, Hope's Y–BOCS score was reduced to 10, and she reported quality improvements in all areas of her life. During a 6-month follow-up visit, Hope reported spending less than 10 minutes with obsessive fears and rituals per day.

Clinical Vignette: Poor outcome with psychotherapy

Josh was a devoutly religious (Christian) 43-year-old man who presented for treatment of OCD symptoms involving scrupulosity and religious compulsions. Obsessive doubts that he might have committed a sin—for example, by being "too proud," or taking the Lord's name in vain without realizing it—were constant; and his rituals involved repeating prayers for forgiveness and compulsively asking for assurances from religious leaders that he had not committed any moral transgressions. Treatment began with a discussion of the rationale for ERP, but Josh was skeptical. At first, he was unwilling to begin exposures because they would entail purposely committing what he believed were serious religious transgressions, such as wearing nice clothes and being proud of how he looked, reading a book written by an atheist, and watching a movie produced by "Hollywood liberals" (things that most Christians do without anxiety). Furthermore, he was unwilling to give up his ritualistic praying, although he recognized that his reassurance-seeking was annoying to those whom he routinely peppered with such questions. After a few weeks, Josh's pastor persuaded Josh to begin therapy. Yet during the first few exposures, it became clear that Josh was "secretly" apologizing to God for committing sins—a direct violation of his response prevention plan. As a result, he was not able to experience the natural increase and habituation of anxiety during these tasks. After a few weeks of arguing with the therapist over the risks of committing sins, and Josh's not being willing to decrease his praying and asking for forgiveness, it was decided that this was not the right time for Josh to receive treatment for his OCD, and therapy was stopped.

COMBINED THERAPY

Three outcomes are possible when one combines pharmacological and psychological treatments for OCD. The first, and most intuitive, is a synergistic effect in which combination treatment is more effective than either type of monotherapy. But it is also possible that medication and ERP add little to each other. For instance, if one is sufficiently powerful, the other would have little more to contribute. And we must also face the third possibility: that one treatment undermines the efficacy of the other. This might occur, for example, if patients attributed their gains to medication and did not adhere to the ERP treatment plan.

Review of Randomized Controlled Trials

Although the concurrent use of medication and psychological treatment is common in clinical settings, relatively few studies have empirically examined whether this approach for OCD affords advantages over either ERP or SRIs alone. For the most part, the available studies suggest that simultaneous treatment with ERP and SRIs yields superior outcome compared to SRI monotherapy, but not compared to ERP alone (Cottraux et al., 1990; Foa et al., 2005; Franklin, Abramowitz, Bux, Zoellner, & Feeny, 2002; Hohagen et al., 1998; Marks et al., 1988; Marks, Stern, Mawson, Cobb, & McDonald, 1980; O'Connor, Todorov, Robillard, Borgeat, & Brault, 1999; van Balkom et al., 1998). That is, adding medication to ERP does not improve the effectiveness of ERP.[1]

Importantly, however, many of the existing studies above have limitations, such as the lack of reliable outcome measures (such as the Y–BOCS), sample sizes too small to detect modest differences between treatments, and complicated designs that obfuscated comparisons between combined treatment and monotherapy. Foa et al.'s (2005) multicenter double-blind RCT provides the most rigorous and easily interpretable evaluation of the effects of combination treatment relative to monotherapy. These authors compared

12 weeks of (1) intensive ERP (4 weeks of therapy followed by eight weekly maintenance sessions), (2) clomipramine, (3) their combination (ER + CMI), and (4) pill placebo. The study was conducted at one center with expertise in pharmacotherapy, another with expertise in ERP, and a third with expertise in both modalities. At week 12, all active treatments were superior to placebo. The effect of ERP (55% Y–BOCS reduction) did not differ from that of ERP + CMI (58% Y–BOCS reduction), and both were superior to clomipramine (31% Y–BOCS reduction) alone. Placebo resulted in an 11% Y–BOCS reduction. Moreover, post-test Y–BOCS scores for ERP and combination treatment fell within the mild range of OCD severity (11.0 and 10.5 respectively), but within the moderate range for clomipramine alone (Y–BOCS = 18.2).

Review of Other Studies

ERP as an adjunct to pharmacotherapy

Given that SRI medications leave the average patient with clinically significant residual OCD symptoms, investigators have examined whether ERP can be used to augment pharmacotherapy following only partial (or no) improvement with one or more adequate SRI trials. Two studies addressing this question are described next.

In the first study, Tenneij, van Megen, Denys, and Westenberg (2005) randomly assigned 96 OCD patients on adequate SRI trials to receive either 6 additional months of their medication, or ERP. Those who received ERP showed greater improvement on the Y–BOCS (19% improvement) compared to those who continued on medication alone (21% worsening; i.e., an *increase* in Y–BOCS scores). Even patients who responded to SRIs benefited further when ERP was added. In the second study, Simpson et al. (2008) randomized 108 OCD patients who remained symptomatic (YBOCS ≥ 16) despite a therapeutic SRI dose for at least 12 weeks to 17 twice-weekly sessions of either ERP or stress management training (SMT) while continuing SRI pharmacotherapy. These authors found that ERP was superior to SMT in reducing OCD symptoms. At the end of psychological treatment (week 8), patients receiving ERP had significantly lower YBOCS scores ($M = 14.3$, $SD = 6.6$) than patients receiving SMT ($M = 22.7$, $SD = 6.3$).

Further analysis of the Simpson et al. (2008) data by Maher et al. (2010) identified the following variables as predictors of poorer ERP augmentation of SRI non-response: female gender, lower pre-treatment quality of life, greater number of comorbid Axis I disorders, and greater number of lifetime SRI trials. Greater pre-treatment OCD symptom severity was not a predictor of attenuated response, suggesting that this alone should not preclude patients who fail SRI trials from trying ERP. Taken together, the findings of these studies indicate that ERP is an effective augmentation strategy for OCD patients who respond either modestly or not at all to SRIs. The clinical implications of these findings are important since medication is the most widely available and most widely used form of treatment for OCD, yet it typically produces only modest improvement.

D-Cycloserine

Given the lack of convincing evidence that SRI medication facilitates the effects of ERP for OCD, researchers have examined whether pharmacologic agents that facilitate the extinction of fear responses might be more powerful adjuncts to ERP. Animal research suggests that the N-methyl-D-aspartate (NMDA) glutamatergic receptors in the basolateral amygdala receptors are important for the expression of conditioned fears (Walker, Ressler, Lu, & Davis, 2002). Because NMDA receptors in the amygdala are critical for fear acquisition, and because fear *extinction*, like fear acquisition, is also a form of learning, researchers have investigated the possibility that NMDA receptors in the amygdala are involved in extinction, and that NMDA agonists facilitate extinction when administered before ERP.

One such NMDA agonist is D-cycloserine (DCS), which has been used for years in humans to treat tuberculosis and is not associated with significant side effects. Animal research has shown that this compound facilitates extinction after either systemic administration or intra-amygdala infusion (Walker et al., 2002). In human adults with OCD, two studies found that DCS administered shortly before an exposure session, facilitated (i.e., sped up) fear extinction and thus the effects of ERP (Kushner et al., 2007; Wilhelm et al., 2008), whereas one study did not (Storch et al., 2007). Further research is needed to understand the reasons for the discrepant results, such as research into the optimal dose of the drug and timing for administration prior to the therapy session, the skill of the therapist in administering ERP, and the way in which treatment progress and outcome are assessed (the benefits of the drug are most apparent in the early sessions of treatment).

Strengths and Benefits of Using a Combined Approach

As we have discussed, pharmacotherapy and ERP each have their individual advantages and disadvantages. Clinically speaking, and considering the empirical data, combining these two treatments enhances neither the advantages nor the disadvantages of the monotherapies. Most patients with OCD will be prescribed medications rather than treated with effective ERP. Accordingly, the major benefit to most OCD patients, therefore, will be that the addition of ERP can improve upon the typically moderate effects of pharmacotherapy.

Clinical Vignette: Combined treatment

Martin, age 47, had suffered with OCD symptoms since he was a teenager. His obsessions concerned the fear that he would lose control and harm family members whom he loved very much; for example, that we would use a knife to stab his wife in her sleep. His rituals included checking for assurances that he was not a violent person. He also avoided items that could be used as "weapons" (e.g., baseball bats, knives) and kept these things locked away. Martin was started on clomipramine for his OCD at the age of 25, but experienced relatively modest improvement. He was also tried on several other SRIs, with similarly disappointing results, before reading about ERP and seeking out this treatment at the age of 40. Martin found a qualified therapist and underwent 18 sessions of ERP. Although the treatment was challenging at first, Martin pushed himself to keep knives and bats out and around the house. He allowed himself to think his obsessive thoughts without trying to neutralize them or seek assurances that he wouldn't murder his family. He even practiced sleeping next to his wife with a knife on his night table. Such experiences helped Martin learn that his obsessive thoughts were merely unwanted intrusions that he had been mistaking for homicidal urges. This knowledge relieved him of the urge to perform rituals, which further solidified his improvement. Martin's psychologist and psychiatrist worked together to reduce Martin's medication while he was still doing ERP so that he could learn that his improvement was not dependent on taking the SRI. Seven years later, Martin continues to have only minimal obsessional thoughts, which he is able to manage without avoidance or compulsive rituals.

FUTURE DIRECTIONS

The effects of ERP and SRI medication are well established. Future research should focus on identifying which patients with OCD will benefit the most from combination treatments. For example, it is possible that combined treatment would enhance the effects of ERP for severely depressed patients who do not fully benefit from ERP monotherapy because of their high emotional reactivity and psychomotor retardation (e.g., Abramowitz, Franklin, Street, Kozak, & Foa, 2000). Given that SRIs are antidepressants in addition to reducing OCD symptom, perhaps such medications would reduce depressive symptoms to the point that it would be possible for patients to engage in and benefit from ERP.

Clinical Points to Remember

1. OCD involves two symptoms: (a) obsessional thoughts that provoke anxiety, and (b) behaviors and mental acts performed to reduce anxiety.
2. Obsessions are not simply repetitive or perseverative thoughts. They are intrusive, unwanted ideas that concern senseless and unrealistic topics that provoke anxiety.
3. Compulsive rituals are not simply repetitive behaviors. They are behaviors (or mental acts) performed to reduce obsessional distress. Compulsive rituals are neutralizing behaviors.
4. There are two forms of treatment that have been scientifically shown to reduce OCD symptoms: cognitive-behavioral therapy (CBT) using exposure and response prevention, and pharmacotherapy using serotonin reuptake inhibitor antidepressants.
5. Whereas it might seem intuitive that combining psychological and pharmacotherapy approaches would be more effective than either treatment alone, it turns out that this is not the case for OCD. While CBT adds to the effectiveness of medications, the addition of medication is not necessarily likely to improve outcome with CBT.

NOTE

1. One exception was reported by Hohagen et al. (1998), who found that combined ERP and fluvoxamine offered an advantage over ERP monotherapy, although this finding was among severely depressed OCD patients.

REFERENCES

Abramowitz, J. S. (1996). Variants of exposure and response prevention in the treatment of obsessive-compulsive disorder: A meta-analysis. *Behavior Therapy, 27,* 583–600.

Abramowitz, J. S. (1997). Effectiveness of psychological and pharmacological treatments for obsessive-compulsive disorder: A quantitative review. *Journal of Consulting and Clinical Psychology, 65,* 44–52.

Abramowitz, J. S. (2006). *Understanding and treating obsessive-compulsive disorder: A cognitive-behavioral approach.* Mahwah, NJ: Lawrence Erlbaum.

Abramowitz, J. S., Deacon, B., Olatunji, B., Wheaton, M. G., Berman, N., Losardo, D., et al. (2010). Assessment of obsessive-compulsive symptom dimensions: Development and evaluation of the Dimensional Obsessive-Compulsive Scale. *Psychological Assessment, 22,* 180–198.

Abramowitz, J. S., & Foa, E. (2000). Does comorbid major depressive disorder influence outcome of exposure and response prevention for OCD? *Behavior Therapy*, *31*, 795–800.

Abramowitz, J. S., Franklin, M. E., Street, G. P., Kozak, M. J., & Foa, E. B. (2000). Effects of comorbid depression on response to treatment for obsessive-compulsive disorder. *Behavior Therapy*, *31*, 517–528.

Abramowitz, J. S., Franklin, M., Zoellner, L., & DiBernardo, C. (2002). Treatment compliance and outcome in obsessive-compulsive disorder. *Behavior Modification*, *26*, 447–463.

Abramowitz, J., Wheaton, M., & Storch, A. (2008). The status of hoarding as a symptom of obsessive-compulsive disorder. *Behaviour Research and Therapy*, *46*, 1026–1033.

American Psychiatric Association (APA). (2000). *Diagnostic and statistical manual of mental disorders* (4th ed., text revision). Washington, DC: APA.

Anderson, R. A., & Rees, C. S. (2007) Group versus individual cognitive-behavioural treatment for obsessive-compulsive disorder: A controlled trial. *Behaviour Research and Therapy*, *45*, 123–137.

Chakrabarty, K., Bhattacharyya, S., Christopher, R., & Khanna, S. (2005). Glutamatergic dysfunction in OCD. *Neuropsychopharmacology*, *30*, 1735–1740.

Cottraux, J., Mollard, E., Bouvard, M., Marks, I., Sluys, M., Nury, A., et al. (1990). A controlled study of fluvoxamine and exposure in obsessive compulsive disorder. *International Journal of Clinical Psychopharmacology*, *5*, 17–30.

DeVeaugh-Geiss, J., Landau, P., & Katz, R. (1989). Treatment of OCD with clomipramine. *Psychiatric Annals*, *19*, 97–101.

Eddy, K., Dutra, L., Bradley, R., & Weston, D. (2004). A multidimensional meta-analysis of psychotherapy and pharmacotherapy for obsessive-compulsive disorder. *Clinical Psychology Review*, *24*, 1011–1030.

Ergovezi, S., Cavallini, M. C., Cavedini, P., Diaferia, G., Locatelli, M., & Bellodi, L. (2001). Clinical predictors of drug response in obsessive-compulsive disorder. *Journal of Clinical Psychopharmacology*, *21*, 488–492.

Fals-Stewart, W., Marks, A. P., & Schafer, J. (1993). A comparison of behavioral group therapy and individual behavior therapy in treating obsessive-compulsive disorder. *Journal of Nervous and Mental Disease*, *181*(3), 189–193.

Foa, E. B. (1979). Failure in treating obsessive-compulsives. *Behaviour Research and Therapy*, *17*, 169–176.

Foa, E. B., Abramowitz, J. S., Franklin, M. E., & Kozak, M. J. (1999). Feared consequences, fixity of belief, and treatment outcome in patients with obsessive-compulsive disorder. *Behavior Therapy*, *30*, 717–724.

Foa, E. B., Grayson, J. B., Steketee, G. S., Doppelt, H. G., Turner, R. M., & Latimer, P. R. (1983). Success and failure in the behavioral treatment of obsessive-compulsives. *Journal of Consulting and Clinical Psychology*, *51*, 287–297.

Foa, E. B., & Kozak, M. J. (1995). DSM-IV field trial: Obsessive-compulsive disorder. *American Journal of Psychiatry*, *152*(1), 90–96.

Foa, E. B., & Kozak, M. J. (1996). Psychological treatment for obsessive-compulsive disorder. In M. R. Mavissakalian, R. F. Prien, M. R. Mavissakalian, & R. F. Prien (Eds.), *Long-term treatments of anxiety disorders* (pp. 285–309). Washington, DC: American Psychiatric Association.

Foa, E. B., Liebowitz, M. R., Kozak, M. J., Davies, S., Campeas, R., Franklin, M. E., et al. (2005). Randomized, placebo-controlled trial of exposure and ritual prevention, clomipramine, and their combination in the treatment of obsessive-compulsive disorder. *American Journal of Psychiatry, 162*, 151–161.

Foa, E. B., Steketee, G., Grayson, J. B., Turner, R. M., & Latimer, P. R. (1984). Deliberate exposure and blocking of obsessive-compulsive rituals: Immediate and long-term effects. *Behavior Therapy, 15*(5), 450–472.

Franklin, M. E., Abramowitz, J. S., Bux, D. A., Jr., Zoellner, L. A., & Feeny, N. C. (2002). Cognitive-behavioral therapy with and without medication in the treatment of obsessive-compulsive disorder. *Professional Psychology: Research and Practice, 33*, 162–168.

Franklin, M. E., Abramowitz, J. S., Foa, E. B., Kozak, M. J., & Levitt, J. T. (2000). Effectiveness of exposure and ritual prevention for obsessive-compulsive disorder: Randomized compared with nonrandomized samples. *Journal of Consulting and Clinical Psychology, 68*(4), 594–602.

Freeston, M. H., Ladouceur, R., Gagnon, F., Thibodeau, N., Rhéaume, J., Letarte, H., & Bujold, A. (1997). Cognitive-behavioral treatment of obsessive thoughts: A controlled study. *Journal of Consulting and Clinical Psychology, 65*(3), 405–413.

Friedman, S., Smith, L. C., Halpern, B., Levine, C., Paradis, C., Viswanathan, R., et al. (2003). Obsessive-compulsive disorder in a multi-ethnic urban outpatient clinic: initial presentation and treatment outcome with exposure and ritual prevention. *Behavior Therapy, 34*, 397–410.

Goodman, W. K., Price, L. H., Rasmussen, S. A., Mazure, C., Delgado, P., Heninger, G. R., & Charney, D. S. (1989b). The Yale–Brown Obsessive Compulsive Scale: Validity. *Archives of General Psychiatry, 46*, 1012–1016.

Goodman, W. K., Price, L. H., Rasmussen, S. A., Mazure, C., Fleischmann, R. L., Hill, C. L., et al. (1989a). The Yale–Brown Obsessive Compulsive Scale: Development, use, and reliability. *Archives of General Psychiatry, 46*, 1006–1011.

Greenberg, B., Benjamin, J., Martin, J., Keuler, D., Huang, S., Altemus, M., & Murphy, D. (2000). Delayed obsessive-compulsive disorder symptom exacerbation after a single dose of serotonin antagonist in fluoxetine-treated but not untreated patients. *Psychopharmacology, 140*, 434–444.

Greist, J. H., Jefferson, J. W., Kobak, K. A., Katzelnick, D. J., & Serlin, R. C. (1995). Efficacy and tolerability of serotonin transport inhibitors in obsessive-compulsive disorder: A meta-analysis. *Archives of General Psychiatry, 52*, 53–60.

Gross, R., Sasson, Y., Chopra, M., & Zohar, J. (1998). Biological models of obsessive-compulsive disorder: The serotonin hypothesis. In R. P. Swinson, M. M. Antony, S. Rachman, & M. A. Richter (Eds.), *Obsessive-compulsive disorder: Theory, research, and treatment* (pp. 141–153). New York: Guilford Press.

Hohagen, F., Winkelmann, G., Rasche-Rauchle, H., Hand, I., Konig, A., Munchau, N., et al. (1998). Combination of behaviour therapy with fluvoxamine in comparison with behaviour therapy and placebo. *British Journal of Psychiatry, 173*, 71–78.

Houghton, S., Saxon, D., Bradburn, M., Ricketts, T., & Hardy, G. (2010) The effectiveness of routinely delivered cognitive behavioral therapy for obsessive-compulsive disorder: A benchmarking study. *British Journal of Clinical Psychology, 49*, 473–489.

Kessler, R., Berglund, P., Demler, O., Jin, R., Merikangas, K., & Walters, E. (2005). Lifetime prevalence and age-of-onset distributions of DSM-IV disorders in the National Comorbidity Survey Replication. *Archives of General Psychiatry, 62*, 593–602.

Kolada, J. L., Bland, R. C., & Newman, S. C. (1994). Obsessive-compulsive disorder. *Acta Psychiatrica Scandinavica, 89*, 24–35.

Kozak, M. J., & Foa, E. B. (1997). *Therapist guide to mastery of obsessive-compulsive disorder: A cognitive-behavioral approach.* San Antonio, TX: Psychological Corporation.

Kushner, M., Kim, S.-W., Donahue, C., Thuras, P., Adson, D., Kotlyar, M., et al. (2007). D-Cycloserine augmented exposure therapy for obsessive-compulsive disorder. *Biological Psychiatry, 62*, 835–838.

Lax, T., Başoğlu, M., & Marks, I. M. (1992). Expectancy and compliance as predictors of outcome in obsessive-compulsive disorder. *Behavioural Psychotherapy, 20*, 257–266.

Lindsay, M., Crino, R., & Andrews, G. (1997). Controlled trial of exposure and response prevention in obsessive-compulsive disorder. *British Journal of Psychiatry, 171*, 135–139.

Maher, M. J., Huppert, J. D., Chen, H., Duan, N., Foa, E. B., Liebowitz, M. R., & Simpson, H. B. (2010). Moderators and predictors of response to cognitive-behavioral therapy augmentation of pharmacotherapy in obsessive-compulsive disorder. *Psychological Medicine, 40*, 2013–2023.

Marks, I. M., Lelliott, P., Başoğlu, M., Noshirvani, H., Monteiro, W., Cohen, D., & Kasvikis, Y. (1988). Clomipramine, self-exposure and therapist-aided exposure for obsessive-compulsive rituals. *British Journal of Psychiatry, 152*, 522–534.

Marks, I. M., Stern, R. S., Mawson, D., Cobb, J., & McDonald, R. (1980). Clomipramine, self-exposure, and therapist-aided exposure for obsessive-compulsive rituals. *British Journal of Psychiatry, 152*, 522–534.

Mataix-Cols, D., Rauch, S., Manzo, P., Jenike, M., & Baer, L. (1999). Use of factor-analyzed symptom dimensions to predict outcome with serotonin reuptake inhibitors and placebo in the treatment of obsessive-compulsive disorder. *American Journal of Psychiatry, 156*, 1409–1416.

McKay, D., Abramowitz, J., Calamari, J., Kyrios, M., Radomsky, A., Sookman, D., et al. (2004). A critical evaluation of obsessive-compulsive disorder subtypes: Symptoms versus mechanisms. *Clinical Psychology Review, 24*, 283–313.

Montgomery, S. A., McIntyre, A., Ostenheider, M., Sarteschi, P., Zitterl, W., Zohar, J., et al. (1993). A double-blind placebo-controlled study of fluoxetine in patients with DSM-III-R obsessive-compulsive disorder. *European Neuropsychopharmacology, 3*, 142–152.

Nakatani, E., Nakagawa, A., Nakao, T., Yoshizato, C., Nabeyama, M., Kudo, A., et al. (2005). A randomized trial of Japanese patients with obsessive-compulsive disorder: Effectiveness of behavior therapy and fluvoxamine. *Psychotherapy and Psychosomatics, 75*, 269–276.

O'Connor, K., Todorov, C., Robillard, S., Borgeat, F., & Brault, M. (1999). Cognitive-behaviour therapy and medication in the treatment of obsessive-compulsive disorder: A controlled study. *Canadian Journal of Psychiatry, 44*, 64–71.

O'Sullivan, G., Noshirvani, H., Marks, I., Monteiro, W., & Lelliott, P. (1991). Six-year follow-up after exposure and clomipramine therapy for obsessive compulsive disorder. *Journal of Clinical Psychiatry, 52*(4), 150–155.

Pato, M., Zohar-Kadouch, R., Zohar, J., & Murphy, D. (1988). Return of symptoms after discontinuation of clomipramine in patients with obsessive-compulsive disorder. *American Journal of Psychiatry, 145*, 1521–1525.

Persons, J. B., & Silberschatz, G. (1998). Are results of randomized controlled trials useful to psychotherapists? *Journal of Consulting and Clinical Psychology, 66*, 126–135.

Price, L. H., Goodman, W. K., Charney, D. S., Rasmussen, S. A., & Heninger, G. R. (1987). Treatment of severe obsessive compulsive disorder with fluvoxamine. *American Journal of Psychiatry, 144*, 1059–1061.

Rasmussen, S. A., & Eisen, J. L. (1992). The epidemiology and clinical features of obsessive-compulsive disorder. *Psychiatric Clinics of North America, 15*, 743–758.

Rasmussen, S. A., & Tsuang, M. T. (1986). Clinical characteristics and family history in DSM-III obsessive-compulsive disorder. *American Journal of Psychiatry, 143*, 317–322.

Rowa, K., Antony, M. M., Summerfeldt, L. J., Purdon, C., Young, L., & Swinson, R. P. (2007). Office-based vs. home-based behavioral treatment for obsessive compulsive disorder: A preliminary study. *Behaviour Research and Therapy, 45*, 1883–1892.

Saiz, P. A., Garcia-Portilla, M., Arango, C., Morales, B., Bascaran, M. T., Martinez-Barrondo, S., et al. (2008). Association study between obsessive-compulsive disorder and serotonin candidate genes. *Progress in Neuropsychopharmacology and Biological Psychiatry, 32*, 765–770.

Simpson, H. B., Foa, E. B., Liebowitz, M. R., Ledley, D. R., Huppert, J. D., Cahill, S., et al. (2008). A randomized, controlled trial of cognitive-behavioral therapy for augmenting pharmacotherapy in obsessive-compulsive disorder. *American Journal of Psychiatry, 165*, 621–630.

Simpson, H. B., Liebowitz, M. R., Foa, E. B., Kozak, M. J., Schmidt, A. B., Rowan, V., et al. (2004). Post-treatment effects of exposure therapy and clomipramine in obsessive-compulsive disorder. *Depression and Anxiety, 19*, 225–233.

Steketee, G. S., Chambless, D. L., & Tran, G. Q. (2001). Effects of Axis I and II comorbidity on behavior therapy outcome for obsessive-compulsive disorder and agoraphobia. *Comprehensive Psychiatry, 42*, 76–86.

Storch, E. A., Merlo, L. J., Bengtson, M., Murphy, T. K., Lewis, M. H., Yang, M. C., Goodman, W. K. (2007). D-Cycloserine does not enhance exposure–response prevention therapy in obsessive-compulsive disorder. *International Clinical Psychopharmacology, 22*, 230–237.

Tenneij, N., van Megen, H., Denys, D., & Westenberg, H. (2005). Behavior therapy augments response of patients with obsessive-compulsive disorder responding to drug treatment. *Journal of Clinical Psychiatry, 66*, 1169–1175.

Tolin, D. F., Abramowitz, J. S., Kozak, M. J., & Foa, E. B. (2001). Fixity of belief, perceptual aberration, and magical ideation in obsessive-compulsive disorder. *Journal of Anxiety Disorders, 15*, 501–510.

van Balkom, A. J. L. M., de Haan, E., van Oppen, P., Spinhoven, P., Hoogduin, K. A. L., & van Dyck, R. (1998). Cognitive and behavioral therapies alone versus in combination with fluvoxamine in the treatment of obsessive compulsive disorder. *Journal of Nervous and Mental Disorders, 186*(8), 492–499.

Vogel, P. A., Stiles, T. C., & Götestam, K. G. (2004). Adding cognitive therapy elements to exposure therapy for obsessive compulsive disorder: A controlled study. *Behavioural and Cognitive Psychotherapy, 32*, 275–290.

Walker, D., Ressler, K., Lu, K., & Davis, M. (2002). Facilitation of conditioned fear extinction by systemic administration or intra-amygdala infusions of D-cycloserine as assessed with fear-potentiated startle in rats. *Journal of Neuroscience, 22,* 2343–2351.

Warren, R., & Thomas, J. C. (2001). Cognitive-behavior therapy of obsessive-compulsive disorder in private practice: an effectiveness study. *Journal of Anxiety Disorders, 15,* 277–285.

Wilhelm, S., Buhlmann, U., Tolin, D. F., Meunier, S. A., Pearlson, G. D., Reese, H. E., et al. (2008). Augmentation of behavior therapy with D-cycloserine for obsessive-compulsive disorder. *American Journal of Psychiatry, 165,* 335–341.

CHAPTER 7

Acute Stress Disorder

Angela Nickerson and Richard A. Bryant

INTRODUCTION

Acute stress disorder (ASD) was introduced in the fourth edition of the *Diagnostic and Statistical Manual of Mental Disorders* (*DSM–IV*, American Psychiatric Association, 1994). The purpose of this diagnosis was twofold: first, to describe severe posttraumatic stress responses within the first month following a trauma (i.e., before a diagnosis of posttraumatic stress disorder [PTSD] could be applied), and second, to identify individuals at risk of developing chronic PTSD reactions following exposure to a traumatic event (Koopman, Classen, Cardeña, & Spiegel, 1995).

Prevalence

Research into psychological reactions following exposure to traumatic experiences has indicated that the majority of trauma survivors experience initial symptoms of distress; however, these generally alleviate over time. For example, in a study examining the responses of rape survivors, the number of individuals meeting criteria for PTSD (initially 94%) halved in the 3 months following the trauma (Rothbaum, Foa, Riggs, Murdock, & Walsh, 1992). This pattern has been observed in survivors of motor vehicle accidents (Blanchard, Hickling, Barton, & Taylor, 1996), non-sexual assault (Riggs, Rothbaum, & Foa, 1995), and terrorist attacks (Galea, 2007). As ASD is only diagnosed in the initial month after trauma exposure, there are currently no population study prevalence rates available. Rates of ASD have been investigated in trauma-exposed populations, and have ranged from 5% to 20% across populations, often depending on the nature of the event. The rates of ASD include 13% for motor vehicle accidents (Harvey & Bryant, 1998), 14% after mild traumatic brain injury (Harvey & Bryant, 1998), 16–19% after assault (Brewin, Andrews, Rose, & Kirk, 1999; Harvey & Bryant, 1999), 10% after burns (Harvey & Bryant, 1999), 6–12% after industrial accidents (Creamer & Manning, 1998;

Harvey & Bryant, 1999), 9% for survivors of the September 11 terrorist attacks (Galea et al., 2002), and 33% after witnessing a mass shooting (Classen, Koopman, Hales, & Spiegel, 1998). A number of studies have also assessed subsyndromal ASD, in which re-experiencing, avoidance, and arousal—but not dissociative—symptoms were required for diagnosis. Higher rates of ASD have been observed when applying this more permissive criterion (Bryant, Creamer, O'Donnell, Silove, & McFarlane, 2008; Dalgleish et al., 2008; Harvey & Bryant, 1998).

Predicting Posttraumatic Stress Disorder from Acute Stress Disorder

Multiple studies have investigated the utility of ASD in identifying those individuals who will go on to develop PTSD 1 month or longer after exposure to the trauma. As already noted, the downward trajectory of psychological distress following exposure to a traumatic event has been well established (Blanchard et al., 1996; Galea, 2007; Riggs et al., 1995; Rothbaum et al., 1992). A systematic review of the capacity of ASD to predict PTSD in trauma survivors indicated that ASD evidenced moderate predictive power for PTSD, but poor sensitivity (Bryant, 2011). This suggests that, while studies indicated that over half of adults with a diagnosis of ASD went on to develop PTSD, there were many trauma survivors who were eventually diagnosed with PTSD who did not meet the full criteria for ASD in the month following the trauma. One possible explanation for this finding is the requirement of dissociative symptoms for a diagnosis of ASD. Studies investigating the capacity of subsyndromal ASD (requiring re-experiencing, avoidance and arousal symptoms, but not symptoms of dissociation) to predict PTSD have yielded higher levels of sensitivity for the ASD diagnosis (Bryant, 2011). As noted by Bryant, Friedman, Spiegel, Ursano, and Strain (2011), this may be accounted for by the fact that re-experiencing, avoidance, and arousal symptom clusters in the ASD diagnosis are directly analogous to those in the PTSD diagnosis, while dissociation is not prominent in the PTSD diagnosis. Overall, the low sensitivity of ASD is problematic, as a key goal of the inception of this disorder was to identify those who were likely to go on to develop PTSD reactions so that early interventions could be implemented to prevent the onset of chronic PTSD.

DSM–IV Criteria for Acute Stress Disorder

The *DSM–IV* criteria for ASD specify that the individual must be exposed to a traumatic event in which there was actual or threatened death or serious injury and they experienced fear, helplessness, or horror (Criterion A). Four clusters of symptoms of symptoms must be present. The first represents dissociative responses, such that the individual must exhibit three or more of the following symptoms: (1) a subjective sense of numbing, detachment, or absence of emotional responsiveness; (2) reduced awareness of surroundings; (3) derealisation; (4) depersonalization; and (5) dissociative amnesia (Criterion B). The survivor must also exhibit one or more re-experiencing symptoms such as intrusive thoughts, images, nightmares, or distress in response to reminders of the event (Criterion C). Marked avoidance of stimuli that remind the individual of the trauma must be present (Criterion D), as well as marked anxiety or arousal symptoms (Criterion E). These symptoms must cause significant distress or impairment (Criterion F), and last for a minimum of 2 days and a maximum of 4 weeks (Criterion G), after which a diagnosis of PTSD should be considered.

There are two primary differences in the conceptualization of ASD as against PTSD reactions. The first concerns the time frame in which the diagnosis can be made: although PTSD can only be diagnosed from 4 weeks following the trauma, ASD refers to symptoms that occur from 2 days to 4 weeks following the traumatic event. The second is the prominence of dissociative symptoms in ASD criteria: while individuals do not need to manifest dissociation for a diagnosis of PTSD, to receive a diagnosis of ASD, trauma survivors must report at least three dissociative symptoms. The prominent role of dissociative symptoms in the diagnosis of ASD has been criticized by theorists, and challenged by findings that the removal of dissociative symptoms as a criterion for ASD results in better prediction of subsequent PTSD (Harvey & Bryant, 1998; 1999). It appears that the requirement of dissociative symptoms for this disorder results in the exclusion of many individuals who are at high risk for developing PTSD (Bryant et al., 2011). However, it has also been noted that dissociative symptoms are common in the aftermath of a traumatic event (Cardeña & Spiegel, 1993; Feinstein, 1989), and predict subsequent PTSD (Ehlers, Mayou, & Bryant, 1998; Koopman, Classen, & Spiegel, 1994; Murray, Ehlers, & Mayou, 2002; Ozer, Best, Lipsey, & Weiss, 2003). It is for this reason that DSM–5 plans to alter the purpose of ASD; while the requirement for symptoms of dissociation will likely be retained, the diagnosis will be describing severe acute stress reactions rather than predicting PTSD (Bryant et al., 2011).

Clinical Considerations with Acute Stress Disorder

A key clinical consideration when working with a survivor of a recent traumatic event is distinguishing normal and pathological stress reactions. It is important to remember that high levels of distress are common in the weeks following a trauma, and are not necessarily indicative of psychopathology. In addition to conducting a thorough assessment to determine the extent of the traumatic stress reactions, it is important to provide psychoeducation to the trauma survivor regarding common psychological reactions and trajectories of response following trauma. In this sense, it is often useful to query whether the stress responses have maintained their severity or are diminishing since the traumatic event. In addition, the context surrounding the traumatic event is extremely important. Most research that has been conducted examining ASD has investigated the effects of single-incident traumatic events in Western countries. In such settings, acute stress symptoms may be expected to reduce as the survivor readjusts to life following the traumatic event and regains a sense of safety and predictability. This may vary considerably from traumatic events that occur in the context of ongoing danger or violence (e.g., in the context of war, domestic violence, or abuse). For example, in a study conducted in Sierra Leone, rates of PTSD were reported as 99% in the context of ongoing civil conflict (de Jong, Mulhern, Ford, van der Kam, & Kleber, 2000); it is likely that exposure to ongoing threat and the realistic prospect of further traumatic events will exacerbate acute stress symptoms, and preclude natural adaptation. Highlighting this point is evidence that found that rates of PTSD actually *increased* over time following Hurricane Katrina (Kessler et al., 2008). Delays in rebuilding infrastructure, lack of housing, and loss of basic infrastructures may have contributed to increasing psychological strain, which led to rising rates of PTSD.

Considering the recent nature of the traumatic event when working with individuals with ASD, it can be expected that the trauma survivors will be experiencing severe psychological distress. Intrusive symptoms related to the trauma are heightened in the immediate aftermath of the event, and the individual is likely to be experiencing intrusive memories as well as nightmares, and possibly even flashback-like memories. Accordingly, patients will generally present with very high levels of anxiety about the possibility of being exposed to a traumatic event again, practical concerns in relation to the event (e.g., providing police statements, undergoing medical examinations), as well as a general sense of lack of safety and trust. Further, avoidance is often pervasive as the person tries to avoid reminders of the event. This may also extend to the therapy environment; for example, the patient may not wish to discuss details of the trauma, or may be reluctant to leave the house to attend sessions. Dissociative responses may be distressing for the participant, particularly the inability to remember important aspects of the trauma, as well as feelings of depersonalization and derealization. For instance, the patient may think that such symptoms indicate that he or she is "going crazy" and that the trauma has changed him or her irreversibly. In such cases it is extremely important to provide psychoeducation to inform the patient about common responses to traumatic events, and to normalize these responses. This is particularly important in light of evidence that catastrophizing about the symptoms that one experiences after trauma exposure is predictive of longer-term PTSD (Ehlers & Clark, 2000).

It is also important to take into consideration the cultural background of the patient when discussing symptoms. Certain symptoms may have different meanings across cultural groups, and accordingly impact differently on the patient's beliefs about his or her internal experiences and the traumatic event (e.g., Hinton, Hinton, Pham, Chau, & Tran, 2003; Schulz, Marovic-Johnson, & Huber, 2006). Familiarizing oneself with cultural beliefs as much as possible or working in conjunction with a cultural consultant will be very useful in understanding and treating psychological distress in patients from varied cultural backgrounds.

SOLITARY TREATMENT APPROACHES

Pharmacological Treatment

Review of randomized controlled trials and other studies

To date, few randomized controlled trials (RCTs) have been undertaken to examine the efficacy of psychopharmacological interventions in treating symptoms of ASD in adults. In a recent study, Shalev and colleagues (2012) randomized 242 patients admitted through an emergency room who subsequently met criteria for either full or subsyndromal ASD to either prolonged exposure, cognitive restructuring, wait list (who were then randomized to exposure or cognitive restructuring after 12 weeks), escitalopram (a serotonin-specific reuptake inhibitor [SSRI]), or placebo. Participants were admitted to the trial if they presented with either ASD or subsydromal ASD approximately 1 month after trauma exposure. At the 9 months follow-up, PTSD rates were comparable across exposure (21%) and restructuring (22%) conditions, relative to the much higher rates in the SSRI (42%) and placebo (47%) conditions. These findings from the largest and most tightly controlled study to date strongly indicate that the merits of pharmacological intervention based on agents traditionally used to treat PTSD may not have substantial gains for patients displaying ASD symptoms.

Multiple approaches have been taken to the treatment of acute stress symptoms. The first approach has focused on the reduction of arousal, anxiety, and agitation following exposure to trauma by using benzodiazepines or high-potency neuroleptics. In one case study, temazepam was administered within 1–3 weeks of the trauma to four trauma survivors over a period of 5 nights, then tapered for 2 nights, before being discontinued. Findings suggested that the use of temazepam reduced sleep difficulties and PTSD severity (Mellman, Byers, & Augenstein, 1998). In a second study, 13 trauma survivors were treated with clonazepman or alprazolam within 2 weeks of the trauma. No difference was observed at 1 or 6 months between these patients and the control group (Gelpin, Bonne, Peri, Brandes, & Shalev, 1996). A second approach has drawn from established literature on the treatment of PTSD, using antidepressant medications. A case series of three patients indicated that tricyclic medications were effective in reducing symptoms of ASD (Blake, 1986). A randomized trial found that 7 days of treatment with imipramine was more effective in treating symptoms of acute stress disorder among 25 child and adolescent burns victims than chloral hydrate (Robert, Blakeney, Villarreal, Rosenberg, & Meyer, 1999). A third strategy, supported by promising initial research, has focused on implementing propranolol within days (or hours) of the traumatic event to reduce noradrenergic activation. It has been hypothesized that this will reduce epinephrine augmentation of fear conditioning, and thus decrease conditioning related to trauma memories (Cahill, Prins, Weber, & McGaugh, 1994). A pilot study found that propanolol was associated with lower reactivity to trauma reminders 3 months after the trauma compared to a placebo condition. However, this did not result in reduced PTSD (Pitman et al., 2002). Another (uncontrolled) study indicated that the administration of propanolol immediately following a traumatic event was related to reduced PTSD after 2 months (Vaiva et al., 2003). In contrast, a review of medical records indicated that propanolol administered in the first 30 days following burns trauma did not reduce ASD symptoms in children who had experienced burns trauma (Sharp, Thomas, Rosenberg, Rosenberg, & Meyer 2010). Another recent study suggests that there may be differential gender effects for the impact of propanolol on traumatic stress symptoms in children (Nugent et al., 2011). Consistent with the goal of reducing norepinephrine in the acute phase, there is also indirect evidence that factors that diminish arousal shortly after trauma exposure may lessen the subsequent PTSD, including natural levels of γ-aminobutyric acid (GABA) (Vaiva et al., 2004) and the administration of morphine in the immediate hours after trauma (Bryant, Creamer, O'Donnell, Silove, & McFarlane, 2009; Holbrook, Galarneau, Dye, Quinn, & Dougherty, 2010; Saxe et al., 2001). These were longitudinal naturalistic studies, rather than RCTs, and so do not provide definitive evidence that agents such as morphine are protective against PTSD development.

Another promising line of research has focused on the role of glucocorticoids in the initial phase after trauma exposure. There is evidence that patients in medical settings who were administered cortisol developed fewer traumatic memories than those who were not (Schelling et al., 2001; Schelling, Kilger et al., 2004). This finding was consistent with evidence that animals administered hydrocortisone immediately after a stressor displayed markedly less anxiety responses than those administered placebo (Cohen, Matar, Buskila, Kaplan, & Zohar, 2008). This raised the possibility that secondary prevention of PTSD may be achieved by cortisol administration (Schelling, Roozendaal, & De Quervain, 2004). A recent pilot randomized controlled trial that administered high-dose hydrocortisone within hours of trauma exposure found that it resulted in less acute stress disorder and later PTSD than placebo (Zohar et al., 2011). These new findings provide some exciting potential for early intervention insofar as the use of cortisol in the acute phase after trauma accords with prevailing models of stress response and animal evidence regarding the role of stress hormones in trauma memories. Although this line of research is in its infancy, it is possible that cortisol administration may play an important role in ameliorating acute stress responses.

Strengths and limitations of pharmacotherapy

To date, there is inadequate research to support definitive recommendations on the use of pharmacotherapy to treat symptoms of ASD and/or prevent the onset of PTSD. Thus, a major limitation of this type of treatment is lack of information regarding the short- and long-term effects of these medications on psychological symptoms. While there are several promising avenues of pharmacotherapy, their use as the sole intervention in the aftermath of a traumatic event is not supported by research evidence. Further, potential side effects of these medications represent significant limitations. For example, the long-term use of benzodiazepines should be avoided, owing to the addictive properties of this class of drugs, as well as potential adverse physical and psychological effects. Similarly, the use of tricyclic antidepressants should be carefully monitored because of a range of potential adverse side effects, including potential lethality when used in high doses, and risks to the elderly and individuals with organ disease.

Clinical Vignette: Good outcome with pharmacotherapy

Martin is a 35-year-old captain in the military who was subjected to intensive combat 1 week ago. He was under fire from enemy fire in Afghanistan after mortar fire hit the convoy he was in and killed a colleague. Martin was subsequently confined in his Humvee for hours as the attack was sustained until darkness permitted them to escape. Although Martin himself was uninjured, he was severely traumatized by the experience. When he was transferred to a hospital base 2 weeks later for management of his stress reaction, he was highly agitated, suffering markedly from nightmares, and had developed intense sleep disturbance. Martin reported problems with onset of sleep as well as frequent awakenings. These awakenings were often caused by nightmares. On the basis that his sleep deprivation was a major cause of immediate distress for Martin, and also that his nightmares were the primary re-experiencing symptom, it was decided to administer a hypnotic medication to facilitate sleep.

Accordingly, he was administered temazepam. Initially he was given 30 mg each night for 5 days, and then 15 mg for the next 2 days. Martin responded rapidly to this medication insofar as he improved from his average of 2 hours' sleep a night to 6 hours of sleep. This afforded Martin considerable relief because the agitation resulting from his sleep deprivation was quickly alleviated. Treating physicians agreed that he should additionally undergo psychotherapy to assist long-term adaptation. However the immediate problem was largely ameliorated by the temazepam.

Clinical Vignette: Poor outcome with pharmacotherapy

Mike is a 57-year-old truck driver who was involved in a traffic accident 2 days ago that involved a fatality. Although Mike suffered some lacerations and a fractured rib, his physical injury healed quickly. On the day of the accident, however, when Mike was admitted to the emergency room, he presented in a highly agitated state. He was in much pain, which was managed with codeine-based medication. Several days later, when he was in a hospital ward, he was still highly anxious, reporting intense flashbacks of the accident, and having vivid nightmares of the other driver's face as she was removed from her mangled car. The physician on duty prescribed the benzodiazepine alprazolam to reduce his arousal level and anxiety. Mike achieved considerable relief with the alprazolam, and was keen to remain on it. Following discharge from hospital, he insisted to the doctors that the prescription be maintained because he was unable to manage the anxiety without the medication. Nine months later, Mike was taking increasingly greater amounts of alprazolam, and it was apparent that he was dependent. On three occasions he has tried to taper off the medication. However, on each occasion he was unable to manage the anxiety. This case highlights a common problem with acute administration of benzodiazepines: it can be extended for excessive periods and dependence can occur. Whereas benzodiazepines have been shown to have some utility in short-term use to manage acute agitation, longer-term reliance can create considerable problems with dependence.

Psychosocial Treatment

Two major psychosocial approaches have been taken to early intervention following exposure to traumatic events. The first represents universal interventions that are provided to all trauma survivors with the aim of preventing the development of psychopathology. The second refers to indicated prevention models that attempt to treat early symptoms identified using certain criteria (e.g., a diagnosis of ASD) to prevent subsequent chronic posttraumatic stress reactions. Hereunder we will review randomized controlled trials and uncontrolled studies evaluating the efficacy and effectiveness of these two approaches.

Review of RCTs: universal interventions

The most popular universal intervention approach over the past three decades has been debriefing, and more specifically critical incident stress debriefing (CISD). This intervention was originally designed to target psychological symptoms following trauma exposure in emergency personnel (Mitchell, 1983), but has since been applied with various other trauma-exposed groups (Adler et al., 2008; Jacobs, Horne-Moyer, & Jones, 2004; Nurmi, 1999; Saarni, Saari, & Hakkinen, 1999; Sacks, Clements, & Fay-Hillier, 2001; Simms-Ellis & Madill, 2001; Townsend & Loughlin, 1998; Wee, Mills, & Koehler, 1999). The original version of the intervention centered on a single session that occurred within a few days of exposure, in which the psychological experience of the trauma survivor is normalized and discussed.

A number of randomized controlled trials have been undertaken to examine the effects of psychological debriefing. Hobbs, Mayou, Harrison, and Worlock (1996) randomized 106 motor vehicle accident survivors to receive either psychological debriefing or an assessment-only control. There were no group differences on PTSD symptoms; however, the psychological debriefing condition was associated with worse general psychiatric symptoms. A follow-up of this study indicated that, while there were no group differences on PTSD symptoms, the psychological debriefing group had significantly worse general psychiatric symptoms, travel anxiety, and overall functioning 3 years after the intervention (Mayou, Ehlers & Hobbs, 2000). Bisson, Jenkins, Alexander, and Bannister (1997) randomly assigned burns victims to receive either CISD or assessment only. Their results indicated that those in the CISD group evidenced greater symptoms of PTSD, depression, and anxiety at 13 months compared to the control group. A study conducted by Conlon, Fahy, and Conroy (1999) found no group differences in PTSD symptoms among 40 motor vehicle accident survivors randomized to either psychological debriefing or an assessment-only control group.

A study conducted by Deahl and colleagues (2000) randomized 106 peacekeepers to receive either debriefing or assessment only. They found that, while the debriefing group had greater reductions in depression and anxiety, the control group had greater reductions in PTSD at the 6-month follow-up. The non-debriefed group also evidenced greater alcohol problems. A second study examining the effects of debriefing on mental health in peacekeepers randomly assigned 952 peacekeepers to receive either CISD, stress management, or assessment only. Findings indicated that CISD was not associated with faster recovery. While those in the CISD experienced slightly greater reductions in PTSD and aggression compared the the stress management condition, they also evidenced more alcohol problems (Adler et al., 2008). Marchand and colleagues (2006) randomly assigned 75 participants to receive either adapted CISD or an assessment-only control condition. Findings suggested that there were no group differences in PTSD 1 and 3 months after the intervention.

Early randomized controlled trials investigating the effect of CBT in reducing psychological distress and preventing PTSD in trauma survivors have been criticized for including all recently distressed trauma survivors, introducing the possibility that natural recovery may confound treatment effects. A study conducted by Kilpatrick and Veronen (1984) of 15 recent rape survivors randomly allocated to repeated assessments, delayed assessments, or a behavioral intervention (including imaginal exposure therapy) found no difference between treatment groups. Limitations of this study included small sample size, varied symptom severity following the assault, and uncertainty about the application of exposure therapy (Kilpatrick & Calhoun, 1988). Resnick, Acierno, Holmes, Kilpatrick, and Jager (1999) investigated the effect of a video psychoeducation intervention on psychological distress. Findings indicated that the video intervention implemented within 72 hours of the rape was associated with reduced distress in the examination compared to the treatment-as-usual control group. Turpin, Downs, & Mason (2005) compared the effectiveness of the provision of self-help information and a control group in reducing psychological distress in trauma survivors. While both groups evidenced decreased PTSD, anxiety, and depression, there were no between-group differences.

Review of controlled studies: indicated interventions

All controlled studies examining the impact of psychological interventions in treating symptoms of ASD and preventing PTSD have investigated the efficacy of cognitive-behavior therapy (CBT). CBT for ASD usually represents an abridged version of CBT for PTSD, taking place over approximately four to six 90-minute sessions. Components of CBT for ASD generally include psychoeducation, anxiety management, imaginal and *in vivo* exposure, and relapse prevention.

Several randomized controlled trials have been undertaken by Bryant and colleagues (Bryant et al., 2008; Bryant, Harvey, Dang, Sackville, & Basten, 1998; Bryant, Moulds, Guthrie, & Nixon, 2003; Bryant, Sackville, Dang, Moulds, & Guthrie, 1999). Bryant et al. (1998) randomly assigned 24 individuals with ASD following exposure to civilian trauma to receive either five sessions of CBT or supportive counseling within two weeks of the trauma. Patients in the CBT condition evidenced lower levels of intrusive and avoidance symptoms, as well as depression and PTSD caseness than those in the supportive counseling con-dition. In a second RCT, Bryant et al. (1999) randomized 45 trauma survivors to receive either (1) prolonged exposure, (2) prolonged exposure and anxiety management, or (3) supportive counseling within 2 weeks of the trauma. Par-ticipants in both of the conditions with prolonged exposure evidenced lower levels of PTSD caseness compared to the supportive counseling group at both 3 and 6 months after the trauma. Those in the supportive counseling also dis-played higher levels of avoidance compared to those in the prolonged exposure conditions. In a 4-year follow-up study, Bryant, Moulds, and Nixon (2003) found that trauma survivors who had been randomly allocated to receive CBT had lower levels of PTSD symptoms (especially avoidance symptoms) than those in the supportive counseling condition. Another study found that both CBT alone and CBT combined with hypnosis were superior to supportive counseling in reducing symptoms of PTSD in 87 trauma survivors who were randomly assigned to one of the three conditions. In addition, the CBT/hypno-sis condition was associated with lower levels of re-experiencing symptoms at post-treatment (Bryant et al., 2005). The relative gains of CBT over supportive counseling were maintained at a 3-year follow-up assessment (Bryant et al., 2006). In another study, 90 trauma survivors were assigned to receive either five weekly sessions of (1) imaginal and *in vivo* exposure, (2) cognitive restruc-turing, or (3) assessment only. Findings indicated that exposure therapy was associated with lower levels of PTSD, depression, and anxiety at post-treatment and follow-up compared to those in the other conditions (Bryant et al., 2008).

Bisson, Shepherd, Joy, Probert, and Newcombe (2004) randomized 152 trauma survivors with physical injuries and psychological distress to receive four sessions of CBT or no intervention 1–3 weeks after the trauma. They found that the intervention group evidenced less pronounced PTSD symptoms at 13 months, although there were no group differences in anxiety or depres-sion. Several other controlled trials that have recruited patients within 3 months of the trauma have applied CBT to acute PTSD, and in this sense these studies do not strictly meet the criteria for ASD (Ehlers et al., 2003; Sijbrandij et al., 2007); they reinforce the conclusion that early provision of CBT results in moderate to large effect sizes.

Not all studies have reported positive findings for CBT. Foa, Zoellner, and Feeny (2006) reported a trial in which 90 female survivors of assault were rand-omized to either CBT, supportive counseling, or an assessment condition. All participants were treated within 4 weeks; however, the entry criterion was PTSD rather than ASD criteria. At 9-month follow-up, all participants had made similar gains in terms of reducing PTSD symptoms; comparable findings were found when only participants who met criteria for ASD were considered. Bugg, Turpin, Mason, and Scholes (2009) conducted a study in which 67 trau-matic injury patients were randomized to either a trauma writing intervention group or an information control group. Findings revealed no differences between the groups at post-treatment and follow-up assessments. In a study conducted by Echeburúa, de Corral, Sarasua, and Zubizaretta (1996), 20 patients exhibiting acute posttraumatic stress symptoms received either cognitive restructuring and coping skills training or progressive relaxation training. While results indicated that there were no group differences at post-treatment, the cognitive restructuring group evidenced greater reductions in PTSD symptoms at the 12-month follow-up assessment.

Review of uncontrolled studies

In a study conducted by Brom, Kleber, and Hofman (1993), 151 survivors of motor vehicle accidents took part in a preventive counseling program or a monitoring group. No between-group differences were observed. Viney, Clarke, Bunn, and Benjamin (1985) found that among 280 patients hospitalized for illness and injury, crisis counseling was associated with reductions in anxiety and depression at the 12-month follow-up assessment. In a study conducted by Foa, Hearst-Ikeda, and Perry (1995), 20 assault victims received either four sessions of CBT or repeated assessments; while the CBT group evidenced greater reductions in PTSD at 2 months than the assessment group, these differences were not maintained at the 5-month follow-up assessment (Foa et al., 1995). A case series investigated the effectiveness of a 5-week CBT intervention utilizing imaginal and *in vivo* exposure techniques to treat three soldiers with PTSD symptoms in the weeks following exposure to traumatic events. Findings indicated that this intervention was associated with substantial reductions in PTSD symptoms.

Strengths and limitations of psychotherapy

Evidence from research to date suggests that psychological debriefing in the aftermath of traumatic events is ineffective in preventing the development of chronic posttraumatic stress reactions, and may even exacerbate symptoms. In contrast, CBT has demonstrated efficacy in reducing psychological distress and preventing the development of chronic PTSD in trauma survivors. The use of trauma-focused psychotherapy in the aftermath of a traumatic event has numerous benefits. First, psychoeducation promotes positive expectations about posttraumatic symptom trajectories. *In vivo* and imaginal exposure therapy reduce negative beliefs about the psychological impact of intrusive memories following traumatic events, and assist the individual with resuming pre-trauma activities. Cognitive therapy directly targets maladaptive assumptions and thougths surrounding the traumatic event and associated symptoms. Relapse prevention equips the individual with the tools to manage future psychological distress.

Clinical Vignette: Good outcome with psychotherapy

John is a 23-year-old student who was recently mugged while walking home from university. He has since been experiencing psychological symptoms, including nightmares and intrusive memories of the muggings. He is jumpy and easily startled, and has been avoiding going to university for fear of being attacked again. Five weeks ago, John presented for treatment at a hospital outpatient unit and, upon meeting clinical criteria for ASD, embarked on a course of CBT. Treatment lasted five sessions and focused on psychoeducation regarding normal posttraumatic psychological responses, imaginal reliving of the trauma memories, *in vivo* exposure to feared situations (including walking alone in safe areas, and returning to university), cognitive therapy related to his maladaptive beliefs (e.g., if I return to university I will be attacked again), and relapse prevention. Initially, John found treatment very emotionally draining as he had to relive the traumatic experience over and over again. Over the past weeks, however, John has noticed a reduction in the frequency of the intrusive memories he has been experiencing. He has been able to return to classes and reengage with his friends. While he is still occasionally fearful, he feels that he has the tools to manage this psychological distress.

Clinical Vignette: Poor outcome with psychotherapy

Jane is a 44-year-old office manager. Two weeks ago there was an incident at her workplace in which a disgruntled former employee presented at the office with a gun, threatening the workplace managers. At one point the gun discharged during a struggle; however, the assailant was subsequently apprehended and no one was injured. In the days following the incident, the organization arranged for counsellors to debrief the staff who had been present at the time. This occurred in a group format; psychoeducation about trauma responses was provided and staff members were strongly encouraged to share their feelings about the incident. Jane had felt highly distressed since the trauma and did not feel comfortable discussing her reactions, but felt obliged to set an example for more junior staff members. Since the event, Jane has been feeling more and more upset. She dreads going to work and wakes up most nights with nightmares. She has moved her office around so she no longer sits with her back facing the door, and is constantly watching for strangers entering the building. Jane feels as though she needs help with these difficulties, but worries that if she seeks assistance from a mental health professional, she will be required to discuss things she doesn't feel comfortable talking about.

COMBINED THERAPY

At the current time there is no reliable research on managing ASD systems with a combination of psychotherapeutic and pharmacological techniques. This dearth of evidence reflects the relative infancy of ASD compared to more complex PTSD responses, where the interactive effects of these two approaches have been explored. As previously noted, the evidence for pharmacological agents in reducing ASD, or preventing PTSD, is not strong, which probably explains the hesitancy of researchers and clinicians to explore potential drugs that might augment the proven effects of psychotherapy.

There are several avenues, however, where combining medication and CBT may show utility, and are worthy of future research. The first scenario is in cases where the person displays clear signs of ASD and most likely would benefit from exposure-based therapy; however, they are experiencing debilitating sleep disturbance and agitation. In such cases it can be difficult for the patient to focus on therapy, comply with homework exercises, and tolerate distress related to the exposure because of the effects of sleep deprivation. For these patients it may be appropriate to administer a short dose of benzodiazepines to facilitate sleep, which has the potential to enhance the patient's motivation and capacity to engage in CBT. Hopefully, the benefits of psychotherapy would assist sleep, thereby reducing the need for benzodiazepines.

A second potential avenue for combination therapy would be to directly augment the effects of CBT with medication. CBT procedures are generally regarded as serving as a form of extinction learning. Extinction learning is observed in the laboratory after fear conditioning in which a neutral stimulus is paired to an aversive stimulus. The individual is then repeatedly exposed to the fear stimulus in the absence of the aversive stimulus (i.e., extinction learning). This latter procedure results in a reliable decline of the fear response as the stimulus is no longer predictive of shock, and has been regarded as parallel to exposure therapy (Davis & Myers, 2002). Extinction shares a dependence on N-methyl-D-aspartate (NMDA) glutamatergic receptors, which suggests that modulating glutamatergic response may influence extinction. Consistent with this proposal, animal studies have shown that giving rats a glutamate agonist in association with extinction results in stronger extinction learning (Ledgerwood, Richardson, & Cranney, 2004; Walker, Ressler, Lu, & Davis, 2002). This observation raises the possibility that exposure therapy may be augmented by increasing glutamate activity at the time of exposure. Administering D-cyloserine (DCS), which is a common antibiotic that has partial glutamate agonist functions, in association with exposure has resulted in greater treatment gains for patients with specific phobia (Ressler et al., 2004), social anxiety disorder (Guastella et al., 2008), panic disorder (Otto et al., 2010), and obsessive-compulsive disorder (Wilhelm et al., 2008), with medium to large effect sizes across studies, relative to placebo (Norberg, Krystal, & Tolin, 2008). ASD is an exemplar disorder of fear conditioning insofar as there is a fear response to a discrete traumatic event, and so it is possible that future research may demonstrate that exposure can be augmented with a glutamate agonist.

CONCLUSION

The body of knowledge regarding psychological and pharmacological interventions to address symptoms of ASD is still relatively small. Evidence to date provides little guidance on the use of medications to reduce psychological distress in the days and weeks following a traumatic event. In contrast, research indicates that CBT approaches are the treatments of choice for alleviating psychological symptoms and preventing the development of PTSD following exposure to a traumatic event. Despite this conclusion, there are promising avenues for secondary prevention via novel pharmacological interventions in the initial days after trauma exposure. At a public health level, however, one of the most demanding challenges is developing and evaluating early interventions for severely distressed people in the short term after a disaster that affects large numbers of people. Tapping into change mechanisms that have been shown to facilitate adaptation, and implementing these in strategies that can be delivered to large numbers of affected people, may result in effective secondary prevention at a population level.

Clinical Points to Remember

1. Research into psychological reactions following exposure to traumatic experiences has indicated that the majority of trauma survivors experience initial symptoms of distress but that these generally lessen over time.
2. A systematic review of the capacity of ASD to predict PTSD in trauma survivors indicated that ASD evidenced moderate predictive power for PTSD, but poor sensitivity.
3. Findings from the largest and mostly tightly controlled study to date strongly indicate that the merits of pharmacological intervention based on agents traditionally used to treat PTSD may not have substantial gains for patients displaying ASD symptoms.
4. A promising line of research has focused on the role of glucocorticoids in the initial phase after trauma exposure.
5. CBT has demonstrated efficacy in reducing psychological distress and preventing the development of chronic PTSD in trauma survivors.

6. Evidence suggests that psychological debriefing in the aftermath of traumatic events is ineffective in preventing the development of chronic posttraumatic stress reactions, and may even exacerbate symptoms.
7. At the current time there is no reliable research on managing ASD systems with a combination of psychotherapeutic and pharmacological techniques.

REFERENCES

Adler, A. B., Litz, B. T., Castro, C. A., Suvak, M., Thomas, J. L., Burrell, L., et al (2008). A group randomized trial of critical incident stress debriefing provided to U.S. peacekeepers. *Journal of Traumatic Stress, 21*, 253–263.

American Psychiatric Association (APA). (1994). *Diagnostic and statistical manual of mental disorders* (4th ed.). Washington, DC: APA.

Bisson, J. I., Jenkins, P. L., Alexander, J., & Bannister, C. (1997). Randomised controlled trial of psychological debriefing for victims of acute burn trauma. *British Journal of Psychiatry, 171*, 78–81.

Bisson, J. I., Shepherd, J. P., Joy, D., Probert, R., & Newcombe, R. G. (2004). Early cognitive-behavioral therapy for post-traumatic stress symptoms after physical injury: Randomised controlled trial. *British Journal of Psychiatry, 184*, 63–69.

Blake, D. J. (1986). Treatment of acute posttraumatic stress disorder with tricylcic antidepressants. *Southern Medical Journal, 79*, 201–204.

Blanchard, E. B., Hickling, E. J., Barton, K. A., & Taylor, A. E. (1996). One-year prospective follow-up of motor vehicle accident victims. *Behaviour Research and Therapy, 34*, 775–786.

Brewin, C. R., Andrews, B., Rose, S., & Kirk, M. (1999). Acute stress disorder and posttraumatic stress disorder in victims of violent crime. *American Journal of Psychiatry, 156*(3), 360–366.

Brom, D., Kleber, R. J., & Hofman, M. C. (1993). Victims of traffic accidents: incidence and prevention of post-traumatic stress disorder. *Journal of Clinical Psychology, 49*, 131–140.

Bryant, R. A. (2011). Acute stress disorder as a predictor of posttraumatic stress disorder: A systematic review. *Journal of Clinical Psychiatry, 72*(2), 233–239.

Bryant, R. A., Creamer, M., O'Donnell, M. L., Silove, D., & McFarlane, A.C. (2008). A multisite study of the capacity of acute stress disorder diagnosis to predict posttraumatic stress disorder. *Journal of Clinical Psychiatry, 69*. 923–292.

Bryant, R. A., Creamer, M., O'Donnell, M., Silove, D., & McFarlane, A. C. (2009). A study of the protective function of acute morphine administration on subsequent posttraumatic stress disorder. *Biological Psychiatry, 65*(5), 438–440.

Bryant, R. A., Friedman, M. J., Spiegel, D., Ursano, R., & Strain, J. (2011). A review of acute stress disorder in DSM-5. *Depression and Anxiety, 28*(9), 802–817.

Bryant, R. A., Harvey, A. G., Dang, S. T., Sackville, T., & Basten, C. (1998). Treatment of acute stress disorder: A comparison of cognitive behavior therapy and supportive counseling. *Journal of Consulting and Clinical Psychology, 66*, 862–866.

Bryant, R. A., Mastrodomenico, J., Felmingham, K. L., Hopwood, S., Kenny, L., Kandris, E., et al. (2008). Treatment of acute stress disorder: A randomized controlled trial. *Archives of General Psychiatry, 65*, 659–667.

Bryant, R. A., Moulds, M. L., Guthrie, R., & Nixon, R. D. V. (2003). Treating acute stress disorder after mild brain injury. *American Journal of Psychiatry, 160*, 585–587.

Bryant, R. A., Moulds, M. A., & Nixon, R. (2003). Cognitive behaviour therapy of acute stress disorder: A four-year follow-up. *Behaviour Research and Therapy, 41*, 489–494.

Bryant, R. A., Moulds, M. L., Nixon, R. D., Mastrodomenico, J., Felmingham, K., & Hopwood, S. (2006). Hypnotherapy and cognitive behaviour therapy of acute stress disorder: a 3-year follow-up. *Behaviour Research and Therapy, 44*, 1331–1335.

Bryant, R. A., Sackville, T., Dang, S. T., Moulds, M., & Guthrie, R. (1999). Treating acute stress disorder: An evaluation of cognitive behavior therapy and supportive counseling techniques. *American Journal of Psychiatry, 156*, 1780–1786.

Bugg, A., Turpin, G., Mason, S., & Scholes, C. (2009). A randomised controlled trial of the effectiveness of writing as a self-help intervention for traumatic injury patients at risk of developing post-traumatic stress disorder. *Behaviour Research and Therapy, 47*, 6–12.

Cahill, L., Prins, B., Weber, M., & McGaugh, J. L. (1994). β-Adrenergic activation and memory for emotional events. *Nature, 371*, 702–704.

Cardeña, E., & Spiegel, D. (1993). Dissociative reactions to the San Francisco Bay Area earthquake of 1989. *American Journal of Psychiatry, 150*, 719–734.

Classen, C., Koopman, C., Hales, R., & Spiegel, D. (1998). Acute stress disorder as a predictor of posttraumatic stress symptoms. *American Journal of Psychiatry, 155*, 620–624.

Cohen, H., Matar, M. A., Buskila, D., Kaplan, Z., & Zohar, J. (2008). Early post-stressor intervention with high-dose corticosterone attenuates posttraumatic stress response in an animal model of posttraumatic stress disorder. *Biological Psychiatry, 64*(8), 708–717.

Conlon, L., Fahy, T. J., & Conroy, R. (1999). PTSD in ambulant RTA victims: A randomized controlled trial of debriefing. *Journal of Psychosomatic Research, 46*, 37–44.

Creamer, M., & Manning, C. (1998). Acute stress disorder following an industrial accident. *Australian Psychologist, 33*(2), 125–129.

Dalgleish, T., Meiser-Stedman, R., Kassam-Adams, N., Ehlers, A., Winston, F., Smith, P., et al. (2008). Predictive validity of acute stress disorder in children and adolescents. *British Journal of Psychiatry, 195*, 392–393.

Davis, M., & Myers, K. M. (2002). The role of glutamate and gamma-aminobutyric acid in fear extinction: Clinical implications for exposure therapy. *Biological Psychiatry, 52*, 998–1007.

De Jong, K., Mulhern, M., Ford, N., van der Kam, S., & Kleber, R. (2000). The trauma of war in Sierra Leone. *Lancet, 355*, 2067–2068.

Deahl, M., Srinivasan, M., Jones, N., Thomas, J., Neblett, C., & Jolly, A. (2000). Preventing psychological trauma in soldiers: The role of operational stress training and psychological debriefing. *British Journal of Medical Psychology, 73*, 77–85.

Echeburúa, E., de Corral, P., Sarasua, B., & Zubizaretta, I. (1996). Treatment of acute posttraumatic stress disorder in rape victims: An experimental study. *Journal of Anxiety Disorders, 10*, 185–199.

Ehlers, A., & Clark, D. M. (2000). A cognitive model of posttraumatic stress disorder. *Behaviour Research and Therapy, 38*(4), 319–345.

Ehlers, A., Clark, D. M., Hackmann, A., McManus, F., Fennell, M., Herbert, C., & Mayou, R. (2003). A randomized controlled trial of cognitive therapy, a self-help booklet, and repeated assessments as early interventions for posttraumatic stress disorder. *Archives of General Psychiatry, 60*(10), 1024–1032.

Ehlers, A., Mayou, R. A., & Bryant, B. (1998). Psychological predictors of chronic posttraumatic stress disorder after motor vehicle accidents. *Journal of Abnormal Psychology, 107*, 508–519.

Feinstein, A. (1989). Posttraumatic stress disorder: A descriptive study supporting DSM-III-R criteria. *American Journal of Psychiatry, 146*, 665–666.

Foa, E. B., Hearst-Ikeda, D., & Perry, K. J. (1995). Evaluation of a brief cognitive behavioral program for the prevention of chronic PTSD in recent assault victims. *Journal of Consulting and Clinical Psychology, 63*, 948–955.

Foa, E. B., Zoellner, L. A., & Feeny, N. C. (2006). An evaluation of three brief programs for facilitating recovery after assault. *Journal of Traumatic Stress, 19*(1), 29–43.

Galea, S. (2007). The long-term health consequences of disasters and mass traumas. *Canadian Medical Association Journal, 176*, 1293–1294.

Galea, S., Resnick, H., Ahern, J., Gold, J., Bucuvalas, M., Kilpatrick, D., et al. (2002). Posttraumatic stress disorder in Manhattan, New York City, after the September 11th terrorist attacks. *Journal of Urban Health, 79*, 340–353.

Gelpin, E., Bonne, O., Peri, T., Brandes, D., & Shalev, A. Y. (1996). Treatment of recent trauma survivors with benzodiazepines: A prospective study. *Journal of Clinical Psychiatry, 57*, 390–394.

Guastella, A. J., Richardson, R., Lovibond, P. F., Rapee, R. M., Gaston, J. E., Mitchell, P., & Dadds, M. R. (2008). A randomized controlled trial of D-cycloserine enhancement of exposure therapy for social anxiety disorder. *Biological Psychiatry, 63*, 544–549.

Harvey, A. G., & Bryant, R. A. (1998). The relationship between acute stress disorder and posttraumatic stress disorder: A prospective evaluation of motor vehicle accident survivors. *Journal of Consulting and Clinical Psychology, 66*, 507–512.

Harvey, A. G., & Bryant, R. A. (1999). Acute stress disorder across trauma populations. *Journal of Nervous and Mental Disease, 186*, 333–337.

Hinton, D. E., Hinton, S., Pham, T., Chau, H., & Tran, M. (2003). "Hit by the wind" and temperature-shift panic among Vietnamese refugees. *Transcultural Psychiatry, 40*, 342–376.

Hobbs, M., Mayou, R., Harrison, B., & Worlock, P. (1996). A randomised controlled trial of psychological debriefing for victims of road traffic accidents. *British Medical Journal, 313*, 1438–1439.

Holbrook, T. L., Galarneau, M. R., Dye, J. L., Quinn, K., & Dougherty, A. L. (2010). Morphine use after combat injury in Iraq and post-traumatic stress disorder. *New England Journal of Medicine, 362*, 110–117.

Jacobs, J., Horne-Moyer, H. L., & Jones, R. (2004). The effectiveness of critical incident stress debriefing with primary and secondary trauma victims. *International Journal of Emergency Mental Health, 6*, 5–14.

Kessler, R. C., Galea, S., Gruber, M. J., Sampson, N. A., Ursano, R. J., & Wessely, S. (2008). Trends in mental illness and suicidality after Hurricane Katrina. *Molecular Psychiatry, 13*(4), 374–384.

Kilpatrick, D. G., & Calhoun, K. S. (1988). Early behavioral treatment for rape trauma: Efficacy or artifact? *Behavior Therapy, 19*, 421–427.

Kilpatrick, D. G., & Veronen, L. J. (1984). Treatment of rape-related problems: Crisis intervention is not enough. In L. Cohen, W. Clairborn, & G. Specter (Eds.), *Crisis intervention* (2nd ed.). New York: Human Services Press.

Koopman, C., Classen, C., Cardena, E., & Spiegel, D. (1995). When disaster strikes, acute stress disorder may follow. *Journal of Traumatic Stress, 8*, 29–46.

Koopman, C., Classen, C., & Spiegel, D. A. (1994). Predictors of posttraumatic stress symptoms among survivors of the Oakland/Berkeley, Calif., firestorm. *American Journal of Psychiatry, 151*, 888–894.

Ledgerwood, L., Richardson, R., & Cranney, J. (2004). D-Cycloserine and the facilitation of extinction of conditioned fear: Consequences for reinstatement. *Behavioral Neuroscience, 118*, 505–513.

Marchand, A., Guay, S., Boyer, R., Iucci, S., Martin, A., & St.-Hilaire, M.-H. (2006). A randomized controlled trial of an adapted form of individual critical incident stress debriefing for victims of an armed robbery. *Brief Treatment and Crisis Intervention, 6*, 122–129.

Mayou, R. A., Ehlers, A., & Hobbs, M. (2000). Psychological debriefing for road traffic accidents: Three-year follow-up of a randomised controlled trial. *British Journal of Psychiatry, 176*, 589–593.

Mellman, T. A., Byers, P. M., & Augenstein, J. S. (1998). Pilot evaluation of hypnotic medication during acute traumatic stress response. *Journal of Traumatic Stress, 11*, 563–569.

Mitchell, J. T. (1983). When disaster strikes … the critical incident stress debriefing process. *Journal of Emergency Medical Services, 8*, 36–39.

Murray, J., Ehlers, A., & Mayou, R. A. (2002). Dissociation and post-traumatic stress disorder: Two prospective studies of road traffic accident survivors. *British Journal of Psychiatry, 180*, 363–368.

Norberg, M. M., Krystal, J. H., & Tolin, D. F. (2008). A meta-analysis of D-cycloserine and the facilitation of fear extinction and exposure therapy. *Biological Psychiatry, 63*, 1118–1126.

Nugent, N. R., Christopher, N. C., Crow, J. P., Browne, L., Ostrowski, S., & Delahanty, D. L. (2011). *Journal of Traumatic Stress, 23*, 282–287.

Nurmi, L. A. (1999). The sinking of the *Estonia*: The effects of critical incident stress debriefing (CISD) on rescuers. *International Journal of Emergency Mental Health, 1*, 23–31.

Otto, M. W., Tolin, D. F., Simon, N. M., Pearlson, G. D., Basden, S., Meunier, S. A., et al. (2010). Efficacy of D-cycloserine for enhancing response to cognitive-behavior therapy for panic disorder. *Biological Psychiatry, 67*, 365–370.

Ozer, E. J., Best, S. R., Lipsey, T. L., & Weiss, D. S. (2003) Predictors of posttrauamtic stress disorder and symptoms in adults: A meta-analysis. *Psychological Bulletin, 129*, 52–73.

Pitman, R. K., Sanders, K. M., Zusman, R. M., Healy, A. R., Cheema, F., Lasko, N. B., et al. (2002). Pilot study of secondary prevention of posttraumatic stress disorder with propranolol. *Biological Psychiatry, 51*, 189–192.

Resnick, H., Acierno, R., Holmes, M., Kilpatrick, D. G., & Jager, N. (1999). Prevention of post-rape psychopathology: Preliminary findings of a controlled acute rape treatment study. *Journal of Anxiety Disorders, 13*, 359–370.

Ressler, K. J., Rothbaum, B. O., Tannenbaum, L., Anderson, P., Graap, K., Zimand, E., et al. (2004). Cognitive enhancers as adjuncts to psychotherapy: Use of D-cycloserine in phobic individuals to facilitate extinction of fear. *Archives of General Psychiatry, 61*, 1136–1144.

Riggs, D. S., Rothbaum, B. O., & Foa, E. B. (1995). A prospective examination of symptoms of posttraumatic stress disorder in victims of nonsexual assault. *Journal of Interpersonal Violence, 10*, 201–214.

Robert, R., Blakeney, P. E., Villarreal, C., Rosenberg, L., & Meyer, W. J. III. (1999). Imipramine treatment in pediatric burns patients with symptoms of acute stress disorder: A pilot study. *Journal of the American Academy of Child and Adolescent Psychiatry, 38*, 873–882.

Rothbaum, B. O., Foa, E. B., Riggs, D. S., Murdock, T., & Walsh, W. (1992). A prospective examination of post-traumatic stress disorder in rape victims. *Journal of Traumatic Stress, 5*, 455–475.

Saarni, H., Saari, S., & Hakkinen, U. (1999). Critical incident stress debriefing (CISD) in a shipping company. *International Maritime Health, 50*, 49–56.

Sacks, S. B., Clements, P. T., & Fay-Hillier, T. (2001). Care after chaos: Use of critical incident stress debriefing after traumatic workplace events. *Perspectives of Psychiatric Care, 37*, 133–136.

Saxe, G., Stoddard, F., Courtney, D., Cunningham, K., Chawla, N., Sheridan, R., et al. (2001). Relationship between acute morphine and the course of PTSD in children with burns. *Journal of the American Academy of Child and Adolescent Psychiatry, 40*(8), 915–921.

Schelling, G., Briegel, J., Roozendaal, B., Stoll, C., Rothenhausler, H. B., & Kapfhammer, H. P. (2001). The effect of stress doses of hydrocortisone during septic shock on posttraumatic stress disorder in survivors. *Biological Psychiatry, 50*(12), 978–985.

Schelling, G., Kilger, E., Roozendaal, B., de Quervain, D. J., Briegel, J., Dagge, A., et al. (2004). Stress doses of hydrocortisone, traumatic memories, and symptoms of posttraumatic stress disorder in patients after cardiac surgery: A randomized study. *Biological Psychiatry, 55*(6), 627–633.

Schelling, G., Roozendaal, B., & De Quervain, D. J. (2004). Can posttraumatic stress disorder be prevented with glucocorticoids? *Annals of the New York Academy of Sciences, 1032*, 158–166.

Schulz, P. M., Marovic-Johnson, D., & Huber, L. C. (2006). Cognitive-behavioral treatment of rape- and war-related posttraumatic stress disorder with a female, Bosnian refugee. *Clinical Case Studies, 5*, 191–208.

Shalev, A. Y., Ankri, Y., Israeli-Shalev, Y., Peleg, T., Adessky, R., & Freedman, S. (2012). Prevention of posttraumatic stress disorder by early treatment: Results from the Jerusalem trauma outreach and prevention study. *Archives of General Psychiatry, 69*(2), 166–176.

Sharp, S., Thomas, C., Rosenberg, L., Rosenberg, M., & Meyer, W. III. (2010). Propranolol does not reduce risk for acute stress disorder in pediatric burn trauma. *Journal of Trauma: Injury, Infection and Critical Care, 1*, 193–197.

Sijbrandij, M., Olff, M., Reitsma, J. B., Carlier, I. V., de Vries, M. H., & Gersons, B. P. (2007). Treatment of acute posttraumatic stress disorder with brief cognitive behavioral therapy: A randomized controlled trial. *American Journal of Psychiatry, 164*(1), 82–90.

Simms-Ellis, R., & Madill, A. (2001). Financial services employees' experience of peer-led and clinician-led critical incident stress debriefing following armed robberies. *International Journal of Emergency Mental Health, 3*, 219–228.

Townsend, C. J., & Loughlin, J. M. (1998). Critical incident stress debriefing in international aid workers. *Journal of Travel Medicine, 5*, 226–227.

Turpin, G., Downs, M., & Mason, S. (2005). Effectiveness of providing self-help information following acute traumatic injury: A randomized controlled trial. *British Journal of Psychiatry, 187*, 76–82.

Vaiva, G., Thomas, P., Ducrocq, F., Fontaine, M., Boss, V., Devos, P., et al. (2004). Low posttrauma GABA plasma levels as a predictive factor in the development of acute posttraumatic stress disorder. *Biological Psychiatry, 55*, 250–254.

Viney, L. L., Clarke, A. M., Bunn, T. A., & Benjamin, Y. N. (1985). The effect of a hospital-based counseling service on the physical recovery of surgical and medical patients. *General Hospital Psychiatry, 7*, 294–301.

Walker, D. L., Ressler, K. J., Lu, K. T., & Davis, M. (2002). Facilitation of conditioned fear extinction by systemic administration or intra-amygdala infusions of D-cycloserine as assessed with fear-potentiated startle in rats. *Journal of Neuroscience, 22*, 2343–2351.

Wee, D. F., Mills, D. M., & Koehler, G. (1999). The effects of critical incident stress debriefing (CISD) on emergency medical services personnel following the Los Angeles Civil Disturbance. *International Journal of Emergency Mental Health, 1*, 33–37.

Wilhelm, S., Buhlmann, U., Tolin, D. F., Meunier, S. A., Pearlson, G. D., Reese, H. E., et al. (2008). Augmentation of behavior therapy with D-cycloserine for obsessive-compulsive disorder. *American Journal of Psychiatry, 165*, 335–341.

Zohar, J., Yahalom, H., Kozlovsky, N., Cwikel-Hamzany, S., Matar, M. A., Kaplan, Z., et al. (2011). High dose hydrocortisone immediately after trauma may alter the trajectory of PTSD: Interplay between clinical and animal studies. *European Neuropsychopharmacology, 21*(11), 796–809.

CHAPTER 8

Posttraumatic Stress Disorder

Amy M. Williams, Greer Richardson, and Tara E. Galovski

INTRODUCTION

The clinical presentation of psychiatric symptoms following exposure to traumatic events, currently categorized in the *Diagnostic Statistical Manual of Mental Disorders, Fourth Edition–Text Revised* (*DSM–IV–TR*; American Psychiatric Association, 2000) as posttraumatic stress disorder (PTSD), has been documented fairly consistently across numerous literary sources spanning the last two centuries. Kraepelin (1896) described the suffering observed in survivors of accidents and injuries as *Schreckneuroses* (translated to *fright neuroses* by Jablensky, 1985, p. 737). Da Costa (1871) described the clinical presentation observed in soldiers during the American Civil War following combat exposure as *irritable heart*, while Myers (1915) used the term *shell shock* to describe similar phenomena. The first edition of the *DSM* (American Psychiatric Association, 1952) described the clinical presentation of survivors of trauma as *gross stress reaction*, while the second edition of the *DSM* omitted the disorder altogether (American Psychiatric Association, 1968). It was not until the third edition of the *DSM* that the disorder was introduced as PTSD (American Psychiatric Association, 1980).

PTSD (as described in *DSM–IV–TR*; APA, 2000) is one of the few psychiatric conditions that occurs secondarily to a specific, external event. According to Criterion A of the diagnosis, this traumatic event must involve actual or threatened death or significant harm to oneself or to others. The traumatic event must be experienced by the individual with fear, helplessness, or horror. Criterion A, in its current form, thus rules out significant psychosocial stressors or events that do not meet the definition of traumatic. The specific symptoms of PTSD are then divided into three separate clusters: re-experiencing symptoms (Cluster B), avoidance and numbing symptoms (Cluster C), and hyperarousal symptoms (Cluster D). In order to meet full diagnostic criteria for PTSD, the trauma survivor must report specific numbers of symptoms experienced at a recurring rate and at a clinical level in each of the clusters. Because it may be normative to experience strong emotional reactions in the immediate aftermath of a traumatic event, the *DSM–IV* further designates that these symptoms must be present for at least 1 month before a diagnosis of PTSD can be made.

The re-experiencing of symptoms is so named as the trauma survivor essentially re-experiences the memory of the trauma over and over again, sometimes on a daily basis, with levels of distress that may mimic or equal the distress experienced during the actual event. Re-experiencing symptoms may be particularly distressing because they are perceived as uncontrollable and attached to significant negative emotion. Specifically, the re-experiencing of symptoms includes intrusive thoughts, nightmares about the event, flashbacks or similar experiences of feeling as if one is right back in the traumatic situation, significant emotional distress when reminded of the trauma, and significant physiological reactivity when reminded of the trauma. In order to meet diagnostic criteria for Cluster B of PTSD, an individual must experience at a clinical level at least one of the five symptoms listed. In an effort to distance themselves from this barrage of re-experiencing symptoms, individuals with PTSD begin to avoid both the actual memory of and reminders of the traumatic event (Resick & Schnicke, 1992). Active avoidance may include avoidance of thoughts, feelings, and conversations associated with the trauma, and avoidance of activities, people, and places reminiscent of the trauma; and it may involve an inability to recall important aspects of the actual event. More passive avoidance symptoms may include anhedonia, feeling detached or estranged from others, emotional numbing or restricted range of affect, or a sense of a foreshortened future. In order to be diagnosed with PTSD, a survivor needs to report at least three out of seven of the Cluster C symptoms. During the actual traumatic event the individual can experience significant physiological reactivity, often described as the fight or flight response. Although this response is adaptive at the time of the traumatic event, people with PTSD continue to experience significant and sustained levels of physiological arousal, even in the absence of identifiable danger. Thus, Cluster C captures the hyperarousal symptoms observed in PTSD, including sleep impairment, irritability and anger, difficulty in concentration, hypervigilance or constantly feeling the need to be on guard, and exaggerated startle response and difficulty recovering physiologically from a startle experience. Individuals with PTSD must endorse at least two out of five hyperarousal symptoms.

Unfortunately, it is not uncommon to experience a traumatic event. Epidemiological research conducted in the United States suggests that the majority of individuals (50–60%) will experience a traumatic event during the course of their lifetime (Kessler, Sonnega, Bromet, Hughes, & Nelson, 1995). The most common outcome following exposure to a traumatic event is recovery. However, for a minority of the total trauma survivor population, PTSD develops. Epidemiological data have been fairly consistent in estimates of prevalence rates of PTSD in the United States as diagnosed by modern criteria (*DSM–III–R* and *DSM–IV*). For example, Kessler et al. (1995) in the original National Comorbidity Study (NCS) reported lifetime prevalence rates of 8%. Prevalence rates remained fairly stable using the revised NCS data, which estimated PTSD prevalence rates at 7% (Kessler, Berglund, Demler, Jin, & Walters, 2005). The conditional risk of developing PTSD varies considerably across different types of traumatic events. Kessler et al. (1995) found that the traumatic event with the highest conditional risk for developing PTSD was rape, while accidents, natural disasters, and witnessing traumas happening to others were associated with lower conditional risk for developing PTSD. The National Vietnam Veterans Readjustment Study (NVVRS) specifically sought to determine the prevalence rates of PTSD within war veterans. The initial study reported lifetime rates of PTSD among Vietnam theater veterans at approximately 31% (Kulka et al., 1990). Membership in the army (as compared to other branches of the military) and longevity of tour were associated with increased PTSD prevalence rates. This is not surprising, as the severity of the exposure to traumatic events has consistently been found to be associated with the development of PTSD, irrespective of the type of trauma experienced (Kessler et al., 1995). Sex differences are also found in exposure to trauma and in the development of PTSD following trauma (Blain, Galovski, & Robinson, 2010). Although men are more likely to experience a traumatic event, women are more likely to develop PTSD. In fact, prevalence rates of PTSD for women (10%) are twice those for men (5%) (Kessler et al., 1995). This sex difference in prevalence rates of PTSD may be explained in part by the differential conditional risk of exposure to specific traumas between men and women. However, women are more likely than men to develop PTSD and, once developed, PTSD may be more likely to develop into a chronic condition in women than men (Blain, Galovski, & Robinson, 2010).

PTSD rarely occurs in isolation (Kessler et al., 1995). As compared to other anxiety and unipolar disorders, PTSD emerged as the psychiatric disorder with the most complex comorbid diagnostic picture (Brown, Campbell, Lehman, Grisham, & Mancill, 2001). Specifically, the vast majority of the community participants (92%) in this study also met criteria for a second current Axis I disorder, with major depressive disorder being the most common (77%), followed by generalized anxiety disorder (38%) and alcohol abuse or dependence (31%). The NVVRS data also revealed high comorbidity rates within the veteran population such that 50% of the PTSD positive veterans were also diagnosed with at least one comorbid Axis I disorder. Elevated rates of Axis II disorders are also observed across studies in PTSD-positive samples, including comorbid diagnoses of borderline, antisocial, avoidant, paranoid, and obsessive-compulsive personality disorders (Bollinger, Riggs, Blake, & Ruzek, 2000).

Exposure to trauma and the subsequent development of PTSD results in significant and excessive societal costs, including medical costs, occupational disability and interruption, and significant functional impairment. Living with

PTSD adversely affects not only the survivor: the burden is shared by family, friends, and society at large (Galovski & Lyons, 2004). Fortunately, over the past several decades several interventions for PTSD have gained substantial empirical support. The fruits of these academic labors are currently being disseminated across a variety of domains and settings in a historic effort both to increase the adoption of these evidence-based practices into clinical settings and to increase the effectiveness of the interventions themselves.

In an effort to guide the clinician in making informed decisions as to which therapy to implement with survivors of trauma suffering from PTSD, a number of national and international organizations have evaluated the available literature to estimate the empirical support accumulated by that intervention. The result has been the development of best-practice guidelines. Forbes et al. (2010) summarized the clinical practice guidelines from seven groups to aid clinicians in deciding which recommendations to follow regarding treatment of PTSD. These interventions will be reviewed in this chapter.

SOLITARY TREATMENT APPROACHES

Pharmacological Treatment

Pharmacotherapies are an effective treatment for PTSD. Clinical practice guidelines differ on medication as an alternative first-line intervention to psychosocial treatment, as a second-line intervention when trauma-focused cognitive-behavioral therapies are not available, acceptable, or suitable, or the Institute of Medicine's rating as failing to meet the requirements to support a recommendation at all (Forbes et al., 2010). Recommendations by different organizations or associations vary according to the literature reviewed and the audience of the particular guidelines (i.e., physicians not trained to practice CBT, primary care settings). The role of pharmacotherapies in reducing the burden of suffering from PTSD will be discussed, with the conclusion that pharmacotherapy offers a welcome treatment option for PTSD.

As with any psychopharmacological treatment, the risks and benefits should be discussed with the patient prior to initiation of treatment. Ideally, monotherapy should be initiated before augmenting with another medication. The proposed plan should be discussed with the patient, including education about the time required to realize a treatment response. Patients should also be educated on the specific symptoms targeted by the medication as well as the need for daily adherence to the medication regimen. The recommended time frame for a trial of medication for the treatment of PTSD is 8 weeks unless the treatment is not tolerated (Department of Veteran Affairs VA/Department of Defense; VA/DoD, 2010). If there is a response by 8 weeks and the treatment is tolerated, then treatment should be continued for at least another 4 weeks. In a recent systematic review of 35 short-term (14 weeks or less) randomized controlled trials (RCTs) including 4597 PTSD-positive participants, a significantly larger proportion of patients responded to medication (59.1%) when compared to placebo (38.5%) (D. J. Stein, Ipser, & Seedat, 2006). A response was defined as a Clinical Global Impression Scale of 1 = very much or 2 = much improved (or similar qualitative scale). The authors also conclude that the evidence for selective serotonin reuptake inhibitors (SSRIs) was more compelling than that for the other classes of medications. Medication was superior to placebo in reducing the severity of PTSD symptom clusters, comorbid depression and disability, but was less tolerated than placebo.

Antidepressants

SELECTIVE SEROTONIN REUPTAKE INHIBITORS (SSRIS)

In the United States, VA/DoD (2010) and the American Psychiatric Association (APA) (Benedek, Friedman, Zatzick, & Ursano, 2009) support and strongly recommend the use of SSRIs for the treatment of PTSD. Contrarily, the Institute of Medicine (IOM, 2007) concludes that the evidence is inadequate to determine the efficacy of SSRIs (or any other medication) in the treatment of PTSD. The IOM differentiated its task (evaluating the scientific evidence) from the task of setting clinical guidelines (developed for those prescribing medications despite inconclusive scientific evidence). The APA reaffirmed its endorsement of SSRIs, saying, "Meta-analyses and several randomized controlled trials ... generally support the superiority of SSRIs and serotonin–norepinephrine reuptake inhibitors (SNRIs) over placebo for non-combat-related PTSD" (Benedek et al., 2009, p. 2). The evidence for SSRIs appears to be strongest for non-combat-related PTSD and when using the medication for at least 10 weeks (Benedek et al., 2009). However, Benedek et al. cite five negative studies (three of fluoxetine and two of sertraline) versus one positive fluoxetine study in combat veterans and conclude that "the SSRIs may no longer be recommended with the same level of confidence for veterans with combat-related PTSD as for patients with non-combat-related PTSD" (2009, p. 2). VA/DoD (2010) recommends the SSRIs with the highest level of confidence, specifically naming fluoxetine, sertraline, and paroxetine as having the strongest support. Friedman, Marmar, Baker, Sikes, and Farfel (2007) studied the efficacy of sertraline (average dose 156mg/day for 12 weeks in completers) in 169 (mostly Vietnam) combat veterans with PTSD recruited from 10 Veterans Affairs (VA) medical centers. Results showed that sertraline did not differ significantly from placebo in reducing PTSD symptoms. The authors argue that the negative findings in this study could be attributed to factors specific to veterans, who comprise a chronic, treatment-refractory cohort not representative of younger veterans of recent wars. In fact, a randomized study of veterans from the Balkan Wars who were treated with fluoxetine did show improvement in PTSD symptoms when compared to a placebo (Martenyi, Brown, Zhang, Koke, & Prakash, 2002). The mean duration from index trauma from the Balkan Wars study was 6–7 years. The VA/DoD study advises that the Friedman et al. (2007) study may not be generalizable to veterans with more recent combat experience. Further, previous studies involving paroxetine have recruited veterans from the general population (rather than from VA hospital treatment settings) and they showed benefit from SSRI treatment comparable to male and female non-veterans (Tucker et al., 2001).

The time needed for a treatment to be effective is an important issue, and most acute studies are 8- to 12-week trials. In a review of the literature on sertraline, Friedman, Davidson, and Stein (2009) note that 30% of participants receiving SSRIs have achieved complete remission after 12 weeks of treatment. If continued, SSRIs can improve PTSD symptoms for months after 12-week trials. Londborg et al. (2001) showed that when sertraline was extended from 12 weeks to 36 weeks, 55% of patients who had not responded or who had shown only partial response converted to medication responders. Marshall et al. (2007) also found continued improvement in PTSD symptoms when patients continued paroxetine for 12 weeks after responding to a 10-week trial.

SSRIs will likely need to be taken indefinitely, given the increased risk of relapse when the medication is discontinued. Davidson et al. (2001) found that over half of patients who responded to a 6-month trial of sertraline relapsed when switched to placebo. Patients who had responded to 6 months of sertraline were more than six times as likely to relapse compared to placebo.

Serotonin–norepinephrine reuptake inhibitors (SNRIs)

Both the VA/DoD (2010) and the APA Guideline Watch (Benedek et al., 2009) support the use of SNRIs for PTSD. There are currently four SNRIs available in the United States: venlafaxine, desvenlafaxine, duloxetine, and milnacipran. Of these, venlafaxine has the strongest evidence, based on two large-scale RCTs with civilian populations. Davidson et al. (2006a) studied venlafaxine extended-release versus placebo in 329 adult outpatients with a CAPS (Clinician-Administered PTSD Scale; Blake et al., 1995) score of 60 or greater and found a mean change in total CAPS score from baseline of −51.7 for venlafaxine compared to −43.9 for placebo. When the three symptom clusters of PTSD were analyzed, the re-experiencing and avoidance/numbing symptom clusters improved compared to placebo, but the hyperarousal symptom cluster did not. Remission rates (CAPS = 20 or below) were 50.9% for venlafaxine and 37.5% for placebo. In a separate 12-week multicenter double-blind trial, venlafaxine extended release was compared to sertraline and placebo. Only venlafaxine indicated significant improvements over placebo (Davidson et al., 2006b). Desvenlafaxine, a metabolite of venlafaxine, has not been studied in PTSD. An open-label preliminary study of duloxetine showed promising results, justifying the need for an RCT (Villarreal, Canive, Calaise, Toney, & Smith, 2010).

NEFAZODONE

It should be noted that nefazodone has a black box warning from the U.S. Food and Drug Administration (FDA) for risk of irreversible liver failure. This significant side effect removes this particular therapy choice as a viable treatment option for a portion of PTSD sufferers. The reported rate of this complication in the United States is about one case of liver failure resulting in death or transplant per 250,000–300,000 patient-years (FDA prescribing information). The brand name Serzone was pulled from the U.S. market in 2004, but generic formulations are available. Serzone has demonstrated efficacy in small to mid-size trials, most open label. One trial demonstrated efficacy compared to placebo in veterans with combat and sexual trauma (Davis et al., 2004), and two trials demonstrated efficacy comparable to that of sertraline (McRae et al., 2004; Saygın, Sungur, Sabol, & Çetinkaya, 2002). Overall, the data for nefazodone are limited and it is recommended by VA/DoD (2010) as a second-line agent for monotherapy for PTSD.

MIRTAZAPINE

Davidson et al. (2003) demonstrated efficacy in a study of 26 patients compared to placebo. Chung et al. (2004) demonstrated that mirtazapine was as effective as sertraline in Korean War veterans. VA/DoD (2010) recommends mirtazapine for the treatment of PTSD.

Tricyclic antidepressants (TCAs)

Friedman et al. (2009) note that concern regarding side effects as well as lack of interest by pharmaceutical companies (due to their waning profitability) likely underscores the lack of any recent interest or research in both TCAs and monoamine oxidase inhibitors (MAOIs). Only amitriptyline (Davidson et al., 1993) and imipramine (Kosten, Frank, Dan, McDougle, & Giller, 1991) have demonstrated efficacy in the treatment of PTSD. Nortriptyline and desipramine, the metabolites of the aforementioned TCAs respectively, have not demonstrated efficacy with core PTSD symptoms (VA/DoD, 2010). VA/DoD recommends amitriptyline and imipramine for the treatment of PTSD.

Monoamine oxidase inhibitors (MAOIs)

In 1988, Frank, Kosten, Giller, and Dan compared phenelzine and imipramine to placebo and both medications outperformed placebo. Kosten et al. (1991) then showed that phenelzine outperformed imipramine and both outperformed placebo. MAOIs have the unfortunate burden of requiring a tyramine-free diet and exhibiting life-threatening interactions with some other medications (e.g., meperidine, serotonergic medications, CNS stimulants, decongestants). VA/ DoD (2010) recommends phenelzine in the treatment of PTSD.

BUPROPION

Bupropion has not demonstrated efficacy in the treatment of PTSD and is not recommended by either major guideline (VA/DoD, 2010; Benedek et al., 2009). The IOM (2007) too does not recommend using buproprion.

Second-generation (atypical) antipsychotics

VA/DoD (2010) and APA Guideline Watch (Benedek et al., 2009) both recommend monitoring for weight gain and metabolic changes when prescribing atypical antipsychotics. At the time that both guidelines came out, there was limited but encouraging data to support the use of adjunctive treatment of PTSD with second-generation antipsychotics, of which risperidone had the most evidence. That optimism has been tempered by the Krystal et al. study (2011), which demonstrated no benefit of risperidone over placebo in veterans with serotonin reuptake–resistant symptoms of chronic military service–related PTSD. This study was a 6-month randomized, double-blind, placebo-controlled multicenter trial. In post-hoc analyses, re-experiencing and hyperarousal symptoms showed statistically significant, but clinically trivial, improvement. Krystal et al. (2011) note that risperidone may be helpful for some patients, calling on its pharmaceutical similarity to other medications (trazodone and prazosin) that act as agonists on similar receptors (5-HT2a and α-1 adrenergic receptor).

Studies of olanzapine have yielded equivocal results in reducing hyperarousal and re-experiencing symptoms (e.g. Butterfield et al., 2001). One small open-label study of quetiapine included 20 patients and showed a significant improvement in PTSD (Hamner, Deitsch, Broderick, Ulmer, & Lorberbaum, 2003) VA/DoD (2010) does not support the use of atypical antipsychotics as monotherapy in the treatment of PTSD.

Antiadrenergic agents

PRAZOSIN

Prazosin is an encouraging medication for hyperarousal symptoms of PTSD, particularly nightmares (Taylor et al., 2006). Taylor et al. (2006) reported that daytime use of prazosin can reduce psychological distress to trauma-specific cues in civilian trauma with PTSD. The APA Guideline Watch (Benedek et al., 2009) notes that further studies need to address the optimal dose and titration of prazosin, which on the basis of current studies appears to be between 3 and 15 mg/night. Clinically, a low dose should be started and then titrated upward, with monitoring of side effects and efficacy. VA/DoD recommends the use of prazosin in the treatment of PTSD. The APA 2009 Guideline Watch suggests that "in certain patient populations new pharmacotherapeutic options, such as prazosin, may be more effective than other widely prescribed medications (e.g., selective serotonin reuptake inhibitors [SSRIs]) indicated for PTSD" (Benedek et al., 2009, p. 1).

GUANFACINE

Two randomized, placebo-controlled trials found that guanfacine had no effect on PTSD symptoms among veterans with chronic PTSD (Neylan et al., 2006; Davis et al., 2008). Both studies, however, included mostly male veterans with chronic PTSD who were already taking additional medication (primarily SSRIs) for PTSD. Given this lack of findings, guanfacine is not recommended in the treatment of PTSD.

Beta-blockers

A 14-day randomized controlled trial of propranolol versus gabapentin versus placebo did not show benefit of either medication over placebo (M. B. Stein, Kerridge, Dimsdale, & Hoyt, 2007). Brunet and colleagues (2008) administered propranolol versus placebo for 1 day after exposure to script-driven imagery. At the 1-week assessment interval, investigators found significantly less physiological hyperarousal in the propranolol group. VA/DoD (2010) is unable to recommend propranolol, citing insufficient evidence.

Benzodiazepines

The Institute of Medicine (IOM) (2007) concluded that the evidence is inadequate and that the available evidence is uninformative in determining the efficacy and primary use of benzodiazepines in the treatment of PTSD. The IOM report did not evaluate the benefit or harm of using benzodiazepines. The VA/DoD Guidelines (2010) place benzodiazepines in Category D Evidence and list benzodiazepines as potentially having harmful effects for PTSD. VA/DoD and the IOM found only one double-blind, placebo-controlled trial (Braun, Greenberg, Dasberg, & Lerer, 1990). Braun et al. (1990) had seven patients in the alprazolam arm and nine patients in the placebo arm. The APA Practice Guidelines (Benedek et al., 2009) cite insufficient quality of evidence to adequately evaluate benzodiazepines for the core symptoms of PTSD. The APA and VA/DoD recommend against using benzodiazepines for the core symptoms of PTSD and caution that discontinuation of benzodiazepines could exacerbate core symptoms of PTSD. Kosten, Fontana, Sernyak, and Rosenheck (2000) studied 370 veterans with PTSD and comorbid substance abuse who were followed for 1 year after discharge from inpatient treatment: 26% of substance abusers with PTSD were pre-scribed benzodiazepines versus 45% of veterans with PTSD without sub-stance abuse. That study did not find adverse effects on outcome for those treated with benzodiazepines.

Pharmacological treatments: benefits and limitations as a sole approach

The pharmacological treatment for PTSD may improve symptoms of posttrau-matic stress disorder, and some patients may experience a remission of PTSD symptoms. The quantitative outcome measure of most studies defines a response as a 20–30% reduction in CAPS scores. The body of evidence suggests that pharmacotherapy can improve symptoms of PTSD but does not usually yield remission of symptoms. The empirical support for pharmacotherapy is not as strong as that for the psychological interventions, particularly cognitive-behavioral treatments (Friedman et al., 2009). Further, pharmacotherapy will likely need to be continued indefinitely unless the side-effect burden is prohibi-tive for long-term treatment: many medications occur with side effects and a discontinuation effect that some patients find difficult to tolerate, causing com-pliance concerns. Therefore, cognitive-behavioral treatments may be more cost-effective in the long run, because there is an increased risk of relapse upon discontinuation of medication. One benefit of pharmacotherapy as a first-line intervention for PTSD is potential patient preference and lack of interest in, or resistance to, psychotherapy.

Clinical Vignette: Good outcome with pharmacotherapy

Jessica, a 33-year-old female, was raped 6 weeks ago and currently meets criteria for PTSD. After reviewing treatment options including medica-tion and psychotherapy, Jessica elects to try sertraline. She understands that she will need 8 weeks for a full trial of this medication. She returns after 1 week to follow-up and reports that she has had some mild nausea and feels mildly tired. Jessica is told that the nausea may go away in a week or two. She elects to continue on the medication and returns 2 weeks later. She notices that she is feeling better in all three symptom clusters and the nausea has gone away, but the mild tiredness has contin-ued. The tiredness is not debilitating and she would like to continue the trial. Five weeks later, she returns for follow-up and reports additional improvement. At that time, Jessica is presented with psychoeducation regarding evidence that people can experience continued improvement if compliant with sertraline.

Clinical Vignette: Poor outcome with pharmacotherapy

Monica is a 23-year-old female who was raped 3 months ago. She meets criteria for posttraumatic stress disorder. After having discussed the risks and benefits of taking a medication and the options for psychotherapy, she elects to try sertraline. She is started on 50 mg of sertraline each morning. She returns in a week and reports that she is feeling nauseated and is sleeping worse. After discussing with her the possibility that these symptoms may improve after continuing at the same dose and the possibility of decreasing the dose to hasten relief from the side effects, she elects to decrease sertraline to 25 mg each day. She returns after another week and reports that she is continuing to have nausea and also reports loose stool. She reports headaches and feeling very tired from insomnia characterized as difficulty staying asleep. She decides not to stay on sertraline, citing how terrible she is feeling. Further, after this experience on sertraline she does not want to take any other medications at this time.

Psychosocial Treatment

Since its inception as a diagnosis in 1980, a burgeoning area of research has resulted in a variety of psychosocial treatments for PTSD. Consensus on first-line treatments for PTSD has been found for cognitive- and exposure-based therapies, which have amassed impressive amounts of empirical support (Forbes et al., 2010). In addition to cognitive processing therapy (CPT) (Resick & Schnicke, 1992), cognitive therapy (Ehlers et al., 2003), and prolonged exposure (PE) (Foa, Hembree, & Rothbaum, 2007), additional treatment approaches are often clustered under this broad category, including stress inoculation training (SIT) (Meichenbaum, 1974) and eye movement desensitization and reprocessing (EMDR) (Shapiro, 1989). Moreover, several other psychosocial treatments demonstrate some evidence of treatment efficacy, although relevant studies did not have all necessary components of a gold standard, randomized trial with comparison groups. These interventions include imagery rehearsal therapy (IRT) (Krakow et al., 2001), psychodynamic psychotherapies, and stress management. Following is a brief description of each, and references for further review.

Cognitive-behavioral therapies (CBT)

EXPOSURE THERAPY

Treatments fitting this description include interventions targeted at helping trauma-exposed clients confront thoughts and reengage in safe situations that are feared or avoided. The combined nature of both imaginal and *in vivo* exposure appears superior to various control conditions such as a wait list, supportive counseling, or relaxation (Cahill, Rothbaum, Resick, & Follette, 2009). PE (Foa et al., 2007) is a specific exposure-based therapy that has widespread use. PE is a manualized intervention typically administered over 10–12 90-minute sessions consisting of psychoeducation, breathing retraining, and imaginal and *in vivo* exposure to activate the traumatic fear structure.

COGNITIVE THERAPY (CT) AND COGNITIVE PROCESSING THERAPY (CPT)

Both CPT and CT for PTSD share a primarily focus on the identification and restructuring of trauma-related beliefs. CPT is based on a social cognitive theory of PTSD that combines elements of information processing and social schema theories (Resick & Schnicke, 1992). CPT is a manualized treatment composed of 12 50-minute sessions that can be delivered in either an individual or a group modality. Although the original version of CPT included a written trauma narrative, a dismantling study indicated the effectiveness of CPT without the written account (Resick et al., 2008). Additional variations of CT have also been shown to be effective in reducing PTSD severity, both alone and combined with exposure interventions (Cahill et al., 2009).

STRESS INOCULATION TRAINING (SIT)

In SIT, individuals are taught to manage anxiety symptoms by using techniques such as muscle relaxation, breathing retraining, guided self-dialogue, and thought stopping (Meichenbaum, 1974). It originally included *in vivo* exposure components, although these have been excluded in some studies because SIT was conducted as part of a comparison treatment. Cahill et al. (2009) note that SIT has received mixed results, having its strongest support for female rape victims, and suggest future research including the *in vivo* component.

EYE MOVEMENT DESENSITIZATION AND REPROCESSING (EMDR)

EMDR (Shapiro, 1989) includes both exposure and cognitive components. While recalling aspects of the trauma, individuals engage in side-to-side eye movements or other alternating movements (i.e., bilateral stimulation). Dismantling studies have not supported unilateral benefit of bilateral stimulation (Spates, Koch, Cusack, Paato, & Waller, 2009), although others suggest that this is due to a lack of power to definitively address this issue (Russell, Lipke, & Figley, 2011). Although EMDR has been found to be as effective as exposure-based therapies, it remains controversial whether EMDR "could be delivered in a more parsimonious manner without detracting from its efficacy" (Spates et al., 2009, p. 298).

IMAGERY REHEARSAL THERAPY (IRT)

Although IRT is included in clinical practice guidelines for PTSD, experts suggest its primary usefulness is as an ancillary treatment for residual nightmares either before or after a course of treatment for PTSD (Foa, Keane, Friedman, & Cohen, 2009; Moore & Krakow, 2010). IRT is a cognitive-behavioral treatment that can be applied individually or in a group. It focuses on nightmares as a learned behavior and invites individuals to change and rehearse the nightmare imagery. Data support its effectiveness in reducing nightmares and improving insomnia in some populations (Moore & Krakow, 2010).

Psychodynamic psychotherapies

Kudler, Krupnick, Blank, Herman, and Horowitz (2009), in a review of psychodynamic psychotherapies for PTSD, stated that an overarching goal of these treatments is to "reengage normal mechanisms of adaptation by addressing what is unconscious and, in tolerable doses, making it conscious" (p. 364). Depending on the type of treatment, duration of individual sessions can range from 12 sessions (i.e., brief psychodynamic psychotherapy) to 7 or more years (i.e., formal psychoanalysis). Because these treatments do not have specific symptom reduction as a primary goal, psychodynamic researchers face difficulties in applying conventional research paradigms to evaluate their work, and the result has been few empirical studies (Foa et al., 2009).

Group therapies

Group therapy is a common treatment modality for PTSD and there are many approaches that have been shown to be effective compared to control or comparison groups (Shea, McDevitt-Murphy, Ready, & Schnurr, 2009). Cognitive-behavioral group therapies such as CPT (Monson et al., 2006) and image rehearsal therapy (Krakow et al., 2001) have shown highest effect sizes. In addition, interpersonal group psychotherapy has demonstrated effectiveness in the treatment of PTSD (Campanini et al., 2010).

Additional treatments for consideration

Several other approaches merit mention when reviewing relevant psychosocial treatments. Most are not considered first-line treatment options, owing to a lack of empirical studies on efficacy, even though early research suggests promising results. These include acceptance and commitment therapy (ACT) (Hayes, Strosahl, & Wilson, 1999), dialectical behavior therapy (DBT) (Linehan, 1993), virtual reality exposure therapy (Rothbaum, Difede, & Rizzo, 2008), and couples and family therapy (Maack, Lyons, Connolly, & Ritter, 2011).

Psychosocial treatments: benefits and limitations as a sole approach

Psychotherapy for PTSD, specifically in the form of cognitive-behavioral treatments, has shown the greatest efficacy in the treatment of PTSD (Foa et al., 2009) when compared to other interventions, including medication. In addition to symptom reduction of PTSD, multiple studies have documented positive effects on secondary measures of depression (Ehlers et al., 2003; Resick et al., 2008), health factors (Galovski, Monson, Bruce, & Resick, 2009), worry, social adjustment (Galovski & Lyons, 2004), emotion regulation, and interpersonal skills (Cloitre, Koenen, Cohen, & Han, 2002). Moreover, long-term follow-ups from cognitive-behavioral RCTs show that treatment gains last even after treatment has ended (Resick, Williams, Suvak, Monson, & Gradus, 2012).

Beyond empirical support for psychotherapy as a sole approach for PTSD, an additional benefit is avoidance of unnecessary side effects due to medication. These may include unwanted side effects reported by patients but also the interfering effects of certain medications (i.e., sedation, numbing) while conducting treatment. For individuals with a history of substance abuse or dependence, avoidance of medications with high addiction potential may be attractive. Last, many individuals seeking treatment from a psychologist or counselor may do so because of personal preferences to avoid medication. Indeed, when given a choice between medication and CBT for PTSD, researchers have found that many PTSD sufferers prefer psychotherapy over medication (Zoellner, Feeny, Cochran, & Pruitt, 2003).

Conversely, there are several limitations to psychotherapy as a sole approach. Access to empirically supported treatments may be limited because of the lack of clinicians adequately trained in providing first-line therapies for PTSD (McLean & Foa, 2011). In addition, owing to the avoidant nature of many individuals suffering from PTSD, direct confrontation with the traumatic memory may be daunting. Although some psychosocial treatments offer treatment without direct confrontation of the traumatic material, even discussing emotions and building insight may be off-putting.

Clinical Vignette: Good outcome with pharmacotherapy

Susan is a 35-year-old female with a history of childhood sexual abuse and mild depression. She self-referred for treatment following the dissolution of a relationship and consequently reported that she has never been able to feel trusting of men. During the intake, Susan admitted that she had never enjoyed sexual intimacy with her former husband and had only married him because he seemed safe. Upon further assessment, it became clear that Susan had long experienced avoidance symptoms surrounding her childhood trauma but that she suffered from ongoing nightmares and intrusive thoughts about the abuse. This was complicated by the fact that her oldest daughter was entering pre-adolescence, the same age at which Susan was abused. Susan and her therapist decided to engage in trauma-focused therapy and proceeded with a course of CPT. Susan identified beliefs, including "I must have done something to make him think I wanted sex" and "It happened because I was trying to be pretty," that led to feelings of guilt and shame. Through worksheets formulated to address and modify these beliefs as well as Susan's willingness to feel her emotions via a written narrative trauma account, Susan reported improvement in her symptoms and self-assessment. Following completion of the 12-session protocol, Susan attended a 1-month follow-up session and reported sustained gains in her ability to trust, as well as in symptoms of PTSD and depression.

Clinical Vignette: Poor outcome with psychotherapy

Nancy is a 65-year-old woman who recently lost her husband of 35 years. She has been grieving for several months, and, rather than getting better, she is becoming more nervous. She is not used to managing the finances and is concerned about having enough money to live on. She has developed insomnia, lost her appetite, and is losing weight. She complains of aches and pains. Her physician recognizes her symptoms and diagnoses her anxiety and developing depression. He suggests some medication for acute relief of the anxiety—specifically, benzodiazepines. But Nancy worries about the side effects, especially the cognitive impairment and risk of falling. She prefers not to take pills. Her doctor arranges for CBT sessions. Although Nancy makes all her appointments, she is not responding well to the behavioral treatment. She has trouble concentrating on the "homework" and finds the effort very fatiguing. For her, CBT is not effective. Eventually, Nancy agrees to try medication. Because she is generally healthy and has no cardiac risk factors, he starts her on venlafaxine. Within a few weeks Nancy feels much better, she has more energy, and finds that she is able to handle her personal affairs more easily than before.

COMBINED THERAPY

The greater part of the current PTSD treatment literature consists of research on monotherapy—either pharmacotherapy alone or psychotherapy alone. There are relatively few RCTs addressing the question of additive benefit of combination approaches to treating PTSD. When discussing treatments that combine a pharmacological and psychosocial approach, one must also consider whether to begin with one or the other as a first-line approach or to begin them both simultaneously. Several of the studies reviewed in this section experimented with addition to or augmentation of either psychotherapy or pharmacotherapy. There are no published RCTs investigating a combined approach at the outset of treatment.

Pharmacotherapy Followed by Psychotherapy

Researchers at Massachusetts General Hospital investigated the combined treatment for PTSD and panic involving Cambodian and Vietnamese refugees (Hinton et al., 2005). Participants were first treated with an SSRI and then randomly assigned to continuation of the SSRI alone or augmentation with a combination cognitive-behavioral treatment (which also addressed panic). Definitive conclusions are limited as no PTSD treatment-only condition was included. In addition, the results from this specific patient population may not be widely generalizable.

Rothbaum et al. (2006) investigated whether adding PE to a regimen of sertraline would prove helpful in treating individuals with PTSD from a community sample. Participants were started on a regimen of sertraline for 10 weeks and individuals who exhibited at least a 20% improvement in their PTSD symptoms were assigned to either PE (10 sessions) with continued sertraline or continued sertraline only for an additional 5 weeks. There was a higher dropout rate among those who received PE augmentation, which the authors attributed to possible hesitancy to delve into memories or reminders once they had experienced some symptom relief. Overall, adding PE did appear to further reduce PTSD severity (but not depression or general anxiety). However, when they partitioned out "partial" medication responders, the augmentation effect for PE was demonstrated.

Campanini et al. (2010) conducted a 16-week interpersonal psychotherapy group with patients who did not respond to a pharmacological intervention for PTSD (generally, antidepressant medication, often combined with atypical antipsychotics or anxiolytic benzodiazepines). Patients received benefit from this add-on treatment, showing significant improvement in PTSD symptoms as well as depression and anxiety. Limitations of the study include the lack of a comparison group, the small sample size, and the fact that not all patients received similar medications.

Psychotherapy Followed by Pharmacotherapy

Recently, Schneier and colleagues (2012) investigated PE combined with either paroxetine or placebo in the treatment of terrorism-related PTSD. Patients underwent 10 sessions of PE over 10 weeks and were then offered 12 additional weeks of continued randomized treatment (either paroxetine or placebo). Patients treated with PE plus paroxetine experienced significantly greater improvement in PTSD symptoms and remission status than patients treated with PE plus placebo. Although the study has several limitations, including a relatively small sample size, the inclusion of only one type of trauma, and the lack of long-term follow-up, it represents an important effort in the field of combined research.

Psychosocial and Pharmacological Combined Treatment: Benefits and Limitations

A combined approach of medication and psychotherapy is likely common in most settings: individuals often receive psychotherapy in conjunction with one or more medications. One potential benefit of a combined approach is related to the high comorbidity with other psychiatric disorders often noted in PTSD. Some of the medications may be helpful in ameliorating some comorbid disorders or associated symptoms. In addition, pharmacotherapy may reduce symptoms that interfere with psychotherapy (Friedman et al., 2009) such as severe depression or suicidality. Finding an optimal combination of alleviating extreme psychological discomfort in order to facilitate engagement with trauma-related material would be the goal of any combined intervention. In the face of the paucity of existing research, the difficulty arises in making a decision regarding when and how to order the treatments and their dose. Combinations do not always augment treatment outcome.

Clinical Vignette: Combined treatment

Mary is a 40-year-old female who presented for psychotherapy following a visit to her local emergency room. She reported that she had recently tried to return to work after a short-term disability absence due to breast cancer and treatment. Mary's cancer was in remission but she reported fears of its return and admitted to avoiding follow-up appointments to her oncologist. Further assessment revealed that during her treatment, Mary had experienced an acute life-threatening procedure in which her lung was punctured; she met criteria for PTSD as a result of this procedure. Mary agreed to participate in cognitive-behavioral therapy (CPT) to address this experience. Initially, her anxiety increased and her physician placed her on an SSRI to address increased frequency of panic attacks and anxiety symptoms. In therapy, Mary and her therapist addressed her thoughts about her cancer (i.e., "I must have done something unhealthy to cause the cancer"), cancer treatment ("I can't go through that again"), and the emergency procedure in which she felt her life was threatened. In response to the procedure, Mary realized that she had been afraid of dying but was also angry at the way in which the emergency physician acted toward her ("The doctor was cold and did not care about me"). Through Socratic dialogue and cognitive restructuring, Mary was able to reframe her understanding of the physician as "focused in the moment" and contrast her experience with other, caring health professionals with whom she had interacted in non-emergency situations. She also addressed her beliefs about her health and cancer diagnosis. Mary's scores on PTSD measures showed a significant decrease in symptoms and her panic attacks remitted. She returned to work part-time. At termination of psychotherapy she reported that she intended to stay on the SSRI while adjusting to her return to work.

FUTURE DIRECTIONS

Pharmacological intervention for a variety of mental health problems (depression, other anxiety disorders) has become increasingly common. In the treatment of PTSD it is likely that patients presenting for evaluation and psychotherapy may already have undergone a trial of medication for their symptoms or a related disorder. This is reflected in current research. Participants in psychotherapy-only RCTs for PTSD are often currently taking a variety of medication and are requested to keep the regimen stable during the provision of the therapy or wait-list condition. Although this is likely a sufficient condition to rule out treatment benefit being attributed to the pharmacological intervention, it complicates the landscape when discussing psychotherapy as a "sole" approach. For instance, in a recent 5-year follow-up community-based treatment outcome study of CPT and PE for physical and sexual assault-related PTSD, 47 (39%) participants reported that they had started to take medication since completing the treatment protocol; it made no difference whether they had participated in CPT or PE (Resick et al., 2012). Of the women who exhibited PTSD 5 years post-treatment, a higher proportion were on medication (29%) than not on medication (15%). Of all the women taking medication 5 years post-treatment, more had a lifetime diagnosis of major depressive disorder (MDD) and endorsed an MDD diagnosis during the follow-up period than those who were not on medication. Results such as these highlight the importance of tracking and understanding medication use and comorbid diagnoses in future studies.

Controlled studies that investigate the combination of psychotherapy and pharmacotherapy are important, given the number of individuals who may have partial rather than complete remissions from PTSD following a particular course of therapy. Clinical trials to assess order of treatments (i.e., psychotherapy or pharmacotherapy first, second, and concurrently) would be helpful in answering questions of best practices and sequencing considerations. Additional data on efficacy of combined approaches could help guide future practice guidelines; current guidelines are often based on limited research.

Clinical Points to Remember

1. PTSD is one of the few psychiatric conditions that occur secondarily to a specific, external event. Individuals with PTSD attempt to avoid both the actual memory of and reminders of the traumatic event.

2. The vast majority of individuals with PTSD also meet criteria for a second current Axis I disorder.

3. The empirical support for psychological interventions in PTSD is stronger than that for pharmacological intervention. First-line psychological treatments include cognitive- and exposure-based therapies, which have considerable empirical support. These treatments are time-limited (usually 10–15 sessions).

4. Psychological interventions tend to have long-lasting effects: individuals who show remission of PTSD symptoms following psychotherapy do not typically "relapse."

5. SSRIs are generally considered the pharmacological therapy of first choice in individuals with non-combat-related PTSD. Several studies involving combat-related PTSD have called the use of SSRIs into question.

6. Pharmacotherapy can improve PTSD symptoms but does not usually yield remission of symptoms. Medication will likely need to be taken indefinitely, given the increased risk of relapse when it is discontinued.

7. Although a combined approach of medication and psychotherapy is probably common, there are no published RCTs investigating the combined approach at the outset of treatment for PTSD.

8. Combined approaches to the treatment of PTSD may be helpful, given the high comorbidity of PTSD with other psychiatric disorders as well as combined approaches' ability to reduce symptoms that interfere with psychotherapy, such as depression and suicidal ideation.

9. Additional research on combined approaches to PTSD treatment is needed to make decisions regarding when and how to order the treatments and their dose.

REFERENCES

American Psychiatric Association (APA). (1952). *The diagnostic and statistical manual: Mental disorders.* Washington, DC: APA.

American Psychiatric Association (1968). *Diagnostic and statistical manual of mental disorders* (2nd ed.). Washington, DC: APA.

American Psychiatric Association (1980). *Diagnostic and statistical manual of mental disorders* (3rd ed.). Washington, DC: APA.

American Psychiatric Association (2000). *The diagnostic and statistical manual of mental disorders* (4th ed., text revision). Washington, DC: APA.

Benedek, D. M., Friedman, M. J., Zatzick, D., & Ursano, R. J. (2009). Practice guideline for the treatment of patients with acute stress disorder and posttraumatic stress disorder. *Psychiatry Online.* Retrieved from www.psychiatryonline.com/content.aspx?aid=156498

Blain, L. M., Galovski, T. E., & Robinson, T. R. (2010). Gender differences in recovery from posttraumatic stress disorder: A critical review. *Aggression and Violent Behavior, 15,* 463–474. doi:10.1016/j.avb.2010.09.001

Blake, D. D., Weathers, F. W., Nagy, L. M., Kaloupek, D. G., Gusman, F. D., Charney, D. S., & Keane, T. M. (1995). The development of a clinician-administered PTSD scale. *Journal of Traumatic Stress, 8,* 75–90.

Bollinger, A., Riggs, D., Blake, D., & Ruzek, J. (2000). Prevalence of personality disorders among combat veterans with posttraumatic stress disorder. *Journal of Traumatic Stress, 13,* 255–270.

Braun, P., Greenberg, D., Dasberg, H., & Lerer, B. (1990). Core symptoms of posttraumatic stress disorder unimproved by alprazolam treatment. *Journal of Clinical Psychiatry, 51,* 236–238.

Brown, T. A., Campbell, L. A., Lehman, C. L., Grisham, J. R., & Mancill, R. B. (2001). Current and lifetime comorbidity of the DSM-IV anxiety and mood disorders in a large clinical sample. *Journal of Abnormal Psychology, 110,* 585–599.

Brunet, A., Orr, S. P., Tremblay, J., Robertson, K., Nader, K., & Pitman, R. K. (2008). Effect of post-retrieval propranolol on psychophysiologic responding during subsequent script-driven traumatic imagery in post-traumatic stress disorder. *Journal of Psychiatric Research, 42*(6), 503–506.

Butterfield, M. I., Becker, M. E., Connor, K. M., Sutherland, S., Churchill, L. E., & Davidson, J. R. (2001). Olanzapine in the treatment of post-traumatic stress disorder: A pilot study. *International Clinical Psychopharmacology, 16,* 197–203.

Cahill, S. P., Rothbaum, B. O., Resick, P. A., & Follette, V. M. (2009). Cognitive-behavioral therapy for adults. In E. B. Foa, T. M. Keane, M. J. Friedman, & J. A. Cohen (Eds.), *Effective treatments for PTSD: Practice guidelines from the International Society for Traumatic Stress Studies* (2nd ed., pp. 139–222). New York: Guilford Press.

Campanini, R. F. B., Schoedl, A. F., Pupo, M. C., Costa, A. C. H., Krupnick, J. L., & Mello, M. F. (2010). Efficacy of interpersonal therapy-group format adapted to post-traumatic stress disorder: An open-label add-on trial. *Depression and Anxiety, 27*(1), 72–77.

Chung, M. Y., Min, K. H., Jun, Y. J., Kim, S. S., Kim, W. C., & Jun, E. M. (2004). Efficacy and tolerability of mirtazapine and sertraline in Korean veterans with posttraumatic stress disorder: A randomized open label trial. *Human Psychopharmacology, 19*(7), 489–494.

Cloitre, M., Koenen, K. C., Cohen, L. R., & Han, H. (2002). Skills training in affective and interpersonal regulation followed by exposure: A phase-based treatment for PTSD related to childhood abuse. *Journal of Consulting and Clinical Psychology, 70,* 1067–1074.

Da Costa, J. M. (1871). Membranous enteritis. *American Journal of Medicine, 124,* 321–338.

Davidson, J., Baldwin, D., Stein, D. J., Kuper, E., Benattia, I., Ahmed, S., et al. (2006a). Treatment of posttraumatic stress disorder with venlafaxine extended release: A 6-month randomized controlled trial. *Archives of General Psychiatry, 63,* 1158–1165.

Davidson, J. R. T., Kudler, H. S., Saunders, W. B., Erickson, L., Smith, R. D., Stein, R. M., et al. (1993). Predicting response to amitriptyline in posttraumatic stress disorder. *American Journal of Psychiatry, 150*(7), 1024–1029.

Davidson, J., Perlstein, T., Londborg, P., Brady, K. T., Rothbaum, B., Bell, J., et al. (2001). Efficacy of sertraline in preventing relapse of posttraumatic stress disorder: Results of a 28-week double-blind, placebo-controlled study. *American Journal of Psychiatry, 158,* 1974–1981.

Davidson, J., Rothbaum, B. O., Tucker, P., Asnis, G., Benattia, I., & Musgnung, J. J. (2006b). Venlafaxine extended release in posttraumatic stress disorder: a sertraline and placebo-controlled study. *Journal of Clinical Psychopharmacology, 26,* 259–267.

Davidson, J. R. T., Weisler, R. H., Butterfield, M. I., Casat, C. D., Connor, K. M., Barnett, S., & van Meter, S. (2003). Mirtazapine vs. placebo in posttraumatic stress disorder: A pilot trial. *Biological Psychiatry, 53*(2), 188–191.

Davis, L. L., Jewell, M. E., Ambrose, S., Farley, J., English, B., Bartolucci, A., & Petty, F. (2004). A placebo-controlled study of nefazodone for the treatment of chronic posttraumatic stress disorder: A preliminary study. *Journal of Clinical Psychopharmacology, 24*(3), 291–297.

Davis, L. L., Ward, C., Rasmusson, A., Newell, J. M., Frazier, E., & Southwick, S. M. (2008). A placebo-controlled trial of guanfacine for the treatment of posttraumatic stress disorder in veterans. *Psychopharmacology Bulletin, 41,* 8–18.

Ehlers, A., Clark, D. M., Hackmann, A., McManus, F., Fennell, M., Herbert, C., & Mayou, R. (2003) A randomized controlled trial of cognitive therapy, a self-help booklet, and repeated assessment as early interventions for posttraumatic stress disorder. *Archives of General Psychiatry, 60,* 1024–1032.

Foa, E. B., Hembree, E. A., & Rothbaum, B. O. (2007). *Prolonged exposure therapy for PTSD: Emotional processing of traumatic experiences.* New York: Oxford University Press.

Foa, E. B., Keane, T. M., Friedman, M. J., & Cohen, J. A. (2009). *Effective treatments for PTSD: Practice guidelines from the International Society for Traumatic Stress Studies* (2nd ed.). New York: Guilford Press.

Forbes, D., Creamer, M., Bisson, J. I., Cohen, J. A., Crow, B. E., Foa, E. B., et al. (2010). A guide to guidelines for the treatment of PTSD and related conditions. *Journal of Traumatic Studies, 23*(5), 537–552.

Frank, J. B.., Kosten, T. R., Giller, E. L. Jr., & Dan, E. (1988) A randomized clinical trial of phenelzine and imipramine for posttraumatic stress disorder. *American Journal of Psychiatry, 145,* 1289–1291.

Friedman, M. J., Davidson, J. R. T., & Stein, D. J. (2009). Psychopharmacotherapy for adults. In E. B. Foa, T. M. Keane, M. J. Friedman, & J. A. Cohen (Eds.), *Effective treatments for PTSD: Practice guidelines from the International Society for Traumatic Stress Studies* (2nd ed., pp. 245–268). New York: Guilford Press.

Friedman, M. J., Marmar, C. R., Baker, D. G., Sikes, C. R., & Farfel, G. M. (2007). Randomized, double-blind comparison of sertraline and placebo for posttraumatic stress disorder in a Department of Veterans Affairs setting. *Journal of Clinical Psychiatry, 68*, 711–720.

Galovski, T. E., & Lyons, J. (2004). The psychological sequelae of exposure to combat violence: A review of the impact on the veteran's family. *Aggression and Violent Behavior, 9*, 477–501.

Galovski, T. E., Monson, C. A., Bruce, S., & Resick, P. A. (2009). Does cognitive-behavioral therapy for PTSD improve perceived health? *Journal of Traumatic Stress, 22*(3), 197–204.

Hamner, M. B., Deitsch, S. E., Broderick, P. S., Ulmer, H. G., & Lorberbaum, J. P. (2003). Quetiapine treatment in patients with posttraumatic stress disorder: An open trial of adjunctive treatment. *Journal of Clinical Psychopharmacology, 23*(1), 15–20.

Hayes, S. C., Strosahl, K. D., & Wilson, K. G. (1999). *Acceptance and commitment therapy: An experiential approach to behavior change.* New York: Guilford Press.

Hinton, D. E., Chhean, D., Pich, V., Safren, S. A., Hofmann, S. G., & Pollack, M. H. (2005). A randomized controlled trial of cognitive-behavior therapy for Cambodian refugees with treatment-resistant PTSD and panic attack: A cross-over design. *Journal of Traumatic Stress, 18*, 617–629.

Institute of Medicine. (2007). *Treatment of PTSD: Assessment of the evidence.* Washington, DC: National Academies Press.

Jablensky, A. (1985). Approaches to the definition and classification of anxiety and related disorders in European psychiatry. In A. H. Tuma & J. D. Maser (Eds.), *Anxiety and the anxiety disorders* (pp. 735–758). Hillsdale, NJ: Lawrence Erlbaum.

Kessler, R. C., Berglund, P., Demler, O., Jin, R., & Walters, E. E. (2005). Lifetime prevalence and age of onset distributions of DSM-IV disorders in the National Comorbidity Survey Replication. *Archives of General Psychiatry, 62*, 593–602.

Kessler, R. C., Sonnega, A., Bromet, E., Hughes, M., & Nelson, C. B. (1995). Posttraumatic stress disorder in the National Comorbidity Survey. *Archives of General Psychiatry, 52*, 1048–1060.

Kosten, T. R., Fontana, A., Sernyak, M. J., & Rosenheck, R. (2000). Benzodiazepine use in posttraumatic stress disorder among veterans with substance abuse. *Journal of Nervous and Mental Disorders, 188*(7), 454–459.

Kosten, T. R., Frank, J. B., Dan, E., McDougle, C. J., & Giller, E. L. (1991). Pharmacotherapy for post-traumatic stress disorder using phenelzine or imipramine. *Journal of Nervous and Mental Disease, 179*(6), 366–370.

Kraepelin, E. (1896). *Psychiatrie: Ein Lehrbuch für Studirende und Aerzte* (5th ed.). Leipzig: Verlag von J. A. Barth.

Krakow, B., Hollifield, M., Johnston, L., Koss, M., Schrader, R., Warner, T. D., et al. (2001). Imagery rehearsal therapy for chronic nightmares in sexual assault survivors with posttraumatic stress disorder: A randomized controlled trial. *JAMA: Journal of the American Medical Association, 296*(5), 537–545.

Krystal, J. H., Rosenheck, R. A., Cramer, J. A., Vessicchio, J. C., Jones, K. M., Vertrees, J. E., et al. (2011). Adjunctive risperidone treatment for antidepressant-resistant symptoms of chronic military service-related PTSD. *Journal of the American Medical Association, 306*(5), 493–502.

Kudler, H. S., Krupnick, J. L., Blank, A. S. Jr., Herman, J. L., & Horowitz, M. J. (2009). Psychodynamic therapy for adults. In E. B. Foa, T. M. Keane, M. J. Friedman, & J. A. Cohen (Eds.), *Effective treatments for PTSD: Practice guidelines from the International Society for Traumatic Stress Studies* (2nd ed., pp. 346–369). New York: Guilford Press.

Kulka, R. A., Schlenger, W. E., Fairbank, J. A., Hough, R. L., Jordan, B. K., Marmar, C. R., et al. (1990). *Trauma and the Vietnam War generation: Report findings from the National Vietnam Veterans Readjustment Study* (Vol. 29). New York: Brunner/Mazel.

Linehan, M. M. (1993). *Cognitive-behavioral treatment of borderline personality disorder.* New York: Guilford Press.

Londborg, P. D., Hegel, M. T., Goldstein S., Goldstein, D., Himmelhoch, J. M., Maddock, R., et al. (2001). Sertraline treatment of posttraumatic stress disorder: Results of 24 weeks of open-label continuation treatment. *Journal of Clinical Psychiatry, 62*(5), 325–331.

Maack, D. J., Lyons, J. A., Connolly, K. M., & Ritter, M. (2011). Couple/family therapy in PTSD. In B. A. Moore & W. E. Penk (Eds.), *Handbook for the treatment of PTSD in military personnel.* New York: Guilford Press.

Marshall, R. D., Lewis-Fernandez, R., Blanco, C., Simpson, H., Lin, S., Vermes, D., et al. (2007). A controlled trial of paroxetine for chronic PTSD, dissociation, and interpersonal problems in mostly minority adults. *Depression and Anxiety, 24*(2), 77–84.

Martenyi, F., Brown, E. B., Zhang, H., Koke, S. C., & Prakash, A. (2002). Fluoxetine versus placebo in posttraumatic stress disorder. *Journal of Clinical Psychiatry, 63,* 199–206.

McLean, C. P., & Foa, E. B. (2011). Prolonged exposure therapy for post-traumatic stress disorder: A review of evidence and dissemination. *Expert Review of Neurotherapeutics, 11*(8), 1151–1163.

McRae, A. L., Brady, K. T., Mellman, T. A., Sonn, S. C., Killeen, T. K., Timmerman, M. A., & Bayles-Dazet, W. (2004). Comparison of nefazodone and sertraline for the treatment of posttraumatic stress disorder. *Depression and Anxiety, 19*(3), 190–196.

Meichenbaum, D. (1974). Self instructional methods. In F. H. Kanfer & A. P. Goldstein (Eds.), *Helping people change* (pp. 357–391). New York: Pergamon Press.

Monson, C. M., Schnurr, P. P., Resick, P. A., Friedman, M. J., Young-Xu, Y., & Stevens, S. P. (2006). Cognitive processing therapy for veterans with military-related posttraumatic stress disorder. *Journal of Consulting and Clinical Psychology, 74*(5), 898–907.

Moore, B. A., & Krakow, B. (2010). Imagery rehearsal therapy: An emerging treatment for posttraumatic nightmares in veterans. *Psychological trauma: Theory, research, practice, and policy, 2*(3), 232–238.

Myers, C. S. (1915). A contribution to the study of shell shock. *Lancet, 188*(4854), 316–320.

Neylan, T. C., Lenoci, M., Samuelson, K. W., Metzler, T. J., Henn-Haase, C., Hierholzer, R. W., et al. (2006). No improvement of posttraumatic stress disorder symptoms with guanfacine treatment. *American Journal of Psychiatry, 163*(12), 2186–2188.

Resick, P. A., Galovski, T. E., Uhlmansiek, M. O., Scher, C. D., Clum, G. A., & Young-Xu, Y. (2008) A randomized clinical trial to dismantle components of cognitive processing therapy for posttraumatic stress disorder in female victims of interpersonal violence. *Journal of Consulting and Clinical Psychology, 76*, 243–258.

Resick, P. A., & Schnicke, M. K. (1992). *Cognitive processing therapy for rape victims: A treatment manual.* Newbury Park, CA: Sage.

Resick, P. A., Williams, L. F., Suvak, M. K., Monson, C. M., & Gradus, J. L. (2012). Long-term outcomes of cognitive-behavioral treatments for posttraumatic stress disorder among female rape survivors. *Journal of Consulting and Clinical Psychology, 80*(2), 201–210. doi:10.1037/a0026602

Rothbaum, B. O., Cahill, S. P., Foa, E. B., Davidson, J. R. T., Compton, J., Connor, K., Astin, M. C., Hahn, C. (2006). Augmentation of sertraline with prolonged exposure in the treatment of posttraumatic stress disorder. *Journal of Traumatic Stress, 19*(5), 625–638.

Rothbaum, B. O., Difede, J., & Rizzo, A. A. (2008). *Therapist treatment manual for virtual reality exposure therapy: Posttraumatic stress disorder in Iraq combat veterans.* Lakewood, WA: Geneva Foundation.

Russell, M. C., Lipke, H., & Figley, C.R. (2011). Eye movement desensitization and reprocessing. In B. A. Moore & W. E. Penk (Eds.), *Handbook for the treatment of PTSD in military personnel.* New York: Guilford Press.

Saygın, M. Z., Sungur, M. Z., Sabol, E. U., & Çetinkaya, P. (2002). Nefazodone versus sertraline in the treatment of posttraumatic stress disorder. *Bulletin of Clinical Psychopharmacology, 12*, 1–5.

Schneier, F. R., Neria, Y., Pavlicova, M., Hembree, E. A., Suh, E. J., Amsel, L. V., & Marshall, R. D. (2011). Combined prolonged exposure therapy and paroxetine for PTSD related to the World Trade Center attack: A randomized controlled trial. *American Journal of Psychiatry, 169*(1), 80–88.

Shapiro, F. (1989). Eye movement desensitization: A new treatment for posttraumatic stress disorder. *Journal of Behavior Therapy and Experimental Psychiatry, 20*(3), 211–217.

Shea, M. T., McDevitt-Murphy, M., Ready, D., & Schnurr, P.P (2009). Group therapy. In E. B. Foa, T. M. Keane, M. J. Friedman, & J. A. Cohen (Eds.), *Effective treatments for PTSD: Practice guidelines from the International Society for Traumatic Stress Studies* (2nd ed.). New York: Guilford Press.

Spates, R. C., Koch, E., Cusack, K., Paato, S., & Waller, S. (2009). Eye movement desensitization and reprocessing. In E. B. Foa, T. M. Keane, M. J. Friedman, & J. A. Cohen (Eds.), *Effective treatments for PTSD: Practice guidelines from the International Society for Traumatic Stress Studies* (2nd ed.). New York: Guilford Press.

Stein, D. J., Ipser, J. C., & Seedat, S. (2006). Pharmaotherapy for post-traumatic stress disorder (PTSD). *Cochran Database Systemic Reviews, 1*, CD002795.

Stein, M. B., Kerridge, C., Dimsdale, J. E., & Hoyt, D. B. (2007). Pharmacotherapy to prevent PTSD: Results from a randomized controlled proof-of-concept trial by physically injured patients. *Journal of Traumatic Stress, 20*, 923–932.

Taylor, F. B., Lowe, K., Thompson, C., McFall, M. M., Peskind, E. R., Kanter, E. D., et al. (2006). Daytime prazosin reduces psychological distress to trauma specific cues in civilian trauma posttraumatic stress disorder. *Biological Psychiatry, 59*(7), 577–581.

Tucker, P., Zaninelli, R., Yehuda, R., Ruggiero, L., Dillingham, K., & Pitts, C. D. (2001). Paroxetine in the treatment of chronic posttraumatic stress disorder: Results of a placebo-controlled, flexible-dosage trial. *Journal of Clinical Psychiatry, 62*, 860–868.

VA/DoD (Department of Veterans Affairs/Department of Defense) (2010). *VA/DoD clinical practice guideline for the management of posttraumatic stress, version 2.0.* Washington, DC: Veterans Health Administration, Department of Defense.

Villarreal, G., Canive, J. M., Calaise, L. A., Toney, G., & Smith, A. K. (2010). Duloxetine in military posttraumatic stress disorder. *Psychopharmacology Bulletin, 43*(3), 26–34.

Zoellner, L., Feeny, N., Cochran, B., & Pruitt, L. (2003). Treatment choice for PTSD. *Behaviour Research and Therapy, 41*, 879–886.

CHAPTER 9

Panic Disorder

Meredith E. Charney, M. Alexandra Kredlow, Eric Bui, and Naomi M. Simon[1]

INTRODUCTION

Panic disorder is an anxiety disorder characterized by recurrent unexpected panic attacks and significant worry around these attacks. Panic can occur with or without agoraphobia. The *DSM–IV–TR* (American Psychiatric Association [APA], 2000) defines a panic attack as a discrete period of intense fear or discomfort in which four or more of 13 symptoms develop abruptly and reach a peak within 10 minutes. These symptoms include: (1) palpitations, pounding heart, or accelerated heart rate; (2) sweating; (3) trembling or shaking; (4) sensations of shortness of breath or smothering; (5) a feeling of choking; (6) chest pain or discomfort; (7) nausea or abdominal distress; (8) feeling dizzy, unsteady, lightheaded, or faint; (9) derealization (feelings of unreality) or depersonalization (being detached from oneself); (10) fear of losing control or going crazy; (11) fear of dying; (12) paresthesias (numbness or tingling sensations); and (13) chills or hot flushes.

Panic disorder (PD), as defined by the *DSM–IV–TR* (APA, 2000), consists of four criteria (A–D) which assess the frequency, impact, characteristics, and cause of the panic attacks. Criterion A includes the presence of recurrent unexpected panic attacks, although panic attacks may become linked to some common triggers over time. In addition, in PD there is 1 month or more of persistent concern ("anticipatory anxiety") about having additional attacks, worry about the implications of the attack or its consequences, and or a significant change in behavior related to the attacks. Criterion B is used to distinguish between PD with or without agoraphobia. Criterion C specifies that the panic attacks are not due to direct physiological effects of a substance (such as intoxication with stimulants or withdrawal from depressants) or a general medical condition (such as vestibular dysfunctions or cardiac conditions). Finally, Criterion D specifies that the panic attacks are not better accounted for by any other mental disorder. Furthermore, in order to meet criteria for a PD diagnosis, the panic attacks have to be recurrent and unexpected, and cause significant interference in daily functioning.

The *DSM–IV–TR* (APA, 2000) considers PD with and without agoraphobia as two separate diagnoses. Agoraphobia is defined by the following three criteria: (A) there is anxiety about being in places or situations from which escape might be difficult or in which help may not be available in the event of having a panic attack or panic-like symptoms; (B) the situations producing this anxiety are avoided, endured with marked distress, or require the presence of a companion; and (C) the anxiety or avoidance is not better accounted for by another mental disorder. Some examples of typical types of situations that may be associated with anxiety and avoidance in individuals with agoraphobia include far travel, being in crowded trains or buses, airplanes, driving in traffic, haircuts, long lines, and, in more severe cases, leaving the house unaccompanied. Further, patients may become fearful of physical sensations that are reminiscent of their panic attacks and avoid activities that replicate sensations such as exercise or being in a warm place. The presence or absence of agoraphobia is significant, as symptom severity, impairment, and comorbidity vary considerably. Symptom severity tends to be higher in panic patients with agoraphobia, demonstrated by higher scores on the Panic Disorder Severity Scale than those for non-agoraphobic panic patients, and greater levels of situational avoidance can clearly impact social and occupational functioning (Kessler et al., 2006). However, the presence or absence of agoraphobia does not seem to affect treatment outcomes (Furukawa, Watanabe, & Churchill, 2006; Gould, Otto, & Pollack, 1995).

Lifetime prevalence rates for PD range from 1.4% to 20.5%. Differences in rates are largely due to the ages of the populations surveyed and whether the *DSM–IV–TR* was used for diagnosis. In the recent National Comorbidity Survey–Replication (NCS–R), which surveyed 9282 U.S. adults across a wide range of age groups, Kessler et al. (2006) found the lifetime prevalence of *DSM–IV–TR*-diagnosed PD with or without agoraphobia to be 4.7%. The 12-month prevalence was 2.8%. In contrast, the lifetime prevalence of having a panic attack was found to be 28.3% and the 12-month prevalence 11.2%.

Prevalence rates for PD are higher in individuals within the 30–44 and 45–59 age brackets (5.7% and 5.9% respectively), with a mean age of onset of 23. Studies have consistently found higher rates of PD among women (Eaton, Kessler, Wittchen, & Magee, 1994; Kessler et al., 2006). In addition, studies suggest that PD may differ across cultures, with prevalence rates of *DSM–IV*-defined PD in the United States being higher than those reported in other countries (Lewis-Fernandez et al., 2009).

There are several important clinical issues to consider when working with patients with PD. First, PD is highly comorbid with other mental health conditions. In the NCS–R, Kessler et al. (2006) found that 83% of PD without agoraphobia and 100% of PD with agoraphobia patients had at least one comorbid disorder in their lifetime. PD is most often comorbid with other anxiety disorders, including generalized anxiety disorder (21% of those with PD without agoraphobia have a lifetime diagnosis of generalized anxiety disorder), specific phobia (34%), social anxiety disorder (31%), posttraumatic stress disorder (22%), and obsessive-compulsive disorder (8%). PD is also highly comorbid with other classes of psychiatric disorders: 50% with mood disorders, 47% with impulse-control disorders, and 27% with substance-use disorders. Comorbidity rates for patients with PD with agoraphobia are higher than for those with PD without agoraphobia, representing the increased difficulties associated with agoraphobia (Kessler et al., 2006). Recent research also suggests that PD may be associated with an elevated risk for suicide attempts (Goodwin & Roy-Byrne, 2006). Second, recent data suggest that the majority of patients with PD seek treatment at some point in their lives. However, it is unclear whether these patients are receiving evidence-based care for their panic symptoms. Kessler et al. (2006) found that 96% of the PD patients with agoraphobia and 85% without agoraphobia had obtained lifetime treatment for psychiatric problems. Treatment however, was broadly defined as "any treatment for any problems with your emotions or nerves or your use of alcohol or drugs." The study indicated that 41–55% of patients obtained treatment which was consistent with basic treatment guidelines (i.e., for pharmacotherapy: at least 2 months of an appropriate medication, defined as antidepressants or anxiolytics, plus at least four visits to any type of medical physician; for psychotherapy: at least eight visits with any healthcare or human services professional lasting an average of at least 30 minutes). This suggested that around half of PD patients may not have received first-line treatment for their PD symptoms.

Another important clinical consideration is that many PD patients present in non-psychiatric medical settings, with medical complaints rather than a psychiatric one. PD prevalence rates have been found to be higher, around 7%, in primary care settings (Kroenke, Spitzer, Williams, Monahan, & Lowe, 2007), and patients with panic utilize medical services more often than other patients with anxiety disorders (Deacon, Lickel, & Abramowitz, 2008). Most patients with panic who present in medical settings do so with somatic complaints, such as cardiac, gastrointestinal, and neurological concerns (Katon, Von Korff, & Lin, 1992). In addition, recent studies have found elevated rates of PD comorbid with documented respiratory disorders, vestibular dysfunction, and hyperthyroidism and hypothyroidism (Simon & Fischmann, 2005). Furthermore, although gains have been made in education of primary care and emergency clinicians about PD, which has anecdotally led to fewer tests and procedures prior to diagnosis, gaps in knowledge of the clinical features and effective treatments for PD continue to be present (Teng, Chaison, Bailey, Hamilton, & Dunn, 2008). It is also worth noting that many large studies of treatment for PD initially focused only on reduction in panic attacks; it has become clear,

however, that a true remission requires elimination of panic attacks and anticipatory anxiety, as well as a return to avoided situations, both to improve quality of life and functioning, and to reduce risk for relapse after treatment
discontinuation.

SOLITARY TREATMENT APPROACHES

Pharmacological Treatment

Because PD shares a pathophysiology with other anxiety disorders involving
fear and anxiety neurocircuitry, including serotonin, norepinephrine, and
γ-aminobutyric acid (GABA) pathways, its pharmacological treatment is mainly
based on agents that target these systems.

Review of randomized controlled trials (RCTs) and other studies

ANTIDEPRESSANTS

Because of their efficacy, safety, favorable side-effect profile, and broad spectrum of efficacy for psychiatric conditions often comorbid with panic,
serotonin-specific reuptake inhibitors (SSRIs) remain the first-line pharmacological treatment of panic. Data from a large number of randomized controlled trials indicate that PD can be effectively treated with fluoxetine
(Michelson et al., 1998), paroxetine (Pollack et al., 2007; Sheehan, Burnham,
Iyengar, & Perera, 2005), and the serotonin–norepinephrine reuptake inhibitor (SNRI) venlafaxine (Liebowitz, Asnis, Mangano, & Tzanis, 2009; Pollack
et al., 2007). In addition, RCTs also indicate that PD can be treated with citalopram (Lepola et al., 1998), escitalopram (Stahl, Gergel, & Li, 2003), fluvoxamine (Asnis et al., 2001), and sertraline (Pollack, Otto, Worthington,
Manfro, & Wolkow, 1998).

More recently, an open-label study provided preliminary support for the efficacy of the SNRI duloxetine in PD (Simon, Kaufman et al., 2009); however,
controlled data are needed. To date, although a few head-to-head comparisons
of SSRIs and SNRIs investigating a variety of outcomes in PD patients have
been conducted (Pollack et al., 2007), there is no compelling evidence suggesting the superiority of one agent or class over another.

TRICYCLIC ANTIDEPRESSANTS

The use of tricyclic antidepressants (TCAs) in the treatment of panic predates
that of SRIs, and a number of RCTs have shown robust efficacy for clomipramine and imipramine in PD (Caillard, Rouillon, Viel, & Markabi, 1999;
Lecrubier, Bakker, Dunbar, & Judge, 1997). Yet while they were the "gold

standard" for treating panic for decades before the advent of SRIs, they should not currently be considered first-line because of their greater side-effect burden, including weight gain, potential cardiac conduction problems, and anticholinergic effects (Papp et al., 1997), toxicity in overdose, and lack of demonstrated superiority over SRIs (Bakker, Van Balkom, & Spinhoven, 2002; Lecrubier et al., 1997; Otto, Tuby, Gould, McLean, & Pollack, 2001). Furthermore, TCAs do not seem to be efficacious for social anxiety disorder, a condition often comorbid with PD (Simpson et al., 1998).

OTHER ANTIDEPRESSANTS

No controlled data are available on the efficacy of monoamine oxidase inhibitors (MAOIs) in PD; however, a few studies on reversible inhibitors of monoamine oxidase A (RIMAs) such as moclobemide or brofaromine (both unavailable in the United States) show similar efficacy compared to SSRIs (Tiller, Bouwer, & Behnke, 1997) or TCAs (Krüger & Dahl, 1999).

There is also some evidence from a small randomized trial (Versiani et al., 2002) that reboxetine, an SNRI not available in the United States, may be effective in PD, although its efficacy compared to that of SSRIs is still unclear (Bertani et al., 2004).

Results from small open-label studies (Sarchiapone et al., 2003) and one small RCT showing no difference in efficacy compared to fluoxetine (Ribeiro et al., 2001) suggest that mirtazapine, a serotonin receptor antagonist, might potentially be effective for PD, though large RCTs are needed to confirm.

Studies investigating the potential efficacy of bupropion, a norepinephrine, serotonin, and dopamine reuptake inhibitor, have yielded conflicting results, with both negative (Sheehan, Davidson, Manschreck, & Wyck Fleet, 1983) and positive (Simon et al., 2003) open-label trials, with the latter suggesting that lower dosing may be better tolerated.

BENZODIAZEPINES

To date, the only two benzodiazepines approved by the U.S. Food and Drug Administration (FDA) in the treatment of PD are alprazolam and clonazepam. A number of RCTs support the efficacy of clonazepam (Moroz & Rosenbaum, 1999; Rosenbaum, Moroz, & Bowden, 1997) and both the immediate and extended-release (Pecknold, Luthe, Munjack, & Alexander, 1994) forms of alprazolam in PD. However, the efficacy of diazepam (Noyes et al., 1996) and other benzodiazepines (Savoldi, Somenzini, & Ecari, 1990) is also well documented by RCTs.

Compared to antidepressants, benzodiazepines have a rapid onset of action and can be used on an as-needed basis. However, their lack of efficacy for comorbid psychiatric conditions such as depression, as well as the increased risk for sedation, memory impairment, fatigue, and dependence, offset the advantage. Further, in the setting of a diagnosis of PD, as-needed dosing of benzodiazepines is rarely indicated and can actually serve to worsen the disorder in some cases (Westra, Stewart, & Conrad, 2002). While there has been concern over the potential development of therapeutic tolerance (i.e., loss of therapeutic efficacy), the evidence suggests that benzodiazepines appear to remain effective in the long term (Pollack et al., 1993), with no significant dose escalation over time in the vast majority of patients (Soumerai et al., 2003).

OTHER MEDICATIONS

Results from a number of small open-label studies suggested that anticonvulsants, including valproic acid (Woodman & Noyes, 1994) and levetiracetam (Papp, 2006), might be efficacious in PD, but results from RCTs have been mixed, with studies failing to show efficacy for carbamazepine (Uhde, Stein, & Post, 1988) or tiagabine (Zwanzger et al., 2009), and one reporting only modest efficacy with gabapentin for a subset of the most severely symptomatic participants (Pande et al., 2000).

Building on promising results from open-label studies (Simon et al., 2006), a recent randomized controlled trial ($n = 56$) reported that low doses of risperidone appear to be as efficacious as paroxetine (Prosser, Yard, Steele, Cohen, & Galynker, 2009).

The potential efficacy of a number of other pharmacological agents, including antihypertensives and buspirone, has been investigated, but, to date, no compelling data suggest that they might be useful in the treatment of panic.

Of interest, the first edition of the APA practice guidelines (APA, 1998), and other (i.e., non-American) guideline recommendations dating from the mid-2000s (National Institute for Health and Clinical Excellence [NICE], 2004; Royal Australian and New Zealand College of Psychiatrists, 2003) recommended that both TCAs and SRIs should be favored over the benzodiazepines, and that the disadvantages of the benzodiazepines did not counterbalance their advantages.

However, according to the recent updated practice guidelines issued by the American Psychiatric Association (2009), there is overall no evidence for the superiority of one of three classes (SRIs, TCAs, and benzodiazepines) in the treatment of PD. While TCAs might not be indicated as a first-line treatment because of the side-effects burden, SRIs and benzodiazepines may be considered as equally reasonable first-line choices, and the choice between these classes should be dictated by cost, potential side effects and drug interactions, prior treatment history, and co-occurring medical and psychiatric conditions. For example, benzodiazepines may be favored in patients for whom the rapid control of the symptoms is critical. On the other hand, SRIs should be the first choice if the patient exhibits comorbid depression, operates machines at work, or has a history of substance abuse and dependence.

Recommendations for the duration of the treatment are at least 12–18 months, as studies have shown long-term therapeutic gains through maintaining pharmacotherapy (Rapaport et al., 2001). Such a time period allows patients sufficient time to experience potential triggers, learn safety, and return to previously avoided situations, and may decrease the risk of relapse with medication discontinuation. Regardless, slow medication discontinuation over weeks to months when possible is preferable and may decrease the likelihood of triggering a return of symptoms or intolerance of medication discontinuation due to medication withdrawal symptoms. It has been reported that combining benzodiazepine and antidepressants early in the treatment resulted in an accelerated response compared to antidepressants alone (Pollack et al., 2003). However, the absence of real long-term advantage of the association (i.e., an additive or synergistic effect) suggests that combination therapy may be best utilized during initiation to improve the speed of response and tolerability of antidepressants, but that benzodiazepines can be tapered after the initial weeks once maintenance antidepressant dosing is achieved.

Strengths and benefits, and weaknesses and limitations, of using pharmacotherapy as sole approach

Compared to psychosocial interventions, pharmacotherapy—and, in particular, benzodiazepines—provides an often rapidly efficacious treatment option and is less time-consuming for patients and clinicians. On the other hand, the benefits of pharmacological agents are often accompanied by some side effects ranging from minor ones such as mouth dryness to more severe ones that might be interfering (e.g., sedation) and may interfere with treatment initiation, and the duration of overall treatment is often longer.

Clinical Vignette: Good outcome with pharmacotherapy

Ben is a 22-year-old man who presents to the emergency room with chest tightness, palpitations, shortness of breath, dizziness, sweating, and a fear he is eventually going to die of a heart attack. He notes that he has been worried about his health, and having a heart attack in particular, for the past 2 months, as he has had multiple "out-of-the-blue" episodes of sudden symptoms and fear. Now he has started to avoid going to the gym because when he starts to sweat or feels his heart pounding, it brings on another episode. After assessing the patient, the emergency-room clinician provides education about panic disorder and its treatment, and assurance about his physical health, which provides initial relief about his safety. The clinician refers the patient to his primary care doctor, who initiates an SSRI at half the usual starting dose for one week, and then gradually titrates the dose every couple of weeks to tolerability and response. By 12 weeks, Mr. B is no longer having panic attacks, has rare anticipatory anxiety, and has begun to return to his usual exercise routine.

Clinical Vignette: Poor outcome with pharmacotherapy

Julia is a 33-year-old woman who has come to her primary care doctor reporting that she suffers from panic disorder and has been afraid to take medication for the past 2 years because she has read about all of the potential side effects, and is certain they will cause her to panic. She notes she has been given a prescription on two prior occasions but never filled it. She also notes that she cannot tolerate any caffeine as it induces panic. Without spending the time to review initiation side effects or Julia's specific concerns, her doctor writes a prescription for 20 mg of fluoxetine (the usual starting dose for depression and individuals without somatic sensitivity) and tells her to go ahead and take it, as it is a very safe and well-tolerated medication. Feeling embarrassed by her previous non-compliance, Julia fills the prescription and starts the medication, but begins to scan herself all day for potential side effects. After 3 days she finds she is having trouble sleeping, is more anxious, nauseous, and beginning to feel herself shake, which brings on additional panic attacks. She stops the medication and does not return to her doctor.

Psychosocial Treatment

Review of RCTs

Cognitive-behavioral therapy (CBT) is a well-established first-line treatment for PD (McHugh, Smits, & Otto, 2009). CBT is a learning-based approach that generally consists of psychoeducation, cognitive restructuring, and behavioral interventions (e.g., exposure techniques). The cognitive and behavioral components of the treatment assist in patients learning how to effectively interpret and respond to internal and external feared situations. Cognitive restructuring helps patients to identify and restructure panic-related thoughts (e.g., "I am having a heart attack"). Patients then learn to see these thoughts as habit based rather than fact based and use rational responses (e.g., "heart racing does not mean a heart attack") when confronted with situations that typically invoke anxiety. Behavioral exercises, such as exposure, help to disconfirm panic-related cognitions, build tolerance of uncomfortable sensations, and enable the patient to learn that avoidance is not necessary to feel less anxious.

RCTs demonstrate that CBT for PD is effective and that treatment gains are maintained over time (e.g., Craske, Maidenberg, & Bystritsky, 1995; Öst, Thulin, & Ramnerö, 2004). For example, Öst and colleagues (2004) evaluated 73 participants randomly assigned to three conditions: (1) *in vivo* exposure only, (2) cognitive-behavioral therapy, and (3) wait-list control. Results indicated that both exposure alone and CBT resulted in clinically significant improvements in panic symptoms compared to the wait-list control group. These results were maintained at 1-year follow-up, when 70% of the exposure group and 63% of the CBT group were panic-free. In addition, Gloster et al. (2011) conducted a multicenter, randomized, controlled trial examining 369 participants with PD. Participants were randomized to two manual-based variants of CBT or a wait-list control group. The primary difference between the CBT groups was that in one condition the therapists planned and supervised the *in vivo* exposures out-side the therapy room, whereas in the other condition therapists planned and discussed exposure but did not accompany the participants. Results indicated that both CBT treatments were effective in treating PD, and gains were main-tained at 6-month follow-up. However, the therapist-guided exposure (i.e., the outside-the-therapy-room condition) demonstrated a quicker and stronger response than the other CBT condition.

Randomized controlled trials for brief CBT for PD have also been shown to be effective. For instance, Craske et al. (1995) evaluated 30 patients with PD who were randomly assigned to four sessions of CBT or non-directive, support-ive therapy. Those who received CBT showed clinically significant improve-ments compared to those who received supportive therapy. In addition, Marchand, Roberge, Primiano, and Germain (2009) conducted a randomized controlled trial of standard (14 sessions), group (14 sessions), and brief (7 ses-sions) CBT for PD compared to wait-list control. Results indicated that all CBT modalities were effective in both the medium and the long term at 2-year fol-low-up.

Randomized controlled trials have begun to look at the role of computers and the Internet in the treatment of PD. Kenardy et al. (2003) evaluated a mult-isite, randomly assigned sample of patients with PD, comparing 12 sessions of CBT, 6 sessions of CBT, and 6 sessions of computer-augmented CBT versus a wait-list control. The computer-augmented CBT consisted of multiple daily prompts to practice therapy as well as modules to enhance the treatment done in session. At 6-month follow-up, all the active CBT treatments demonstrated significant levels of clinical improvement. In addition, a follow-up study by Kenardy, Robinson, and Dob (2005) indicated that 6–8 years after the end of the treatment study, gains were maintained. Furthermore, Bergström et al. (2010)

compared internet- and group-administered CBT for PD and found significant improvements across both treatment conditions, with no differences between the two conditions. The study also found that the group CBT used significantly more clinician time. In a cost-effectiveness analysis of therapist time, the study found that internet treatment had superior cost-effectiveness ratios in relation to group treatment both at post-treatment and at follow-up.

Although the RCT literature has predominantly focused on CBT programs for panic, there is a small body of literature providing support for psychodynamic psychotherapy to treat PD (Milrod et al., 2007). Panic-focused psychodynamic psychotherapy is a twice-weekly, 12-week manualized therapy that focuses on psychodynamic conflicts commonly found in PD. Milrod and colleagues found that in a sample of 49 patients with PD, those who received psychodynamic psychotherapy had superior outcomes compared to those who received applied relaxation training, with a 73% response rate compared with 39% found in the relaxation condition.

Review of other studies (open label, case)

Although there is a wealth of controlled trials supporting the use of CBT to treat PD, evidence to support alternative psychosocial treatments is more limited. There is emerging evidence, however, that treatments such as biofeedback, exercise, and a mindfulness-based approach may be beneficial in treating PD. In a study involving 37 patients with PD, Meuret, Wilhelm, Ritz, and Roth (2008) compared breathing training therapy to a delayed treatment. Results suggested that panic severity, agoraphobic avoidance, anxiety sensitivity, disability, and respiratory measures all improved. At 12-month follow-up, 68% of participants in the treatment condition no longer reported panic attacks.

In addition, several studies have demonstrated that brief exercise programs consisting of repeated short periods of moderate to vigorous exercise result in lower anxiety sensitivity (a fear of anxiety and related sensations), a precursor to panic attacks and PD. For instance, Broman-Fulks, Berman, Rabian, and Webster (2004) examined the impact of aerobic exercise on anxiety sensitivity. Results indicated that both high- and low-intensity exercise reduced anxiety sensitivity, with high-intensity exercise causing more rapid reductions and producing more treatment responders. In addition, only high-intensity exercise reduced fear of anxiety-related bodily sensations. Furthermore, a randomized controlled trial involving 46 patients with PD found that a 10-week treatment protocol of regular exercise was associated with significant clinical improvement in panic symptoms compared to placebo (Broocks et al., 1998). Exercise may be conceptualized as one component of exposure therapy, with exposure to overlapping physical sensations commonly present in panic attacks, but may have other benefits on biological systems that contribute to panic as well.

Kim et al. (2009) examined the effectiveness of a mindfulness-based cognitive therapy (MBCT) compared to an anxiety disorder education program, and found significantly greater reduction in panic and related anxiety scales with MBCT.

Strengths and benefits, and weaknesses and limitations, of using psychotherapy as sole approach

The above-referenced studies provide strong support for the use of evidence-based psychotherapy in treating PD. One area of strength for the use of psychotherapy alone is that CBT has been shown to be more cost-effective than pharmacotherapy and combined therapies (McHugh et al., 2009). However, the widespread availability of clinicians trained in evidence-based psychotherapy for PD is limited. Psychotherapy may be less accessible than medication, particularly given that medication may be prescribed across multiple services (psychiatry and primary care). Dissemination of evidence-based clinical care is limited across the mental health field, a state of affairs not unique to PD (McHugh et al., 2009). In addition, there may be patient-related factors that prevent engagement in weekly psychotherapy, such as work or childcare schedules, transportation issues, language barriers, or some comorbid disorders.

Clinical Vignette: Good outcome with psychotherapy

Gail is a 20-year-old college student who began experiencing her first panic attacks 2 years ago without a clear trigger, but noted an increase in frequency, growing focus and anxiety about recurrent attacks, and increasing avoidance of crowds, travel, driving in traffic, and exercise. She has become aware that she is beginning to avoid parties and small seminar classes because leaving as a result of a panic attack would be embarrassing. She is also avoiding haircuts, and can only go to the cafeteria at off hours when there are no lines. Gail's counselor refers her to a cognitive-behavioral therapist, who begins with education about the fear of fear cycle, and explains how avoidance enhances rather than prevents anxiety and panic. Although initially skeptical, after support and encouragement Gail creates an exposure hierarchy with her therapist, and is able to start both within and outside session retuning to avoided situations, starting with the least "risky" ones. After 12 weeks, Gail reports an almost full resolution of her symptoms and is able to sign up for her favorite teacher's eight-person seminar.

> ### Clinical Vignette: Poor outcome with psychotherapy
>
> Yvonne is a 32-year-old woman with panic disorder with agoraphobia who has been treated off and on with pharmacotherapy for many years by her primary care doctor but has never participated in psychotherapy, as she believes panic is solely a medical problem that must be handled with medication to avoid adverse outcomes. After pressure from her husband, she begins to see a CBT therapist, who fails to inquire about her other treatments. After 10 sessions, Yvonne is completing her homework assignments, yet not improving. She remains fully convinced there is nothing she can do with the therapist that will improve her symptoms. After calling her primary care doctor, the therapist discovers that the latter was unaware the patient had begun psychotherapy, and when the patient called 6 weeks ago with increased anxiety, she increased her as-needed alprazolam, with which the patient has been pre-medicating herself with prior to every exposure assignment to "make sure" she does not panic.

COMBINED THERAPY

Review of RCTs

The above studies demonstrate that there is substantial evidence that pharmacotherapy and CBT offer benefit to patients with PD. There has been hope that the combination of these two types of treatment would lead to a powerful intervention. However, the results of combination treatments have been variable, providing only limited support for the use of combined treatment in patients with PD. In a meta-analysis of 23 randomized comparisons (incorporating data from 1709 patients across 21 trials), Furukawa et al. (2006) found that acute combined treatment with antidepressants and CBT was superior to monotherapy (i.e., either pharmacotherapy or CBT); however, the advantage was lost after medication discontinuation. In addition, McHugh et al. (2007) found that the cost–benefit ratio for combined treatment is substantially less favorable than for CBT alone.

Review of other studies (open label, case)

The variable findings of combination treatments and the overall cost-effectiveness of CBT have led researchers to begin to investigate novel ways to combine pharmacotherapy and CBT. In recent years, in part driven by evidence that benzodiazepines may interfere with extinction learning and retention, novel approaches to pharmacotherapy have been applied as a strategy to enhance the retention of the therapeutic learning provided by exposure-based CBT. This approach is based on studies which found that D-cycloserine (DCS) can be utilized as an agent capable of enhancing extinction learning (Otto et al., 2010). In a small randomized, double-blind, placebo-controlled augmentation trial, Otto et al. examined the addition of DCS or pill placebo to brief-exposure-based CBT for patients with PD. Doses of the study drug were administered 1 hour before CBT sessions 3–5. Results indicated large effect sizes for the additive benefit of DCS administration compared to placebo in the enhancement of CBT, with statistically significant differences at post-treatment and 1-month follow-up.

Strengths and benefits of using a combined approach: recommendations for future studies and research

The varying evidence for using a combined treatment approach makes it difficult to recommend it as a first-line treatment for uncomplicated PD at this time. The literature clearly supports the efficacy of monotherapies, and in particular CBT, as cost-effective treatment approaches for PD. Further research is needed to more clearly understand best practices for PD (i.e., combined versus monotherapy versus the use of agents such as DCS to enhance panic treatment). In addition, more widespread dissemination of evidence-based treatments, particularly psychotherapy, is needed for the general population to have access to the most effective treatments for PD. Much less is understood about what to do next if an initial intervention is unsuccessful. Options include switching or combining approaches. One RCT has suggested that CBT and clonazepam augmentation of SSRIs may be equally efficacious (Simon, Otto et al., 2009). In addition, more closely examining reasons for treatment failure in panic, which may include insufficient psychoeducation, excessively rapid medication dosing, non-compliance, incorrect dosing, intolerance of initiation side effects, and comorbid disorders that, unaddressed, interfere with engagement in CBT.

Clinical Vignette: Combined treatment

Candida is a 30-year-old woman with panic disorder with agoraphobia comorbid with major depressive disorder. She has so little energy and motivation, and is so fearful of driving alone, that she has difficulty leaving the house without her husband. She has been unable to work for the past 9 months, causing financial stress for the couple, and her husband is having difficulty taking time off work on a regular basis to drive her to regular therapy appointments. She has been fearful of medications but has started and stopped CBT three times, canceling sessions at the last minute. Her psychotherapist spends time explaining to her the role of medication, and she agrees to see a psychiatrist. After 2 months of antidepressant treatment, Candida's depression has begun to lift, her panic attacks are somewhat less frequent, and she is no longer napping during the day. She feels more motivated, and energized to return to a full program of 12 weekly sessions of CBT, with an agreement with her husband and therapist that she will begin driving after the first few sessions, which she does after directly addressing this concern in treatment. Eighteen months later, Candida is in full remission and wishes to discontinue her medication before becoming pregnant. With the help of a few intermittent "booster" sessions from her CBT therapist, she is able to successfully discontinue her antidepressant after a slow taper despite some mild discontinuation-related dizziness, and remains in full remission.

Clinical Points to Remember

1. Panic disorder affects about 5% of the population in the United States, is highly comorbid with other mental health conditions, and is associated with increased medical services utilization.
2. Patients with panic disorder frequently present to primary care with somatic complaints, such as cardiac, gastrointestinal, and neurological concerns.
3. Serotonin reuptake inhibitors (both SSRIs and SNRIs) are the first-line pharmacological treatment of panic disorder with no evidence suggesting the superiority of one agent or class over another.
4. Tricyclic antidepressants used to be the "gold standard" for treating panic disorder, but are no longer used as first-line agents, owing to the greater side-effect burden and lack of demonstrated superiority over serotonin reuptake inhibitors.
5. Although benzodiazepines can be used on an as-needed basis, this practice is rarely indicated for a full panic disorder diagnosis and can serve to worsen the disorder in some cases.
6. Randomized controlled trials demonstrate that cognitive-behavioral therapy (CBT) for panic disorder is effective and treatment gains are maintained over time.
7. CBT can be effectively delivered in standard form (approximately 12 sessions), brief form (approximately 6 sessions), or using computer-augmented approaches.

8. CBT has shown to be more cost-effective than pharmacotherapy and combined therapies; however, access to clinicians trained in evidence-based therapies is limited.
9. A combined treatment approach is not recommended as a first-line treatment for uncomplicated panic disorder at this time.

NOTE

1. Work on this manuscript by Meredith E. Charney, M. Alexandra Kredlow, Eric Bui, and Naomi Simon has been supported in part by the Highland Foundation.

REFERENCES

American Psychiatric Association (APA). (1998). *Practice guideline for the treatment of patients with panic disorder.* Washington, DC: American Psychiatric Press.
American Psychiatric Association. (2000). *Diagnostic and statistical manual of mental disorders* (4th ed., text revision). Washington, DC: APA.
American Psychiatric Association. (2009). *Practice guideline for the treatment of patients with panic disorder* (2nd ed.). Washington, DC: APA.
Asnis, G. M., Hameedi, F. A., Goddard, A. W., Potkin, S. G., Black, D., Jameel, M., et al. (2001). Fluvoxamine in the treatment of panic disorder: A multi-center, double-blind, placebo-controlled study in outpatients. *Psychiatry Research, 103*(1), 1–14. doi:10.1016/S0165-1781(01)00265-7
Bakker, A., Van Balkom, A. J., & Spinhoven, P. (2002). SSRIs vs. TCAs in the treatment of panic disorder: A meta-analysis. *Acta Psychiatrica Scandinavica, 106*(3), 163–167. doi:10.1034/j.1600-0447.2002.02255.x
Bergström, J., Andersson, G., Ljótsson, B., Rück, C., Andréewitch, S., Karlsson, A., et al. (2010). Internet- versus group-administered cognitive behaviour therapy for panic disorder in a psychiatric setting: A randomised trial. *BMC Psychiatry, 10*, 54. doi:1471-244X-10-54
Bertani, A., Perna, G., Migliarese, G., Di Pasquale, D., Cucchi, M., Caldirola, D., & Bellodi, L. (2004). Comparison of the treatment with paroxetine and reboxetine in panic disorder: a randomized, single-blind study. *Pharmacopsychiatry, 37*(5), 206–210. doi:10.1055/s-2004-832593
Broman-Fulks, J. J., Berman, M. E., Rabian, B. A., & Webster, M. J. (2004). Effects of aerobic exercise on anxiety sensitivity. *Behaviour Research and Therapy, 42*(2), 125–136. doi:10.1016/S0005-7967(03)00103-7
Broocks, A., Bandelow, B., Pekrun, G., George, A., Meyer, T., Bartmann, U., et al. (1998). Comparison of aerobic exercise, clomipramine, and placebo in the treatment of panic disorder. *American Journal of Psychiatry, 155*(5), 603–609. Retrieved from http://ajp.psychiatryonline.org/article.aspx?articleid=172822
Caillard, V., Rouillon, F., Viel, J. F., & Markabi, S. (1999). Comparative effects of low and high doses of clomipramine and placebo in panic disorder: A double-blind

controlled study. French University Antidepressant Group. *Acta Psychiatrica Scandinavica, 99*(1), 51–58. doi:10.1111/j.1600-0447.1999.tb05384.x

Craske, M. G., Maidenberg, E., & Bystritsky, A. (1995). Brief cognitive-behavioral versus nondirective therapy for panic disorder. *Journal of Behavior Therapy and Experimental Psychiatry, 26*(2), 113–120. doi:10.1016/0005-7916(95)00003-I

Deacon, B., Lickel, J., & Abramowitz, J. S. (2008). Medical utilization across the anxiety disorders. *Journal of Anxiety Disorders, 22*(2), 344–350. doi:10.1016/j.janxdis.2007.03.004

Eaton, W. W., Kessler, R. C., Wittchen, H. U., & Magee, W. J. (1994). Panic and panic disorder in the United States. *American Journal of Psychiatry, 151*(3), 413–420. Retrieved from http://ajp.psychiatryonline.org

Furukawa, T. A., Watanabe, N., & Churchill, R. (2006). Psychotherapy plus antidepressant for panic disorder with or without agoraphobia. *British Journal of Psychiatry, 188*, 8. doi:10.1192/bjp.188.4.305

Gloster, A. T., Wittchen, H. U., Einsle, F., Lang, T., Helbig-Lang, S., Fydrich, T., et al. (2011). Psychological treatment for panic disorder with agoraphobia: A randomized controlled trial to examine the role of therapist-guided exposure in situ in CBT. *Journal of Consulting and Clinical Psychology, 79*(3), 406–420. doi:10.1037/a0023584

Goodwin, R. D., & Roy-Byrne, P. (2006). Panic and suicidal ideation and suicide attempts: results from the National Comorbidity Survey. *Depression and Anxiety, 23*(3), 124–132. doi:10.1002/da.20151

Gould, R. A., Otto, M. W., & Pollack, M. H. (1995). A meta-analysis of treatment outcome for panic disorder. *Clinical Psychology Review, 15*(8), 819–844. doi:10.1016/0272-7358(95)00048-8

Katon, W. J., Von Korff, M., & Lin, E. (1992). Panic disorder: Relationship to high medical utilization. *American Journal of Medicine, 92*(1A), 7S–11S. doi:10.1016/0002-9343(92)90130-4

Kenardy, J. A., Dow, M. G., Johnston, D. W., Newman, M. G., Thomson, A., & Taylor, C. B. (2003). A comparison of delivery methods of cognitive-behavioral therapy for panic disorder: An international multicenter trial. *Journal of Consulting and Clinical Psychology, 71*(6), 1068–1075. doi:10.1037/0022-006X.71.6.1068

Kenardy, J., Robinson, S., & Dob, R. (2005). Cognitive behaviour therapy for panic disorder: Long-term follow-up. *Cognitive Behaviour Therapy, 34*(2), 75–78. doi:10.1080/16506070410005410

Kessler, R. C., Chiu, W. T., Jin, R., Ruscio, A. M., Shear, K., & Walters, E. E. (2006). The epidemiology of panic attacks, panic disorder, and agoraphobia in the National Comorbidity Survey Replication. *Archives of General Psychiatry, 63*(4), 415–424. doi:10.1001/archpsyc.63.4.415

Kim, Y. W., Lee, S. H., Choi, T. K., Suh, S. Y., Kim, B., Kim, C. M., et al. (2009). Effectiveness of mindfulness-based cognitive therapy as an adjuvant to pharmacotherapy in patients with panic disorder or generalized anxiety disorder. *Depression and Anxiety, 26*(7), 601–606. doi:10.1002/da.20552

Kroenke, K., Spitzer, R. L., Williams, J. B., Monahan, P. O., & Lowe, B. (2007). Anxiety disorders in primary care: Prevalence, impairment, comorbidity, and detection. *Annals of Internal Medicine, 146*(5), 317–325. Retrieved from http://www.annals.org

Krüger, M. B., & Dahl, A. A. (1999). The efficacy and safety of moclobemide compared to clomipramine in the treatment of panic disorder. *European Archives of Psychiatry and Clinical Neuroscience, 249* (Suppl. 1), S19–S24. Retrieved from http://www.springerlink.com/content/7kx9m2wj6k4uehfl

Lecrubier, Y., Bakker, A., Dunbar, G., & Judge, R. (1997). A comparison of paroxetine, clomipramine and placebo in the treatment of panic disorder. Collaborative Paroxetine Panic Study Investigators. *Acta Psychiatrica Scandinavica, 95*(2), 145–152. doi:10.1111/j.1600-0447.1997.tb00388.x

Lepola, U. M., Wade, A. G., Leinonen, E. V., Koponen, H. J., Frazer, J., Sjodin, I., et al. (1998). A controlled, prospective, 1-year trial of citalopram in the treatment of panic disorder. *Journal of Clinical Psychiatry, 59*(10), 528–534. doi:10.4088/JCP.v59n1006

Lewis-Fernandez, R., Hinton, D. E., Laria, A. J., Patterson, E. H., Hofmann, S. G., Craske, M. G., et al. (2009). Culture and the anxiety disorders: Recommendations for DSM-V. *Depression and Anxiety, 27*(2), 212–229. doi:10.1002/da.20647

Liebowitz, M. R., Asnis, G., Mangano, R., & Tzanis, E. (2009). A double-blind, placebo-controlled, parallel-group, flexible-dose study of venlafaxine extended release capsules in adult outpatients with panic disorder. *Journal of Clinical Psychiatry, 70*(4), 550–561. doi:10.4088/JCP.08m04238

Marchand, A., Roberge, P., Primiano, S., & Germain, V. (2009). A randomized, controlled clinical trial of standard, group and brief cognitive-behavioral therapy for panic disorder with agoraphobia: A two-year follow-up. *Journal of Anxiety Disorders, 23*(8), 1139–1147. doi:10.1016/j.janxdis.2009.07.019

McHugh, R. K., Otto, M. W., Barlow, D. H., Gorman, J. M., Shear, M. K., & Woods, S. W. (2007). Cost-efficacy of individual and combined treatments for panic disorder. *Journal of Clinical Psychiatry, 68*(7), 1038–1044. doi:10.4088/JCP.v68n0710

McHugh, R. K., Smits, J. A., & Otto, M. W. (2009). Empirically supported treatments for panic disorder. *Psychiatric Clinics of North America, 32*(3), 593–610. doi:10.1016/j.psc.2009.05.005

Meuret, A. E., Wilhelm, F. H., Ritz, T., & Roth, W. T. (2008). Feedback of end-tidal pCO_2 as a therapeutic approach for panic disorder. *Journal of Psychiatric Research, 42*(7), 560–568. doi:10.1016/j.jpsychires.2007.06.005

Michelson, D., Lydiard, R. B., Pollack, M. H., Tamura, R. N., Hoog, S. L., Tepner, R., et al. (1998). Outcome assessment and clinical improvement in panic disorder: Evidence from a randomized controlled trial of fluoxetine and placebo. The Fluoxetine Panic Disorder Study Group. *American Journal of Psychiatry, 155*(11), 1570–1577. Retrieved from http://ajp.psychiatryonline.org

Milrod, B., Leon, A. C., Busch, F., Rudden, M., Schwalberg, M., Clarkin, J., et al. (2007). A randomized controlled clinical trial of psychoanalytic psychotherapy for panic disorder. *American Journal of Psychiatry, 164*(2), 265–272. doi:10.1176/appi.ajp.164.2.265

Moroz, G., & Rosenbaum, J. F. (1999). Efficacy, safety, and gradual discontinuation of clonazepam in panic disorder: A placebo-controlled, multicenter study using optimized dosages. *Journal of Clinical Psychiatry, 60*(9), 604–612. Retrieved from http://www.psychiatrist.com

National Institute for Health and Clinical Excellence. (2004). *Management of anxiety (panic disorder, with or without agoraphobia, and generalised anxiety disorder) in adults*

in primary, secondary and community care. Retrieved from http://guidance.nice.org.
uk/CG22

Noyes, R. Jr., Burrows, G. D., Reich, J. H., Judd, F. K., Garvey, M. J., Norman, T. R.,
et al. (1996). Diazepam versus alprazolam for the treatment of panic disorder. *Journal of Clinical Psychiatry, 57*(8), 349–355. Retrieved from http://www.psychiatrist.
com

Öst, L.-G., Thulin, U., & Ramnerö, J. (2004). Cognitive behavior therapy vs exposure
in vivo in the treatment of panic disorder with agoraphobia (corrected from agrophobia). *Behaviour Research and Therapy, 42*(10), 1105–1127. doi:10.1016/j.
brat.2003.07.004

Otto, M. W., Tolin, D. F., Simon, N. M., Pearlson, G. D., Basden, S., Meunier, S. A.,
et al. (2010). Efficacy of D-cycloserine for enhancing response to cognitive-behavior
therapy for panic disorder. *Biological Psychiatry, 67*(4), 365–370. doi:10.1016/j.
biopsych.2009.07.036

Otto, M. W., Tuby, K. S., Gould, R. A., McLean, R. Y., & Pollack, M. H. (2001). An
effect-size analysis of the relative efficacy and tolerability of serotonin selective
reuptake inhibitors for panic disorder. *American Journal of Psychiatry, 158*(12),
1989–1992. doi:10.1176/appi.ajp.158.12.1989

Pande, A. C., Pollack, M. H., Crockatt, J., Greiner, M., Chouinard, G., Lydiard, R. B.,
et al. (2000). Placebo-controlled study of gabapentin treatment of panic disorder.
Journal of Clinical Psychopharmacology, 20(4), 467–471. doi:10.1176/appi.
ajp.158.12.1989

Papp, L. A. (2006). Safety and efficacy of levetiracetam for patients with panic disorder: Results of an open-label, fixed-flexible dose study. *Journal of Clinical Psychiatry,
67*(10), 1573–1576. Retrieved from http://www.psychiatrist.com

Papp, L. A., Schneier, F. R., Fyer, A. J., Leibowitz, M. R., Gorman, J. M., Coplan, J.
D., et al. (1997). Clomipramine treatment of panic disorder: Pros and cons. *Journal
of Clinical Psychiatry, 58*(10), 423–425. Retrieved from http://www.psychiatrist.
com

Pecknold, J., Luthe, L., Munjack, D., & Alexander, P. (1994). A double-blind, placebo-controlled, multicenter study with alprazolam and extended-release alprazolam in
the treatment of panic disorder. *Journal of Clinical Psychopharmacology, 14*(5),
314–321. doi:10.1097/00004714-199410000-00005

Pollack, M. H., Lepola, U., Koponen, H., Simon, N. M., Worthington, J. J., Emilien,
G., et al. (2007). A double-blind study of the efficacy of venlafaxine extended-release, paroxetine, and placebo in the treatment of panic disorder. *Depression and
Anxiety, 24*(1), 1–14. doi:10.1002/da.20218

Pollack, M. H., Otto, M. W., Tesar, G. E., Cohen, L. S., Meltzer-Brody, S., & Rosenbaum, J. F. (1993). Long-term outcome after acute treatment with alprazolam or
clonazepam for panic disorder. *Journal of Clinical Psychopharmacology, 13*(4),
257–263. doi:10.1097/00004714-199308000-00005

Pollack, M. H., Otto, M. W., Worthington, J. J., Manfro, G. G., & Wolkow, R. (1998).
Sertraline in the treatment of panic disorder: A flexible-dose multicenter trial.
Archives of General Psychiatry, 55(11), 1010–1016. doi:10.1001/archpsyc.55.11.1010

Pollack, M. H., Simon, N. M., Worthington, J. J., Doyle, A. L., Peters, P., Toshkov,
F., & Otto, M. W. (2003). Combined paroxetine and clonazepam treatment strategies compared to paroxetine monotherapy for panic disorder. *Journal of Psychopharmacology, 17*(3), 276–282. doi:10.1177/02698811030173009

Prosser, J. M., Yard, S., Steele, A., Cohen, L. J., & Galynker, I. I. (2009). A comparison of low-dose risperidone to paroxetine in the treatment of panic attacks: A randomized, single-blind study. *BMC Psychiatry, 9*, 25. doi:10.1186/1471-244X-9-25

Rapaport, M. H., Wolkow, R., Rubin, A., Hackett, E., Pollack, M., & Ota, K. Y. (2001). Sertraline treatment of panic disorder: Results of a long-term study. *Acta Psychiatrica Scandinavica, 104*(4), 289–298. doi:10.1111/j.1600-0447.2001.00263.x

Ribeiro, L., Busnello, J. V., Kauer-Sant'Anna, M., Madruga, M., Quevedo, J., Busnello, E. A., & Kapczinski, F. (2001). Mirtazapine versus fluoxetine in the treatment of panic disorder. *Brazilian Journal of Medical and Biological Research, 34*(10), 1303–1307. doi:10.1590/S0100-879X2001001000010

Rosenbaum, J. F., Moroz, G., & Bowden, C. L. (1997). Clonazepam in the treatment of panic disorder with or without agoraphobia: A dose–response study of efficacy, safety, and discontinuance. Clonazepam Panic Disorder Dose–Response Study Group. *Journal of Clinical Psychopharmacology, 17*(5), 390–400. Retrieved from http://journals.lww.com/psychopharmacology

Royal Australian and New Zealand College of Psychiatrists (2003). Australian and New Zealand clinical practice guidelines for the treatment of panic disorder and agoraphobia. *Australian and New Zealand Journal of Psychiatry, 37*(6), 641–656. doi:10.1111/j.1440-1614.2003.01254.x

Sarchiapone, M., Amore, M., De Risio, S., Carli, V., Faia, V., Poterzio, F., et al. (2003). Mirtazapine in the treatment of panic disorder: An open-label trial. *International Clinical Psychopharmacology, 18*(1), 35–38. doi:10.1097/00004850-200301000-00006.

Savoldi, F., Somenzini, G., & Ecari, U. (1990). Etizolam versus placebo in the treatment of panic disorder with agoraphobia: A double-blind study. *Current Medical Research and Opinion, 12*(3), 185–190. doi:10.1185/03007999009111500

Sheehan, D. V., Burnham, D. B., Iyengar, M. K., & Perera, P. (2005). Efficacy and tolerability of controlled-release paroxetine in the treatment of panic disorder. *Journal of Clinical Psychiatry, 66*(1), 34–40. doi:10.4088/JCP.v66n0105

Sheehan, D. V., Davidson, J., Manschreck, T., & Wyck Fleet, J. V. (1983). Lack of efficacy of a new antidepressant (bupropion) in the treatment of panic disorder with phobias. *Journal of Clinical Psychopharmacology, 3*(1), 28–31. doi:10.1097/00004714-198302000-00006

Simon, N. M., Emmanuel, N., Ballenger, J., Worthington, J. J., Kinrys, G., Korbly, N. B., et al. (2003). Bupropion sustained release for panic disorder. *Psychopharmacology Bulletin, 37*(4), 66–72. Retrieved from http://www.medworksmedia.com

Simon, N. M., & Fischmann, D. (2005). The implications of medical and psychiatric comorbidity with panic disorder. *Journal of Clinical Psychiatry, 66* (Suppl. 4), 8–15. Retrieved from http://www.psychiatrist.com

Simon, N. M., Hoge, E. A., Fischmann, D., Worthington, J. J., Christian, K. M., Kinrys, G., & Pollack, M. H. (2006). An open-label trial of risperidone augmentation for refractory anxiety disorders. *Journal of Clinical Psychiatry, 67*(3), 381–385. doi:10.4088/JCP.v67n0307

Simon, N. M., Kaufman, R. E., Hoge, E. A., Worthington, J. J., Herlands, N. N., Owens, M. E., & Pollack, M. H. (2009). Open-label support for duloxetine for the treatment of panic disorder. *CNS Neuroscience and Therapeutics, 15*(1), 19–23. doi:10.1111/j.1755-5949.2008.00076.x

Simon, N. M., Otto, M. W., Worthington, J. J., Hoge, E. A., Thompson, E. H., Lebeau, R. T., et al. (2009). Next-step strategies for panic disorder refractory to initial pharmacotherapy: A 3-phase randomized clinical trial. *Journal of Clinical Psychiatry, 70*(11), 1563–1570. doi:10.4088/JCP.08m04485blu

Simpson, H. B., Schneier, F. R., Campeas, R. B., Marshall, R. D., Fallon, B. A., Davies, S., et al. (1998). Imipramine in the treatment of social phobia. *Journal of Clinical Psychopharmacology, 18*(2), 132–135. doi:10.1097/00004714-199804000-00005

Soumerai, S. B., Simoni-Wastila, L., Singer, C., Mah, C., Gao, X., Salzman, C., & Ross-Degnan, D. (2003). Lack of relationship between long-term use of benzodiazepines and escalation to high dosages. *Psychiatric Services, 54*(7), 1006–1011. doi:10.1176/appi.ps.54.7.1006

Stahl, S. M., Gergel, I., & Li, D. (2003). Escitalopram in the treatment of panic disorder: A randomized, double-blind, placebo-controlled trial. *Journal of Clinical Psychiatry, 64*(11), 1322–1327. Retrieved from http://www.psychiatrist.com

Teng, E. J., Chaison, A. D., Bailey, S. D., Hamilton, J. D., & Dunn, N. J. (2008). When anxiety symptoms masquerade as medical symptoms: What medical specialists know about panic disorder and available psychological treatments. *Journal of Clinical Psychology in Medical Settings, 15*(4), 314–321. doi:10.1007/s10880-008-9129-4

Tiller, J. W., Bouwer, C., & Behnke, K. (1997). Moclobemide for anxiety disorders: A focus on moclobemide for panic disorder. *International Clinical Psychopharmacology, 12* (Suppl. 6), S27–S30. Retrieved from http://journals.lww.com/intclinpsychopharm

Uhde, T. W., Stein, M. B., & Post, R. M. (1988). Lack of efficacy of carbamazepine in the treatment of panic disorder. *American Journal of Psychiatry, 145*(9), 1104–1109. Retrieved from http://ajp.psychiatryonline.org.

Versiani, M., Cassano, G., Perugi, G., Benedetti, A., Mastalli, L., Nardi, A., & Savino, M. (2002). Reboxetine, a selective norepinephrine reuptake inhibitor, is an effective and well-tolerated treatment for panic disorder. *Journal of Clinical Psychiatry, 63*(1), 31–37. doi:10.4088/JCP.v63n0107

Westra, H. A., Stewart, S. H., & Conrad, B. E. (2002). Naturalistic manner of benzodiazepine use and cognitive behavioral therapy outcome in panic disorder with agoraphobia. *Journal of Anxiety Disorders, 16*(3), 233–246. doi:10.1016/S0887-6185(02)00091-9

Woodman, C. L., & Noyes, R. Jr. (1994). Panic disorder: treatment with valproate. *Journal of Clinical Psychiatry, 55*(4), 134–136. Retrieved from http://www.psychiatrist.com

Zwanzger, P., Eser, D., Nothdurfter, C., Baghai, T. C., Moller, H. J., Padberg, F., & Rupprecht, R. (2009). Effects of the GABA-reuptake inhibitor tiagabine on panic and anxiety in patients with panic disorder. *Pharmacopsychiatry, 42*(6), 266–269. doi:10.1055/s-0029-1241798

CHAPTER 10

Social Anxiety Disorder

Catherine M. Kariuki and Dan J. Stein

INTRODUCTION

Social anxiety disorder, or social phobia, has been reported as one of the most common anxiety disorders, with a lifetime prevalence of between 3% and 16% in the United States, depending on the criteria used to confirm the diagnosis (American Psychiatric Association [APA], 1995; Kessler et al., 1994; Schneier, Johnson, Hornig, Liebowitz, & Weissman, 1992; Wancata, Fridl, & Friedrich, 2009). A recent systematic review of European studies found 12-month prevalence rates similar to those in the United States (Wancata et al., 2009; Weiller, Bisserbe, Boyer, Lepine, & Lecrubier, 1996). Many epidemiological studies have demonstrated a female preponderance, but in clinical samples, males and females are equally affected (Kessler et al., 1994; Schneier et al., 1992; Wancata et al., 2009). Typically, individuals begin to experience symptoms in middle childhood or early adolescence (Schneier et al., 1992). There is strong evidence to suggest that children with SAD may have an underlying trait characterized by a habitual pattern of behavioral inhibition and severe shyness (Turner, Beidel, & Wolff, 1996). Despite its high prevalence, SAD is underdiagnosed and undertreated (Schneier et al., 1992; Weiller et al., 1996). Symptoms of SAD tend to persistent into adulthood if untreated (Liebowitz, Gelenberg, & Munjack, 2005; Weiller et al., 1996).

Characteristically, individuals with SAD experience intense persistent anxiety or fear of drawing attention to themselves in social or performance situations, believing they will be evaluated negatively (APA, 1994; Davidson, 2006). This core feature is understood to occur in circumstances in which the individual is observed by others, in the company of unfamiliar persons, or exposed to the possible scrutiny of others. The individual then fears that he or she may seem visibly anxious, do something to appear stupid or unfriendly, or offend others. As described in the text revision of the fourth edition of the *Diagnostic and Statistical Manual of Mental Disorders* (*DSM–IV–TR*), socially anxious individuals experience subjective and somatic symptomatology which may include blushing, trembling, palpitations, sweating, dry mouth, and inarticulate speech

(Davidson, 2006). These symptoms may cluster together as a panic attack evoked by the feared situation, prompting the affected individual to avoid the phobic situation or to endure it with intense distress. The anticipatory anxiety or distress, distorted thinking patterns, and avoidance behaviour significantly impair the person's social and occupational functioning (APA, 1994).

Individuals with SAD tend to avoid social relationships and are often unmarried (Liebowitz et al., 2005; Veale, 2003; Weiller et al., 1996). They commonly drop out of academic institutions, and may reject potentially lucrative work promotions. Numerous studies have confirmed the association of SAD with considerable social and occupational impairment (Kessler, Stein, & Berglund, 1998; Schneier et al., 1992; Wancata et al., 2009). Economic and healthcare costs cut across upper-, lower-, and middle-income countries alike, and are high. Costs incurred relate to health service uptake, loss of production, and out-of-pocket expenses to the individual (Liebowitz et al., 2005).

While adults may recognize this phobic distress as out of proportion with the actual danger posed by the social situation, children with SAD may not. In addition, children who meet the *DSM–IV* diagnostic criteria for this disorder must be able to form social relationships with people familiar to them, and must experience this anxiety in interactions with both adults and their peers. Crying, appearing paralyzed, emotional outbursts, and shrinking from social engagement may be evidence of SAD in children (APA, 1994).

Diagnostic criteria according to the *DSM–IV–TR* (APA, 1994) are as follows:

1. Marked, persistent fear of one or more social or performance situations in which the person is exposed to unfamiliar people or possible scrutiny by others. The individual fears that he or she will act in a way (or show anxiety symptoms) that will be humiliating or embarrassing. In children, there must be evidence of the capacity for age-appropriate social relationships with familiar people, and the anxiety must occur in peer settings, not only in interactions with adults.
2. Exposure to the feared social situation almost invariably provokes anxiety, which may take the form of a situationally bound or situationally predisposed panic attack. In children, the anxiety may be expressed by crying, tantrums, freezing, or shrinking from social situations with unfamiliar people.
3. The person recognizes that the fear is excessive or unreasonable. In children, this feature may be absent.
4. The feared social or performance situations are avoided or else are endured with intense anxiety or distress.
5. The avoidance, anxious anticipation, or distress in the feared social or performance situation(s) interferes significantly with the person's normal routine, occupational (academic) functioning, or social activities or relationships, or there is marked distress about having the phobia.

6. In individuals under age 18 years, the duration is at least 6 months.
7. The fear or avoidance is not due to the direct physiological effects of a substance (e.g., a drug of abuse, a medication) or a general medical condition and is not better accounted for by another mental disorder (e.g., panic disorder with or without agoraphobia, separation anxiety disorder, body dysmorphic disorder, a pervasive developmental disorder, or schizoid personality disorder).
8. If a general medical condition or another mental disorder is present, the social or performance fear is unrelated to it—for example, the fear is not of stuttering, trembling in Parkinson's disease, or exhibiting abnormal eating behavior in anorexia nervosa or bulimia nervosa.

A *DSM–5* Work Group is responsible for addressing revisions to the *DSM–IV–TR*. Proposed changes include terminology that is consistent, less ambiguous, and relevant to the sociocultural context (Bogels et al., 2010). The definition of various social situations has been broadened and clarified. For instance, the words "observation" and "interaction" have been added to reflect research demonstrating the different types of social anxiety situations. The criterion regarding "humiliation and embarrassment" has been replaced with the statement "cause negative evaluation." The concept of offending others has also been included to enhance cultural sensitivity, as found in *taijin kyofusho*, a condition in Japanese populations. Here the focus is on causing offense to others, rather than embarrassing oneself (Davidson, 2006). Some authors argue that this condition encompasses aspects of a delusional disorder, somatic type, which would differentiate it from SAD (D. J. Stein, Le Roux, Bouwer, & Van Heerden, 1998).

In the *DSM–IV–TR*, SAD has been subtyped into a generalized form, in which the phobic situation includes most social interactions, and a nongeneralized form (APA, 1994). The generalized subtype is more severe and is associated with greater comorbidity and impairment (Bogels et al., 2010). Selective mutism is a discrete clinical entity that has been described predominantly in children who consistently refuse to speak in specific social situations where there is an expectation to speak (e.g., in a school setting) despite speaking in other situations (APA, 1994).

SAD has significant comorbidities, most notably with depression and substance use disorders, especially alcohol use disorders (Schneier et al., 1992; Weiller et al., 1996). Other co-occurring conditions include other anxiety disorders, bulimia nervosa, general medical illnesses, and certain personality disorders (Davidson, 2006).

It is important to differentiate the symptoms in SAD from normal shyness and psychotic disorders (the anxiety in SAD is not of a delusional intensity). In SAD, the anxiety symptoms precede any comorbid depressive features.

Decreased rates of treatment-seeking are evident in SAD, with fewer than 50% of those with SAD presenting to a healthcare provider (Thompson, Hunt, & Issakidis, 2004; Wancata et al., 2009; Weiller et al, 1996). An Australian study identified a lack of knowledge about mental illness and available treatment as the predominant reason for delayed presentation to services (Thompson et al., 2004). Another possible barrier to help-seeking may be self-consciousness at having to undergo an evaluation, and the fear of not being taken seriously. The primary care practitioner is often the first contact for patients with SAD, and time to presentation can be decades long (Thompson et al., 2004; Weiller et al., 1996). Owing to the nature of the disorder, individuals may be reluctant to volunteer symptoms. Self-report measures such as the Liebowitz Social Anxiety Scale, the Brief Social Phobia Scale, and the Social Phobia Inventory may facilitate the assessment process by quantifying severity (Veale, 2003).

An emerging evidence base is helping to inform the compilation and publication of treatment guidelines and algorithms. Options for management of SAD include medication alone, psychotherapeutic measures, or combination treatment. There is no evidence at present to indicate what factors could be used to determine response to treatment.

SOLITARY TREATMENT APPROACHES

Pharmacological Treatment

The pharmacotherapy of SAD was given significant impetus by the early finding that monoamine oxidase inhibitors (MAOIs) were more efficacious than tricyclic antidepressants (TCAs).

The introduction of selective serotonin reuptake inhibitors (SSRIs) led to a marked increase in clinical trials in SAD, and these agents were found to be safe and effective. Indeed, first-line medication in the treatment of SAD currently comprises an SSRI or a serotonin–norepinephrine reuptake inhibitor (SNRI) (Guastella, Howard, Dadds, Mitchell, & Carson, 2009).

A systematic review of randomized controlled trials (RCTs) on the pharmacotherapy of SAD suggests that SSRIs are generally well tolerated, safe, and effective for the anxiety symptoms as well as for the associated comorbidities in SAD (Bandelow, Seidler-Brandler, Becker, Wedekind, & Rüther, 2007). Response rates of up to 60% have been reported with SSRIs (Allgulander, 1999; Baldwin, Bobes, Stein, Scharwächter, & Faure, 1999; Davidson, 2006; Katzelnick, 1995; van Vliet, den Boer, & Westenberg, 1994). Sertraline and paroxetine have received approval by the U.S. Food and Drug Administration (FDA) for the treatment of SAD. There may be some evidence for differences in efficacy between groups, but the lack of within-group direct comparisons between these SSRIs prevents a firm conclusion (Van Ameringen et al., 2001).

Several short-term RCTs showed paroxetine to be more effective than placebo in reducing social anxiety (Allgulander, 1995; Baldwin et al., 1999; Book, Thomas, Randall, & Randall, 2008). Sexual side effects and a discontinuation syndrome were some of the adverse effects reported in these trials. One RCT which included patients with co-occurring alcohol use disorders noted superiority of paroxetine over placebo in improving SAD symptoms but not in reducing drinking outcomes (Book et al., 2008; Randall et al., 2001). An open-label study of controlled-release formulation of paroxetine also confirmed its efficacy over placebo in the more severe generalized subtype of SAD (M. B. Stein et al., 1996).

Three large RCTs indicated that sertraline is more effective than placebo in the treatment of fear, avoidance, and physiological arousal in SAD (Blomhoff et al., 2001; Katzelnick et al., 1995; Van Ameringen et al., 2001). Sertraline also led to significant improvement in occupational function (Van Ameringen et al., 2001).

Fluvoxamine was studied in a small number of RCTs, all of which demonstrated its separation from placebo on multiple outcome measures (Asakura, Tajima, & Koyama, 2007; Davidson, Yaryura-Tobias et al., 2004; M. B. Stein, Fyer, Davidson, Pollack, & Wiita, 1999; Westenberg, Stein, Yang, Li, & Barbato, 2004). Studies in which controlled-release formulation of fluvoxamine was used recommended that a longer treatment period was needed to achieve and sustain symptom remission, as most of the fluvoxamine-treated patients remained symptomatic at the end point of the study (Davidson, Yaryra-Tobias et al., 2004; Westenberg, 2004).

Several open trials have indicated the efficacy of fluoxetine in the treatment of SAD (Fairbanks et al., 1997; Perugi et al., 1995; Van Ameringen, Mancini, & Streiner, 1993), but one short-term RCT found that it failed to separate from placebo (Kobak, Greist, Jefferson, & Katzelnick, 2002). A case report and an open trial of citalopram also suggested that this agent is more effective than placebo (Bouwer & Stein, 1998). Escitalopram was found to be effective, safe, and well tolerated in three trials (Bouwer & Stein, 1998; Kasper, Stein, Loft, & Nil, 2005; Montgomery, Nil, Durr-Pal, Loft, & Boulenger, 2005).

Very few direct comparisons have been made within the SSRI group or with other medication classes in the treatment of SAD. A longer trial comparing escitalopram and paroxetine demonstrated the statistically significant superiority of both agents over placebo. The escitalopram doses were flexible (5–20 mg), with the highest dose being more efficacious than a fixed 20 mg dose of paroxetine (in most secondary outcome measures in both short and long-term treatment; Lader, Stender, Bürger, & Nil, 2004). A short RCT evaluating venlafaxine extended release (ER) and paroxetine found that while venlafaxine ER was more efficacious than paroxetine and placebo in the short term (weeks 1 and 2), paroxetine was superior to both venlafaxine ER and placebo in the longer term (week 3 onwards) (Allgulander et al., 2004; Liebowitz et al., 2005).

The SNRI venlafaxine has also been approved by the FDA for treatment of SAD, and has evidence to suggest its efficacy and tolerability over placebo in the acute phase and short-term treatment (Rickels, Mangano, & Khan, 2004). A discontinuation syndrome has also been described with venlafaxine.

A highly selective noradrenaline reuptake inhibitor, atomoxetine, used in the treatment of attention deficit hyperactivity disorder, was not found to be superior to placebo in the treatment of generalized social anxiety disorder (Ravindran, Kim, Letamendi, & Stein, 2009).

In the past, four studies established the efficacy of the irreversible monoamine oxidase inhibitor phenelzine in the treatment of SAD (Blanco, Antia, & Liebowitz, 2002). Dietary restrictions and concerns about the development of a tyrosine-driven hypertensive crisis have limited its use in clinical practice. Nevertheless, comparisons with atenolol have shown phenelzine to be superior to the beta-blocker as well as to pill placebo (Liebowitz et al., 1992). The reversible, selective monoamine oxidase inhibitor (RIMA) moclobemide is effective in treating symptoms of SAD but is not available in all countries.

Benzodiazepines are known to possess anxiolytic properties. Alprazolam, bromazepam, and clonazepam have all been studied in double-blind trials and found to alleviate physiological symptoms of SAD. Owing to concerns about their potential for abuse and dependence, diversion, and toxicity in overdose, benzodiazepines are not considered first-line therapies for SAD (Connor et al., 1998; Stahl, 2008; D. J. Stein et al., 2010).

Although they are often recommended for specific phobia, there is relatively little evidence to support the use of the cardioselective beta-blockers atenolol and propranolol in this condition (D. B. Clark & Agras, 1991).

Other antidepressants studied less commonly in SAD include the tetracyclic mirtazapine and nefazodone (Muehlbacher et al., 2005; Van Ameringen et al., 2007). Mirtazapine may be efficacious in the treatment of SAD on the basis of one RCT conducted in a female population, but more work is required in this area (Muehlbacher et al., 2005). While three open trials suggested that nefazodone may be efficacious in treating generalized SAD, a recent RCT identified a lack of superiority over placebo, as well as a high risk of hepatotoxicity (Van Ameringen et al., 2007).

While a few open trials have suggested that the 5HT1A-agonist buspirone may be modestly efficacious in the pharmacotherapy of SAD, an RCT did not support the findings of these open trials (van Vliet, den Boer, Westenberg, & Pian, 1997).

Studies of the second-generation antipsychotics olanzapine and quetiapine produced mixed results in SAD. A pilot study and placebo-controlled trial of olanzapine in SAD showed its efficacy on some primary outcomes. A pilot study of quetiapine monotherapy failed to show statistically significant on primary outcome measures but produced some improvement on secondary endpoint measures. There is some evidence that these agents are useful in treatment-resistant SAD (Barnett, Kramer, Casat, Connor, & Davidson, 2002; Vaishnavi, Alamy, Zhang, Connor, & Davidson, 2007).

Novel compounds such as the alpha-2-delta calcium channel blockers pregabalin and gabapentin, and the anticonvulsant topiramate, appear promising in the treatment of generalized SAD but require more studies in order for robust conclusions to be drawn (Pande et al., 1999; 2004).

While preclinical evidence has suggested that a neurokinin-1 receptor antagonist may produce substantial anxiolysis, a clinical trial comparing it to paroxetine and placebo showed that paroxetine was superior to both (Tauscher et al., 2009).

Two pilot studies of the anticonvulsant levetiracetam found that, while it was well tolerated, it failed to separate from placebo (M. B. Stein et al., 2010).

Tiagabine, a selective γ-aminobutyric acid (GABA) reuptake inhibitor, was studied in a pilot trial with an open-label design for 12 weeks, after which responders could enter a relapse withdrawal prevention arm (Dunlop et al., 2007). Tiagabine is understood to inhibit the GABA transporter, thereby blocking GABA reuptake selectively from the synaptic cleft and increasing its availability in the cleft (Allgulander et al., 2004).

A Cochrane review of medications for SAD concluded that SSRIs are the most studied and efficacious for the treatment of SAD (Bandelow et al., 2007), and RIMAs, to a lesser extent. At present there is limited evidence for the use of other agents (Stein, Ipser, & van Balkom, 2009).

Benefits of sole pharmacological interventions for SAD are a relatively rapid reduction in symptom severity and cost effectiveness (Sadock & Sadock, 2003). Delayed onset of action of some medications, potential side effects, and relapse after treatment discontinuation may all be viewed as limitations of pharmacotherapy.

Clinical Vignette: Good outcome with pharmacotherapy

Steven was a happily married 46-year-old man who had enjoyed his position as a university laboratory technician for 10 years. He had written textbooks and papers in his field, but had never been expected to teach the students directly. However, 18 months ago a more senior colleague took partial retirement, and Steven's duties expanded to include giving lectures and demonstrations to students. These expectations caused him great distress, as he would be required to stand in front of a group of 8–10 students at a time, explaining and demonstrating the intricacies of chemical experiments. Steven was concerned about his hands visibly shaking, and appearing incompetent. His psychiatrist advised a reduction in caffeine and nicotine use, and initiated an SSRI, escitalopram, at a low dose. Steven was fortunate not to experience any side effects, and was able to manage the somatic symptoms of his performance anxiety. He chose to remain on the medication for a year, during which time his confidence in his ability to lecture in public improved. Thereafter the medication was successfully tapered off, and Steven was able to continue his job without psychotropic agents.

Clinical Vignette: Poor outcome with pharmacotherapy

Theresa was a 29-year-old woman who decided to commit to full-time stand-up comedy after years of consistent work attendance at a customer call center. Though Theresa was aware of her social discomfort around others, she felt that this comedy act was a calling which she wanted to explore. On her first few impromptu appearances, she was too nervous to attempt her skit, fearing being heckled and humiliated. She did, however, observe the reception some of the other comedians received. These observations evoked palpitations, tremulousness, sweaty palms, and a tremendous loss of confidence. After approaching her general practitioner for assistance, Theresa was prescribed a short course of the beta-blocker propranolol to take as needed. Over the next few evenings she took to the stage after ingesting first 30 mg of propranolol, and then 60 mg. In both instances, Theresa was paralyzed, lightheaded, and unable to recall her lines. She remained very worried about embarrassing herself. While the crowd jeered, she fled the stage and reluctantly returned to her previous position as a call centre agent, where she was not expected to face customers directly.

Psychosocial Treatment

There is a growing knowledge base regarding psychosocial treatments for social anxiety disorder. Of the evidence available, behavioral and cognitive-behavioral therapies (CBT) are the best-studied and most widely practiced non-pharmacological treatments for SAD (D. M. Clark et al., 2003; Sadock & Sadock, 2003). While most of the work is non-comparative, several studies have shown CBT to be as efficacious as pharmacotherapy in both the short term and the longer term (D. M. Clark et al., 2003; Heimberg, 2002). Recent research suggests that individual CBT is superior to that in a group setting (Heimberg,

2002). CBT is a short-term, highly structured, and manualized psychotherapy that focuses on the present. This goal-oriented approach to interpersonal and intrapsychic difficulties seeks to identify, challenge, and modify thinking patterns in order to effect mood and behavior changes. The therapist and client form a collaborative team, employing various techniques over a period of 12–16 weeks. Sessions typically last for 45–60 minutes. Components of CBT include (Sadock & Sadock, 2003):

1. *Situational and implosion exposure.* In situational exposure therapy a hierarchy of feared situations is compiled and systematically mastered, from the least to the most anxiety-provoking. The goal is for the client to tolerate increasing levels of anxiety in order to encourage the natural conditioning process to result in extinction. The therapist makes use of imagery, role play, or gradual, serial exposure to the actual, feared stimulus to desensitize the client to each stimulus on the scale. Flooding therapy involves exposing the client to the actual phobic stimulus in its full intensity in order for the client to learn to tolerate the feared situation. Medication and progressive muscle relaxation techniques can be used to augment the process.

2. *Cognitive restructuring.* People with SAD often overestimate the danger involved in social situations and underestimate their ability to cope in such situations. Additionally, they personalize others' social responses, affording these responses more significance than they might truly carry in relation to their performance. Cognitive retraining seeks to identify such dysfunctional thoughts, evaluate the evidence in support of these thoughts using a range of behavioral experiments (e.g., self-monitoring diaries), and replace these with more balanced, rational cognitions.

3. *Relaxation training.* The physiological symptoms of SAD can be attenuated by progressive muscle relaxation after identification and recognition of these symptoms by the individual. Coupled with breathing exercises, relaxation can be induced *in vivo* to enable the anxious individual to cope in the event that they cannot avoid or escape the feared situation.

4. *Social skills training (SST).* The premise of this intervention is based on the hypothesis that individuals with social anxiety disorder display impaired socialization skills such as aversive eye contact. Techniques include education and enhancement of awareness, modeling of appropriate social behavior by the therapist, role play and rehearsal during sessions, constructive audiovisual feedback, and a range of homework assignments. There is little evidence to support the use of SST in the treatment of SAD (Ponniah & Hollon, 2008).

While cognitive-behavioral group therapy has been compared with various pharmacotherapeutic agents and wait-list controls in robust trials, only two head-to-head comparisons appear to have been made between CBT and other

psychotherapeutic measures (Cottraux et al., 2000; Stangier, Schramm, Heidenreich, Berger, & Clark, 2011).

One open study compared the efficacy of CBT with educational-supportive
therapy, proving that CBT is superior (Heimberg et al., 1998). A large recent
RCT found CBT to be more efficacious than interpersonal therapy, with both
therapies maintaining improvement in symptoms of SAD at 1-year follow-up
(Stangier et al., 2011).

Individuals with SAD are understood to have heightened sensitivity to, and
negative cognitions about, perceived socially threatening cues in the form of
facial expression and social behaviours (Sadock & Sadock, 2003). Attentional
training is a treatment modality that attempts to reduce emotional reactivity by
distracting the affected person from these anxiety-inducing cues. Neutral, non-
threatening stimuli are employed to facilitate this emotional disengagement.
The findings of a recent small RCT comparing an attention modification program with an attention control condition indicated a possible reduction in
social anxiety associated with attention training, which was maintained at
16-week follow-up (Amir et al., 2009).

An open trial conducted more than a decade ago examined the efficacy of
interpersonal psychotherapy in a small sample. This type of therapy is time-
limited and based on the assumption that psychiatric disorders arise and are
maintained within an interpersonal environment. It is administered to patients
with mood and eating disorders. This therapy was found to be well accepted by
individuals with SAD and to have an efficacy comparable to that of CBT (Lipsitz, Markowitz, Cherry, & Fyer, 1999). However, the improvement noted was
not as rapid as that obtained with phenelzine.

Although effect sizes of the most psychotherapies of CBT are moderate in
comparison to pharmacotherapy, they appear to be maintained during the follow-up period (Hofmann, 2004). The advantages of psychotherapy include
better tolerability, greater likelihood of maintaining response after treatment
has been terminated, and cost-effectiveness in some settings (Sadock & Sadock,
2003; Veale, 2003). Limitations of psychotherapy encompass structural barriers
to treatment such as language and transportation, lack of access to psychotherapeutic services and long wait lists, a slower response of symptom to treatment,
and the time-consuming nature of these treatments.

Clinical Vignette: Good outcome with psychotherapy

Angela was a 19-year-old unmarried university student who was pursuing
a Bachelor's degree with a major in English literature. Once a semester,
each student would be expected to recite a short piece of prose to a class
of approximately 25 others. Despite a history of feeling unable to speak in

public, Angela had not sought treatment until it became evident that a large percentage of her end-of-year mark would be determined by these regular prose recitals. She reported feeling increasingly nervous whenever she thought of the impending recital in 3 months' time. She confided being afraid of saying something stupid or freezing up in front of her classmates. Angela recalled feeling this way throughout her school career, and during the test for her driving license. On presentation to the campus wellness center she impressed as very motivated and committed to addressing these fears, recognizing them as extreme and impairing. The student counselor suggested a brief intervention based on the cognitive model. After a few individual sessions, Angela had identified and challenged her inaccurate beliefs that nothing she had to say was worth listening to, and had learned methods of relaxation. Her self-esteem and confidence were noted to be improved and she was able to recite her piece with only some discomfort. Since Angela was fortunate enough to have received recordings of the therapy sessions, she was able to refer repeatedly to these in preparation for subsequent recitals.

Clinical Vignette: Poor outcome with psychotherapy

Mary was a fairly successful sales executive working in a large company that specialized in carpet manufacture. Since starting her job 2 years ago, she had coped with marketing and selling her merchandise to clients over the telephone. Prior to making these calls, Mary would attempt to steady her nerves by smoking cigarettes and drinking copious cups of strong coffee. Six months ago her job description was expanded to include face-to-face sales in which she was expected to secure appointments with potential retailers, and present samples to interested parties in order to complete the sale. Mary had noted a growing sense of dread every morning before work, which had often resulted in lateness and even absenteeism from work. On the days when she forced herself to attend these appointments, she would blush furiously, stammer through her sales pitch, and sweat profusely and visibly. Mary declined the offer of medication from her general practitioner, but agreed to see a therapist. After almost 3 months of individual CBT she denied feeling any better, and in fact began to despair. She resigned from her position at work a short time thereafter.

COMBINED THERAPY

There are relatively few direct comparisons of pharmacotherapy and psychotherapy in SAD (Bandelow et al., 2007). Some studies have compared a drug with a placebo condition while others have compared a psychological treatment with a psychological placebo, a wait-list control, or another psychosocial treatment.

Of the eight RCTs directly comparing the two treatment modalities in SAD, all psychosocial interventions administered were CBT based. Two RCTs compared the monoamine oxidase inhibitor phenelzine and cognitive-behavioral group therapy (CBGT) (Allgulander et al., 2004; Blanco et al., 2010). In the first study, phenelzine was superior to CBGT and both were more efficacious than placebo. When the two modalities were compared to each other alone, against a pill placebo, against an educational-supportive psychotherapy, and in combination, combined phenelzine and CBGT proved superior to either modality on its own, and to the control conditions on some measures, including response rate (Cottraux et al., 2000).

The efficacy of social skills training combined with the cardioselective beta-blocker propranolol was compared with social skills training plus inert placebo under controlled conditions (Heimberg, 2002). Both subgroups showed similar improvements on outcome measures, with both groups maintaining treatment gains at 6-month follow-up.

Another RCT examined whether busipirone alone or in combination with CBT was superior to CBT or pill placebo alone, but yielded disappointing results for buspirone. CBT alone, however, resulted in improvement in SAD symptoms in the same study.

A fourth study looked at efficacy of CBT versus fluoxetine and found that patients treated with CBT alone improved significantly more than those who received self-exposure instructions combined with either fluoxetine or pill placebo. The fact that self-exposure alone did not prove as effective as CBT suggests the importance of the cognitive restructuring component. In addition, treatment gains in the CBT-only group were maintained a year later (D. M. Clark et al., 2003).

Sertraline and exposure therapy were compared in a Scandinavian study conducted in a general practice setting. Sertraline was well tolerated and superior to placebo when used either alone or in combination with exposure therapy, while exposure therapy alone failed to separate from placebo in the short term. Combined sertraline and exposure therapy was superior to medication alone and to placebo. Patients treated with either exposure therapy alone or placebo showed further improvement in SAD symptoms up to a year after treatment cessation, while the sertraline-only and combined sertraline–exposure groups deteriorated in the longer term. This strengthens the evidence for the role of CBT in long-term relapse prevention of SAD (Blomhoff et al., 2001).

Lastly, a study in which clonazepam and cognitive-behavioral group therapy were compared found that both were effacious treatments in the acute phase of SAD (Otto et al., 2000).

In one trial, flooding was shown to be superior to both placebo and the beta-blocker atenolol in the reduction of negative cognitions and symptoms of SAD (Turner, Beidel, & Jacob, 1994).

Research has examined the novel agents intranasal oxytocin and D-cycloserine in the augmentation of exposure therapy for SAD (Guastella et al., 2009; Hofmann et al., 2006). Oxytocin is thought to mediate social behavior by facilitating emotional attachment. Patients with SAD treated with oxytocin augmentation of exposure therapy showed improvement in the speech performance measures compared with the placebo group, although this improvement was lost at follow-up (Guastella et al., 2009). The partial NMDA-receptor agonist D-cycloserine is postulated to be instrumental in enhancing memory and learning associated with the fear circuit by modifying the extinction process. A pilot study suggested the superiority of D-cycloserine over placebo in short-term augmentation of exposure therapy in SAD (Hofmann et al., 2006).

Future research should focus on patients with significant comorbidities, and combination therapies. Longer trials are required to confirm the role of different therapies in the maintenance of treatment gains found in short-term and relapse prevention studies. More work on the role of atypical antipsychotic agents and other medication classes in treatment-resistant SAD needs to be undertaken. Psychotherapeutic modalities other than CBT for the treatment of SAD require investigation. Larger studies are required to further elucidate the efficacy of D-cycloserine and other adjuncts (such as oxytocin) to exposure-based therapy. Treatment of SAD in special groups such as children, elderly people, and pregnant women continues to pose a unique challenge.

Clinical Vignette: Combined treatment

Brad was a 42-year-old divorced father of four who was self-employed as an engineer. When his company expanded to employ five junior engineers, he described extreme discomfort whenever he had to address his employees. His heart would pound, his voice would start to shake, and he would worry that the other engineers were laughing at him behind his back. On one occasion, Brad was even sure that he would faint. Spurred on by the desire to improve working relations, he approached his family doctor for assistance. Given the severity of symptoms, the presence of subsyndromal depression, and the need for an immediate and sustained response, Brad's doctor decided to combine medical and psychosocial treatments. The patient accepted a course of citalopram, coupled with CBT administered by the trained therapist at the practice. Within a month, Brad was able to sit in the company lunchroom with his employees, and felt able to hold short conversations with the group. He felt hopeful that his anxiety would be significantly reduced after a prolonged period of treatment.

Clinical Points to Remember

1. Social anxiety disorder (SAD) is a highly prevalent psychiatric illness that is associated with significant impairment if left untreated.
2. Onset frequently occurs at adolescence, and thereafter the course is chronic.
3. SAD is often under-recognized and undertreated, with many affected individuals reluctant to seek medical attention.
4. This common anxiety disorder carries great comorbidity, thus complicating symptom presentation and treatment response.
5. Individuals with social anxiety disorder shrink from social contact for fear of humiliating or embarrassing themselves.
6. Two types of social anxiety disorder have been identified: generalized and non-generalized. The generalized type is more pervasive and more severe.
7. There is robust evidence for effective treatments, both pharmacological and non-pharmacological.
8. Of the medications shown to be efficacious, SSRIs are the best studied, and are an accepted first-line treatment in the short term and in the longer term.
9. Of the psychotherapies shown to be efficacious, cognitive-behavioral therapy is the best studied and is an accepted first-line treatment.
10. There are clinical indications for combining or sequencing SSRIs or CBT; for example, it is possible that CBT is useful in preventing relapse during pharmacotherapy withdrawal.

REFERENCES

Allgulander, C. (1999). Paroxetine in social anxiety disorder: A randomized placebo-controlled study. *Acta Psychiatrica Scandinavica, 100,* 193–198.

Allgulander, C., Mangano, R., Zhang, J., Dahl, A. A., Lepola, U., Sjödin, I., & Emilien, G. (2004). Efficacy of Venlafaxine ER in patients with social anxiety disorder: A double-blind, placebo-controlled, parallel-group comparison with paroxetine. *Human Psychopharmacology: Clinical and Experimental, 19,* 387–396.

American Psychiatric Association (APA). (1994). *Diagnostic and statistical manual of mental disorders* (4th ed.). Washington, DC: APA.

Amir, N., Beard, C., Taylor, C. T., Klumpp, H., Elias, J., Burns, M., & Chen, X. (2009). Attention training in individuals with generalized social phobia: A randomized controlled trial. *Journal of Consulting and Clinical Psychology, 77,* 961–973.

Asakura, S., Tajima, O., & Koyama, T. (2007). Fluvoxamine treatment of generalized social anxiety disorder in Japan: A randomized double-blind, placebo-controlled study. *International Journal of Neuropsychopharmacology, 10,* 263–274.

Baldwin, D., Bobes, J., Stein, D. J., Scharwächter, I., & Faure, M. (1999). Paroxetine in social phobia/social anxiety disorder: Randomised, double-blind, placebo-controlled study. Paroxetine Study Group. *British Journal of Psychiatry, 175,* 120–126.

Bandelow, B., Seidler-Brandler, U., Becker, A., Wedekind, D., & Rüther, E. (2007). Meta-analysis of randomized controlled comparisons of psychopharmacological and psychological treatments for anxiety disorders. *World Journal of Biological Psychiatry, 8,* 175–187.

Barnett, S. D., Kramer, M. L., Casat, C. D., Connor, K. M., & Davidson, J. R. T. (2002). Efficacy of olanzapine in social anxiety disorder: A pilot study. *Journal of Psychopharmacology, 16,* 365–368.

Blanco, C., Antia, S. X., & Liebowitz, M. R. (2002). Pharmacotherapy of social anxiety disorder. *Biological Psychiatry, 51,* 109–120.

Blanco, C., Heimberg, R. G., Schneier, F. R., Fresco, D. M., Chen, H., Turk, C. L., et al. (2010). A placebo-controlled trial of phenelzine, cognitive behavioral group therapy, and their combination for social anxiety disorder. *Archives of General Psychiatry, 67,* 286–295.

Blomhoff, S., Haug, T. T., Hellström, K., Holme, I., Humble, M., Madsbu, H. P., & Wold, J. E. (2001). Randomised controlled general practice trial of sertraline, exposure therapy and combined treatment in generalised social phobia. *British Journal of Psychiatry, 179,* 23–30.

Bogels, S. M., Alden, L., Beidel, D. C., Clark, L. A., Pine, D. C., Stein, M. B., & Voncken, M. (2010). Social anxiety disorder: questions and answers for the DSM-V. *Depression and Anxiety, 27,* 168–189.

Book, S. W., Thomas, S. E., Randall, P. K., & Randall, C. L. (2008). Paroxetine reduces social anxiety in individuals with co-occurring alcohol use disorder. *Journal of Anxiety Disorders, 22,* 310–318.

Bouwer, C., & Stein, D. J. (1998). Use of the selective serotonin reuptake inhibitor citalopram in the treatment of generalized social phobia. *Journal of Affective Disorders, 49,* 79–82.

Clark, D. B., & Agras, W. S. (1991). The assessment and treatment of performance anxiety in musicians. *American Journal of Psychiatry, 148,* 598–605.

Clark, D. M., Ehlers, A., McManus, F., Hackmann, A., Fennell, M., Campbell, H., et al. (2003). Cognitive therapy versus fluoxetine in generalized social phobia: A randomized placebo-controlled trial. *Journal of Consulting and Clinical Psychology, 71,* 1058–1067.

Connor, K. M., Davidson, J. R. T., Potts, N. L. S., Tupler, L. A., Miner, C. M., Malik, M. L., et al. (1998). Discontinuation of clonazepam in the treatment of social phobia. *Journal of Clinical Psychopharmacology, 18*, 373–378.

Cottraux, J., Note, I., Albuisson, E., Yao, S. N., Note, B., Mollard, E., et al. (2000). Cognitive behavior therapy versus supportive therapy in social phobia: A randomized controlled trial. *Psychotherapy and Psychosomatics, 39*, 137–146.

Davidson, J. R. T. (2006). Pharmacotherapy of social anxiety disorder: What does the evidence tell us? *Journal of Clinical Psychiatry, 67*, 20–26.

Davidson, J. R. T., Foa, E. B., Huppert, J. D., Keefe, F. J., Franklin, M. E., Compton, J. S., et al. (2004). Fluoxetine, comprehensive cognitive behavioral therapy, and placebo in generalized social phobia. *Archives of General Psychiatry, 61*, 1005–1013.

Davidson, J., Yaryura-Tobias, J., DuPont, R., Stallings, L., Barbato, L. M., van der Hoop, R. G., & Li, D. (2004). Fluvoxamine-controlled release formulation for the treatment of generalized social anxiety disorder. *Journal of Clinical Psychopharmacology, 24*, 118–125.

Dunlop, B. W., Papp, L., Garlow, S. J., Weiss, P. S., Knight, B. T., & Ninan, P. T. (2007). Tiagabine for social anxiety disorder. *Human Psychopharmacology: Clinical and Experimental, 22*, 241–244.

Fairbanks, J. M., Pine, D. S., Tancer, N. K., Dummit, E. S. III, Kentgen, L. M., Martin, J., et al. (1997). Open fluoxetine treatment of mixed anxiety disorders in children and adolescents. *Journal of Child and Adolescent Psychopharmacology, 7*, 17–29.

Guastella, A. J., Howard, A. L., Dadds, M. R., Mitchell, P., & Carson, D. S. (2009). A randomized controlled trial of intranasal oxytocin as an adjunct to exposure therapy for social anxiety disorder. *Psychoneuroendocrinology, 34*, 917–923.

Heimberg, R. G. (2002). Cognitive-behavioral therapy for social anxiety disorder: Current status and future directions. *Society of Biological Psychiatry, 51*, 101–108.

Heimberg, R. G., Liebowitz, M. R., Hope, D. A., Schneier, F. R., Holt, C. S., Welkowitz, L. A., et al. (1998). Cognitive behavioral group therapy vs phenelzine therapy for social phobia 12-week outcome. *Archives of General Psychiatry, 55*, 1133–1141.

Hofmann, S. G. (2004). Cognitive mediation of treatment change in social phobia. *Journal of Consulting and Clinical Psychology, 72*, 392–399.

Hofmann, S. G., Meuret, A. E., Smits, J. A. J., Simon, N. M., Pollack, M. H., Eisenmenger, K., et al. (2006). Augmentation of exposure therapy with D-cycloserine for social anxiety disorder. *Archives of General Psychiatry, 63*, 298–304.

Kasper, S., Stein, D. J., Loft, H., & Nil, R. (2005). Escitalopram in the treatment of social anxiety disorder: Randomised, placebo-controlled, flexible-dosage study. *British Journal of Psychiatry, 186*, 222–226.

Katzelnick, D. J., Kobak, K. A., Greist, J. H., Jefferson, J. W., Mantle, J. M., & Serlin, R. C. (1995). Sertraline for social phobia: A double-blind, placebo-controlled crossover study. *American Journal of Psychiatry, 152*, 1368–1371.

Kessler, R. C., McGonagle, K. A., Zhao, S., Nelson, C. B., Hughes, M., Eshleman, S., et al. (1994). Lifetime and 12-month prevalence of *DSM-III-R* psychiatric disorders in the United States: Results from the National Comorbidity Survey. *Archives of General Psychiatry, 51*, 8–19.

Kessler, R. C., Stein, M. B., & Berglund, P. (1998). Social phobia subtypes in the National Comorbidity Survey. *American Journal of Psychiatry, 155*, 613–619.

Kobak, K. A., Greist, J. H., Jefferson, J. W., & Katzelnick, D. J. (2002). Fluoxetine in social phobia: A double-blind, placebo-controlled pilot study. *Journal of Clinical Psychopharmacology, 22*, 257–262.

Lader, M., Stender, K., Bürger, V., & Nil, R. (2004). Efficacy and tolerability of escitalopram in 12- and 24-week treatment of social anxiety disorder: Randomised, double-blind, placebo-controlled, fixed-dose study. *Depression and Anxiety, 19*, 241–248.

Liebowitz, M. R., Gelenberg, A. J., & Munjack, D. (2005). Venlafaxine extended release vs placebo and paroxetine in social anxiety disorder. *Archives of General Psychiatry, 62*, 190–198.

Liebowitz, M. R., Schneier, F. R., Campeas, R., Hollander, E., Hatterer, J., Fyer, A., et al. (1992). Phenelzine vs atenolol in social phobia: A placebo-controlled comparison. *Archives of General Psychiatry, 49*, 290–300.

Lipsitz, J. D., Markowitz, J. C., Cherry, S., & Fyer, A. J. (1999). Open trial of interpersonal psychotherapy for the treatment of social phobia. *American Journal of Psychiatry, 156*, 1814–1816.

Montgomery, S. A., Nil, R., Durr-Pal, N., Loft, H., & Boulenger, J. P. (2005). A 24-week randomized, double-blind, placebo-controlled study of escitalopram for the prevention of generalized social anxiety disorder. *Journal of Clinical Psychiatry, 66*, 1270–1278.

Muehlbacher, M., Nickel, M. K., Nickel, C., Kettler, C., Lahmann, C., Gil, F. P., et al. (2005). Mirtazapine treatment of social phobia in women: a randomized, double-blind, placebo-controlled study. *Journal of Clinical Psychopharmacology, 25*, 580–583.

Otto, M. W., Pollack, M. H., Gould, R. A., Worthington, J. J., McArdle, E. T., Rosenbaum, J. F., & Heimberg, R. G. (2000). A comparison of the efficacy of clonazepam and cognitive-behavioral group therapy for the treatment of social phobia. *Journal of Anxiety Disorders, 14*, 345–358.

Pande, A. C., Davidson, J. R., Jefferson, J. W., Janney, C. A., Katzelnick, D. J., Weisler, R. H., et al. (1999). Treatment of social phobia with gabapentin: A placebo-controlled study. *Journal of Clinical Psychopharmacology, 19*, 341–348.

Pande, A. C., Feltner, D. E., Jefferson, J. W., Davidson, J. R. T., Pollack, M., Stein, M. B., et al. (2004). Efficacy of novel anxiolytic pregabalin in social anxiety disorder: A placebo-controlled, multicenter study. *Journal of Clinical Psychopharmacology, 24*, 141–149.

Perugi, G., Nassini, S., Lenzi, M., Simonini, E., Cassano, G. B., & McNair, D. M. (1995). Treatment of social phobia with fluoxetine. *Anxiety, 1*, 282–286.

Ponniah, K., & Hollon, S. D. (2008). Empirically supported psychological interventions for social phobia in adults: A qualitative review of randomized controlled trials. *Psychological Medicine, 38*, 3–14.

Randall, C. L., Johnson, M. R., Thevos, A. K., Sonne, S. C., Thomas, S. E., Willard, S. L., et al. (2001). Paroxetine for social anxiety and alcohol use in dual-diagnosed patients. *Depression and Anxiety, 14*, 255–262.

Ravindran, L. N., Kim, D. S., Letamendi, A. M., & Stein, M. B. (2009). A randomized controlled trial of atomoxetine in generalized social anxiety disorder. *Journal of Clinical Psychopharmacology, 29*, 561–564.

Rickels, K., Mangano, R., & Khan, A. (2004). A double-blind, placebo-controlled study of a flexible dose of venlafaxine ER in adult outpatients with generalized social anxiety disorder. *Journal of Clinical Psychopharmacology, 24,* 488–496.

Sadock, B. J., & Sadock, V. A. (2003). *Kaplan and Sadock's synopsis of psychiatry: Behavioral sciences/clinical psychiatry* (9th ed.). Philadelphia: Lippincott Williams & Wilkins.

Schneier, F. R., Johnson, J., Hornig, C. D., Liebowitz, M. R., & Weissman, M. M. (1992). Social phobia: Comorbidity and morbidity in an epidemiologic sample. *Archives of General Psychiatry, 49,* 282–288.

Stahl, S. M. (2008). *Stahl's essential psychopharmacology: Neuroscientific basis and practical applications* (3rd ed.). New York: Cambridge University Press.

Stangier, U., Schramm, E., Heidenreich, T., Berger, M., & Clark, D. M. (2011). Cognitive therapy vs interpersonal psychotherapy in social anxiety disorder: A randomized controlled trial. *Archives of General Psychiatry, 68,* 692–700.

Stein, D. J., Baldwin, D. S., Bandelow, B., Blanco, C., Fontenelle, L. F., Lee, S., et al. (2010). A 2010 evidence-based algorithm for the pharmacotherapy of social anxiety disorder. *Current Psychiatric Reports, 12,* 471–477.

Stein, D. J., Ipser, J. C., & van Balkom, A. J. (2009). *Pharmacotherapy for social anxiety disorder (review).* The Cochrane Library.

Stein, D. J., Le Roux, L., Bouwer, C., & Van Heerden, B. (1998). Is olfactory reference syndrome an obsessive-compulsive spectrum disorder? Two cases and a discussion. *Journal of Neuropsychiatry and Clinical Neuroscience, 10,* 96–99.

Stein, M. B., Chartier, M. J., Hazen, A. L., Kroft, C. D., Chale, R. A., Cote, D., & Walker, J. R. (1996). Paroxetine in the treatment of generalized social phobia: Open-label treatment and double-blind placebo-controlled discontinuation. *Journal of Clinical Psychopharmacology, 16,* 218–222.

Stein, M. B., Fyer, A. J., Davidson, J. R. T., Pollack, M. H., & Wiita, B. (1999). Fluvoxamine treatment of social phobia (social anxiety disorder): A double-blind, placebo-controlled study. *American Journal of Psychiatry, 156,* 756–760.

Stein, M. B., Ravindran, L. N., Simon, N. M., Liebowitz, M. R., Khan, A., Brawman-Mintzer, O., et al. (2010). Levetiracetam in generalized social anxiety disorder: A double-blind, randomized controlled trial. *Journal of Clinical Psychiatry, 71,* 627–631.

Tauscher, J., Kielbasa, W., Iyengar, S., Vandenhende, F., Peng, X., Mozley, D., et al. (2009). Development of 2nd generation neurokinin-1 receptor antagonist LY686017 for social anxiety disorder. *European Neuropsychopharmacology, 20,* 80–87.

Thompson, A., Hunt, C., & Issakidis, C. (2004). Why wait? Reasons for delay and prompts to seek help for mental health problems in an Australian clinical sample. *Social Psychiatry and Psychiatric Epidemiology, 39,* 810–817.

Turner, S. M., Beidel, D. C., & Jacob, R. G. (1994). Social phobia: A comparison of behavioral therapy and atenolol. *Journal of Consulting and Clinical Psychology, 62,* 350–358.

Turner, S. M., Beidel, D. C., & Wolff, P. L. (1996). Is behavioural inhibition related to the anxiety disorders? *Clinical Psychological Review, 16,* 157–172.

Vaishnavi, S., Alamy, S., Zhang, W., Connor, K. M., & Davidson, J. R. T. (2007). Quetiapine as monotherapy for social anxiety disorder: A placebo-controlled study. *Progress in Neuro-Psychopharmacology and Biological Psychiatry, 31,* 1464–1469.

Van Ameringen, M., Mancini, C., Oakman, J., Walker, J., Kjernisted, K., Choppa, P., et al. (2007). Nefazodone in the treatment of generalized social phobia: A randomized, placebo-controlled trial. *Journal of Clinical Psychiatry, 68*, 288–295.

Van Ameringen, M., Mancini, C., & Streiner, D. L. (1993). Fluoxetine efficacy in social phobia. *Journal of Clinical Psychiatry, 54*, 27–32.

Van Ameringen, M. A, Lane, R. M., Walker, J. R., Bowen, R. C., Chokka, P. R., Goldner, E., Swinson, R. P. (2001). Sertraline treatment of generalized social phobia: A 20-week, double-blind, placebo-controlled study. *American Journal of Psychiatry, 158*, 275–281.

van Vliet, I. M., den Boer, J. A., & Westenberg, H. G. M. (1994). Psychopharmacological treatment of social phobia: A double blind placebo controlled study with fluvoxamine. *Psychopharmacology, 115*, 128–134.

van Vliet, I. M., den Boer, J. A., Westenberg, H. G. M., & Pian, K. L. (1997). Clinical effects of buspirone in social phobia: A double-blind placebo-controlled study. *Journal of Clinical Psychiatry, 58*, 164–168.

Veale, D. (2003). Treatment of social phobia. *Advances in Psychiatric Treatment, 9*, 258–264.

Wancata, J., Fridl, M., & Friedrich, F. (2009). Social phobia: Epidemiology and health care. *Psychiatria Danubina, 21*, 520–524.

Weiller, E., Bisserbe, J. C., Boyer, P., Lepine, J. P., & Lecrubier, Y. (1996). Social phobia in general health care: An unrecognised undertreated disabling disorder. *British Journal of Psychiatry, 168*, 169–174.

Westenberg, H. G. M., Stein, D. J., Yang, H., Li, D., & Barbato, L. M. (2004). A double-blind placebo-controlled study of controlled release fluvoxamine for the treatment of generalized social anxiety disorder. *Journal of Clinical Psychopharmacology, 24*, 49–55.

CHAPTER 11

Specific Phobia

David S. Shearer, S. Cory Harmon, Robert D. Younger, and
Christopher S. Brown

INTRODUCTION

Specific phobia (SP), formerly called simple phobia (APA, 1980; 1987), is classified in the *DSM–IV–TR* as an anxiety disorder (APA, 2000). The hallmark of SP
is an irrational fear of a specific object or situation that the person realizes is
unreasonable. Exposure to this object or situation results in an intense anxiety
response, which sometimes results in a panic attack. The individual may avoid
the feared stimulus or tolerate it with significant anxiety and distress. Common
specific phobias include fear of spiders, flying, heights, tunnels, dental procedures, cramped spaces, seeing blood, having an injection by needle, and others.
The phobias are organized into five different subtypes: Animal Type, Natural
Environment Type, Blood-Injection-Injury (B-I-I) Type, Situational Type, and
Other (APA, 2000).

The onset of SP is typically in childhood or early adolescence; Situational
phobia and Natural Environment phobia may have a later onset ranging from
adolescence to young adulthood (Craske, Antony & Barlow, 2006; Becker et
al., 2007; Lipsitz, Barlow, Mannuzza, Hoffman, & Fyer, 2002). Several authors
have attempted to identify pathways to the development of SP, which may
include associative conditioning (direct, vicarious, or verbal acquisition), non-
associative (no direct or indirect association with feared stimulus), biological
(e.g., genetic), and informational or cognitive (e.g., being warned about stimulus by others) (Gamble, Harvey, & Rapee, 2010; Craske et al., 2006, Rachman,
1977). Variables that may predispose one to development of SP include exposure to traumatic events, being in the presence of others expressing fearfulness,
the occurrence of an unexpected panic attack while in the presence of the stimulus, or exposure to information that engenders fear of the stimulus (APA,
2000). Craske et al. (2006) suggest that given the right combination of experiences and individual factors, fears are likely to develop. Learning experiences,
both general and specific, may combine with genetics and other biological
variables to produce a specific phobia (Antony & Barlow, 2002).

Having one SP increases the likelihood that a person will have other phobias in their lifetime (Wittchen, Lecrubier, Beesdo, & Nocon, 2003; Curtis, Magee, Eaton, Wittchen, & Kessler, 1998). Natural-environment and animal phobias are less associated with comorbid psychopathology than situational phobias (Depla, ten Have, van Balkom, & de Graaf, 2008). Persons with situational phobias may be more likely to experience substance use disorders, affective disorders, and disorders with onset in childhood (Becker et al., 2007). One study suggests that B-I-I-phobic persons have greater comorbidity rates for a number of other disorders when compared to non-B-I-I-phobic individuals; these include anxiety disorders, depression, and marijuana abuse (Bienvenu & Eaton, 1998).

Prevalence

Lifetime prevalence rates of SP appear to vary by subtype. A comprehensive review of recent SP literature reports the following lifetime prevalence estimates: animal phobia (3.3–7%), natural environment phobia (8.9–11.6%), situational phobia (5.2–8.4%), and B-I-I phobia (3.2–4.5%) (LeBeau et al., 2010). Females overall have higher prevalence rates of SP than males, with the exception of the B-I-I subtype, for which findings vary (e.g., Fredrikson, Annas, Fisher, & Wik, 1996; Bienvenu & Eaton, 1998).

SOLITARY TREATMENT APPROACHES

Pharmacological Treatment

Reviews of pharmacologic monotherapy for specific phobias have been mostly discouraging. In an early review, Fyer (1987) reported that no psychotropic medication has adequate evidence to suggest its use in the treatment of specific phobias. In a more recent review, Grös and Anthony (2006) report that benzodiazepines have not convincingly been shown to improve treatment outcomes for specific phobias, although they are often used. They further cite the dearth of research on antidepressant use in specific phobias and conclude that "these findings provide little support for the use of medications in the treatment of this disorder" (p. 301). In a book on SP treatment, Craske et al. (2006) state that "it is widely believed that medication is not necessary to treat clients with specific phobias" (p. 13) and conclude that medication studies for SP suggest limited benefit. However, some authors have suggested that medication has potential utility, at least in the acute treatment of phobias (Choy, Fyer, & Lipsitz, 2007; Hayward & Wardle, 1997; Whitehead, Blackwell, & Robinson, 1978).

Randomized clinical trials

Benjamin, Ben-Zion, Karbofsky and Dannon (2000) report the results of a pilot study comparing paroxetine to placebo for patients meeting the *DSM–IV* (APA, 2000) specific phobia criteria. Eleven patients were randomized in this double-blind study to either placebo or medication treatment for 4 weeks. Paroxetine (up to 20 mg once daily) was superior to placebo in this small-scale pilot study.

Whitehead et al. (1978) report on a small double-blind study in which 14 individuals with phobias of cats or roaches were randomly assigned to diazepam (10 mg) or placebo treatment conditions. Four individuals with SP were in the active treatment group, and outcome measures included the participants' willingness to approach the feared stimulus and their subjective ratings of anxiety while in the presence of the feared stimulus. Comparison of pre- and post-treatment measures indicates that diazepam was superior to placebo in terms of the subjects' willingness to approach the feared stimulus and their subjective rating of anxiety. This study suggests the utility of benzodiazepines in the acute reduction of anxiety in the presence of the phobic stimulus.

Bernadt, Silverstone, and Singleton (1980) compared the results of a single treatment with a beta-blocker (tolamolol, 200 mg), benzodiazepine (diazepam, 10 mg) or placebo for 22 female spider- or snake-phobic patients. The results of this double-blind, crossover trial suggest that tolamolol did not improve subjective anxiety or behavioral approach to the feared stimulus as compared to placebo. Behavioral performance was somewhat improved over placebo in the diazepam condition, but subjective anxiety was not. The authors note that subjective ratings of anxiety in this study were more influenced by order effect than by medication.

Other studies

Thom, Sartory, and Jöhren (2000) compared the effects of a single treatment session for 50 dental-phobic patients. Treatment conditions included a psychological treatment, a benzodiazepine treatment (midazolam), and a placebo group. Both treatment conditions were superior to placebo in reducing anxiety during the dental procedure. However, while patients in the psychological treatment condition continued to show improvement up to 2 months later, the patients in the benzodiazepine condition were more likely to relapse and discontinue further dental treatment.

Abene and Hamilton (1998) provide two case reports of fluoxetine treatment for depression having the unintended effect of resolving a comorbid fear of flying that predated the onset of depression in both cases.

Benefits and limitations of pharmacotherapy as the sole approach

In sum, there is a paucity of research on the use of medication as monotherapy for specific phobias. Although there is some limited evidence, and clinical experience suggests, that benzodiazepines may have some utility in the acute treatment of specific phobia, they may not yield improvement in long-term outcomes. For patients unable or unwilling to engage in exposure/extinction therapy, benzodiazepines may be a reasonable short-term solution. Outcomes with antidepressants and beta-blockers have not been encouraging, or the few studies have too few participants to allow confidence in the results. In most cases, medication alone appears to be moderately effective at best, and in some cases ineffective, as compared to the robust response reported for behavioral and cognitive therapies.

Clinical Vignete: Good outcome with pharmacotherapy

Michael is a 40-year-old Chinese American male who works in sales for an agricultural supplier in New York. He is married and has a daughter in elementary school. He underwent brief psychiatric treatment several years ago. At that time he responded well to acute treatment with a benzodiazepine as a means of reducing anxiety related to some medical procedures. He is not taking any medications currently. Michael now presents for treatment related to a fear of air travel, in which he engages once a year to visit family in China.

Michael's distress while flying began 10 years ago when he experienced extreme turbulence during a flight and feared for his life. Memories of that event are not clinically re-experienced. However, since then Michael has felt very anxious whenever he must fly, particularly over water. Although he has not altered his pattern of yearly visits to family in China, he now tolerates hours of significant anxiety during travel, during which he cannot stop thinking about ways in which the flight could end in disaster. He reports that if family connections were not so important to him, he would not subject himself to such distress.

Michael presented to his primary care physician for anxiety treatment after researching his options online. The physician used a structured interview and diagnosed Michael with specific phobia, situational type. The physician initially recommended that Michael pursue psychotherapy as a first-line treatment; however, the patient declined this suggestion on the basis that there were no qualified therapists within several hours' drive of his residence, making such treatment impractical. The physician recommended acute use of clonazepam (0.5–1 mg) every 8 hours just prior to and during flight, given Michael's prior positive response to benzodiazepines, lack of alcohol or other substance abuse, and the infrequent nature of his airline flights.

Michael took the clonazepam as directed and felt only transient and minimal distress during his flights to and from China. Upon returning to the United States, he spoke with the physician by phone and expressed satisfaction with the treatment. Michael has no plans to use a benzodiazepine again until he flies the same route next year, at which time he plans to again use clonazepam.

Clinical Vignette: Poor outcome with pharmacotherapy

Justin is a 28-year-old biracial male who works as a network engineering contractor. His work takes up much of his time, although he maintains an active social network, with frequent contact through the internet. He has no history of mental health treatment. Historically, much of his contract work has been regional, but he was recently given a project that will require nationwide travel several times per month. Justin is very apprehensive about this travel, owing to anxiety related to flying.

Justin's first flight occurred when he was a young teenager, and although it was objectively routine, he described the experience as "awful." He was preoccupied with thoughts of the plane crashing, and analyzed each mechanical noise during the flight for indications of problems. He felt trapped by the tight confines of the plane and could not stop thinking about how difficult escape would be in an emergency. This pattern continued through adolescence, and after leaving for college, Justin avoided air travel entirely. In some cases he opted for interstate train trips lasting several days. He has been intensely anxious about the requirement to fly for his new project, and has been unable to sleep soundly since learning about it.

Justin expressed his anxiety during a routine visit to his primary care provider. The primary care physician administered a computerized anxiety assessment measure and diagnosed Justin with specific phobia, situational type, on the basis of his answers to the screening questions. Justin was uncomfortable with receiving a mental health diagnosis, and the physician attempted to reassure him that the condition was treatable and should not be a source of shame. Initially the provider strongly encouraged a referral to a therapist with specialization in treating anxiety disorders. Justin adamantly rejected this option and stated, "I'm not crazy; I just don't like to fly." Justin agreed to a trial of diazepam (5 mg) to be taken 45–60 minutes prior to the flight. The provider ordered 15 tablets of clonazepam at this dose, with three refills.

After his first flight, Justin called the physician and excitedly related that he was able to fly with minimal anxiety. This pattern was repeated twice more, but on the fourth flight Justin had packed his diazepam in a pill carrier rather than the prescription bottle, and was not allowed to carry them through the security checkpoint. His anxiety on the flight was the worst it had ever been, and while he was in his destination city he missed a work appointment while securing more medication from an urgent care clinic for the return flight.

Several months later, Justin returned to the physician after the diazepam refills ran out. He reported only taking the medication while on flights, and although the physician was suspicious that the patient would have flown that often, time pressure led to this avenue of inquiry being ignored. Three weeks later the physician received a call from Justin's pharmacist informing him that the patient was filling identical prescriptions from two other prescribers. The physician spoke by phone with Justin, who stated that he had begun taking up to 10 mg of diazepam before stressful work meetings as well as before flying. The physician canceled Justin's prescription pending an in-person meeting, and the next week Justin ran out of medication before a flight and experienced a panic attack at the airport. He quit his job and sought work that did not involve travel by air.

Psychological Treatment

Psychological treatments of SP mainly comprise behaviorally based exposure and/or cognitive interventions. Other less studied and less well-accepted treatments include supportive therapy and hypnotherapy. Behavioral treatment is considered by many to be the first-line treatment.

The centerpiece of behavioral treatment is exposure-based exercise. Exposure consists of intentionally "approaching" the feared stimulus rather than avoiding the phobic object or situation, the latter of which increases anxiety through negative reinforcement conditioning. For example, an exposure task for cockroach phobia could consist of gradually increasing contact, from viewing a picture of cockroaches to eventually holding a cockroach in one's hand while monitoring subjective experience of anxiety. Exposure can be completed gradually, through intensifying the amount of exposure over time (i.e., graded exposure) or through flooding, in which the subject is exposed to a high-anxiety task (e.g., beginning treatment by holding the cockroach in their hand). Exposure is based on the principle of *habituation*, which is simply the reduction in anxiety following repeated exposure to the feared object. The goal of exposure treatment is habituation and eventual extinction of the phobic response.

The success of exposure techniques is typically measured via a Behavior Avoidance Test (BAT) and self-report measures of anxiety. A BAT consists of a series of behavioral tasks in which the subject is rated by an observer while approaching the feared object or situation (e.g., number of steps taken toward a feared object). Subjective feelings of anxiety are frequently monitored during a BAT via a Subjective Units of Distress Scale (SUDS). SUDS monitoring consists of the phobic individual assigning a numeric value, typically between 0 and 100, to their level of anxiety at predetermined intervals during the exposure exercise. Anxiety is also measured through self-report questionnaires.

Exposure is conducted through a variety of methods: imaginal/systematic desensitization, *in vivo*, virtual reality/augmented reality, interoceptive, and applied tension. Each method has been widely studied and validated, with the various methods demonstrating differential effectiveness.

Cognitive treatment for SP consists of cognitive restructuring in which cognitive distortions and/or the fear appraisals of phobic individuals are systematically examined and modified. For example, a patient with flying phobia may learn about aviation accident base rates by reviewing flight safety data. Cognitive treatment is rarely offered as a sole intervention for SP (Chambless & Gillis, 1993); rather, if utilized, it is offered in tandem with exposure treatments. Research suggests that exposure treatment is effective regardless of whether cognitive modification strategies are directly added to the treatment (Emmelkamp & Felten, 1985; Booth & Rachman, 1992).

In addition to treatment type, duration of treatment has varied from one session, typically lasting 3 hours or more, to treatment spanning multiple hour-long sessions. Öst's (1989) one-session treatment consists of *in vivo* exposure and modeling with successive exposure tasks until the patient's anxiety level has been reduced by at least 50%. Psychoeducation, skills training, reinforcement, and a cognitive component are also frequently included in general practice (Zlomke & Davis, 2008). Patients are expected to carry on with exposure to the phobic stimulus in naturalistic settings after the one-session treatment in order to maintain or extend therapeutic gains.

Randomized clinical trials

A number of RCTs have compared the efficacy of different treatment approaches. Wolitzky-Taylor, Horowitz, Powers, & Telch (2008) conducted a meta-analytic review of studies of psychological treatment of SPs published between 1977 and 2004. Thirty-three randomized treatment studies, representing 1193 subjects and 90 treatments, were included in the final analysis. Exposure approaches included *in vivo*, systematic desensitization, imaginal, virtual reality (VR), eye movement desensitization therapy, applied tension, and applied relaxation. Non-exposure therapies included cognitive therapy and progressive muscle relaxation. Nearly half of the studies utilized one-session treatment interventions. Follow-up ranged from 2 weeks to 14 months. Effect-size comparisons yielded the following broad conclusions: (1) exposure treatment is superior to non-exposure treatment, wait list, and placebo; (2) non-exposure treatment is superior to wait list; (3) *in vivo* exposure is superior to other forms of exposure at post-treatment (but there is no difference at follow-up); (4) adding cognitive components to exposure treatment is not superior to exposure alone; (5) multiple-session treatment is superior to single-session treatment; and (6) exposure treatments do not have differential efficacy based on phobia type.

Looking more specifically at the outcomes, Wolitzky-Taylor et al. reported the average exposure-treated person is better off than approximately 64% of subjects randomly assigned to an active non-exposure treatment. Data from six studies comparing non-exposure treatment (e.g., cognitive treatment, relaxation) to wait list or placebo indicated that the average treated patient is better off than approximately 84% of participants not receiving an active treatment. This is significant in view of the large number of patients who refuse to engage in an exposure-based treatment. Results indicate that even though exposure-based treatments are more effective than those without an exposure component, phobic individuals can still derive a degree of benefit from other treatments, though this effect may not be greater than placebo (Wolitzky-Taylor et al., 2008).

Further, analysis of seven studies comparing *in vivo* exposure to other types of exposure indicated superiority of *in vivo* at post-treatment and no difference at follow-up. This suggests *in vivo* may be more effective at bringing about rapid change, whereas other exposure treatments assist in more gradual change and / or change that occurs in naturalistic settings after treatment has been completed. Four studies were utilized to compare multiple-session to single-session exposure treatments, with results indicating no significant difference at post-treatment and limited support for the superiority of multiple sessions at follow-up based on questionnaires (no difference was found for behavioral avoidance measures). Because of the mixed findings and small number of studies in the comparison, the authors suggest that this result must be interpreted with caution. Analysis of effect-size moderators indicated that phobia type was not a significant moderator of treatment outcome, indicating that phobia subtypes did not respond differentially to specific treatment types (for example, height phobia is not best treated by systematic desensitization as opposed to other exposure modalities).

Choy et al.'s (2007) review of SP treatment studies published between 1960 and 2005 yielded many similar conclusions. To be included in the review, the study was required to have had at least 10 subjects per treatment group and a controlled study design in which at least two treatment groups were compared to each other. The researchers concluded that *in vivo* exposure has the strongest support for most of the SPs that have been studied. VR exposure was concluded to be comparable to *in vivo* for certain phobia types, namely height and flying phobia. Systematic desensitization was described as possibly helpful in lowering anxiety, with less robust evidence that it reduces avoidant behavior. They further concluded that owing to a dearth of controlled trials, there is little evidence for the effectiveness of imaginal exposure alone (i.e., when it is not offered as an adjunct to other exposure-based techniques), as well as treatments that were not cognitively or behaviorally based (e.g., supportive psychotherapy, hypnotherapy).

VR has received significant attention, perhaps in part owing to the belief that the procedures are more acceptable to patients. Numerous studies have shown VR to be an effective exposure method for treating SP (e.g., Rothbaum et al., 1995; Rothbaum, Hodges, Smith, Lee & Price, 2000), with some studies indicating that it is equally effective as *in vivo* exposure (Emmelkamp, Bruynzeel, Drost, & van der Mast, 2001; Emmelkamp et al., 2002). Emmelkamp et al. (2002) randomly assigned 33 height-phobic patients to either three sessions of VR exposure or three sessions of *in vivo*. In order to ensure comparability of exposure, the researchers recreated the exact locations of the *in vivo* exposure in the virtual world and utilized a BAT to examine whether improvements in treatment correspond to decreased avoidance in real-world settings. Patients in the VR environment viewed VR images of a mall with four stories, a fire escape approximately 50 feet (15 meters) high, and a roof garden at the top of a 65-foot (20-meter) building. To enhance the feeling of looking down from a great height, a physical railing was available for the VR patients to hold on to as they were instructed continually to look over the railing to ground level. In the *in vivo* condition, participants went to the physical locations described above and participated in graduated exposure (e.g., riding the escalator at the mall with the therapist, then alone; looking over railings to the ground from successively greater heights). In the VR condition the therapist controlled the VR world seen by the patient via a joystick. In both conditions the therapist guided the patients in gradual exposure utilizing verbal guidance and regular ratings of anxiety levels (e.g., SUDS). Participants were exposed to successively greater heights as they experienced anxiety reduction and/or habituated. Results indicated that participants in both conditions reported reduced anxiety and decreased avoidance, and these gains were maintained up to 6 months.

RCTs assessing multiple-session versus single-session treatments have suggested promising results with single-session treatments (Öst, 1989; Öst, Alm, Brandberg, & Breitholtz, 2001). In their review of one-session treatment studies, Zlomke and Davis (2008) utilized empirically supported treatment criteria (see Task Force on Promotion and Dissemination of Psychological Procedures, 1995) and concluded that one-session exposure treatments as described by Öst

(1989; 1997) can be considered "probably efficacious," but because of a lack of enough carefully controlled studies, the treatment does not at this time merit classification as a "well-established treatment." A meta-analysis examining a subset of RCTs guardedly concluded that multiple-session treatment is preferable (Wolitzky-Taylor et al., 2008). Single-session treatments may be a good option for some patients, especially when resources are limited.

Other studies

There are a number of case studies and treatment studies utilizing non-randomized designs to assess newer forms of SP treatments. Botella, Bretón-López, Quero, Baños, and García-Palacios (2010) utilized augmented reality (AR) in the treatment of six cockroach-phobic individuals who completed a one-session treatment protocol created by Öst, Salkovskis, and Hellström (1991). Computerized images designed to look like real cockroaches were superimposed on the participant's real-world environment. The patient utilized a head-mounted display that projected the computer image of the cockroach onto the environment. The therapist viewed the images seen by the patient via a computer monitor and led the patient through exposures of graduating intensity. Results indicate that the AR system succeeded in stimulating anxiety in all of the participants, and the exposure treatment decreased avoidance for all participants. At post-treatment, all participants demonstrated the ability to enter a room where a cockroach was in a jar, open the jar, and keep their hands in the jar for a few seconds. Additionally, half were able to complete the task of killing a real cockroach with a fly swatter or their feet.

Benefits and limitations of psychological treatment as a sole approach

The effectiveness of exposure-based treatments is so well established that there is very little disagreement among experts regarding best practices for treatment; most agree exposure is both necessary and sufficient to achieve a positive treatment outcome (Antony & Barlow, 2002). More recent research has focused on fine-tuning exposure exercises, such as by determining the ideal length of an exposure, whether exposure should be therapist directed or can be completed through self-guided interventions, how far apart to space sessions, and ways to increase patient engagement and retention. In particular, efficacious one-session treatments may be particularly beneficial for patients with limited time or financial resources. In addition to their strong efficacy, when compared to pharmacological treatment psychological treatments for SP pose less risk of adverse effects. Medication side effects, as well as evidence that medication is of limited utility for the treatment of SP, further strengthen the case for utilizing psychological treatments.

Clinical Vignette: Good outcome with psychotherapy

Cara is an 18-year-old African American female who recently has moved from Chicago to a rural community in Illinois in order to begin working as a firefighter. She is an introverted person who did well in school and has a core group of close friends. She met with a social worker for several sessions after the death of a grandparent during her childhood, and that treatment was helpful. Cara self-referred to a community mental health clinic after she experienced several panic attacks at home after seeing spiders.

During an intake session with a therapist, Cara reported that she has always felt afraid of insects, and particularly spiders. She described several encounters with spiders during early childhood that she found "terrifying," including bumping into one under the covers of her bed. These encounters triggered panic that alarmed her parents. She stated that she avoids environments where spiders are likely to be present, such as basements, garages, and sheds. Cara's new community has more spiders than her previous urban environment, and there are areas of her apartment (such as the closet and pantry) in which they can often be found. The therapist diagnosed her with specific phobia, animal type.

The therapist first carefully explained the rationale for exposure therapy to Cara to the point that she could paraphrase it in her own words without any assistance. This included discussion of the anxiety response and relaxation strategies to counteract it. The therapist began by introducing imaginal exposure exercises around spider imagery, using a 1–100 Subjective Units of Distress Scale (SUDS) to track the patient's anxiety and continuing exercises to the point of habituation. This treatment plan included daily homework, which Cara initially avoided completing because of the unpleasant increase in her anxiety. With the successful use of motivational interviewing techniques during the next session, Cara began doing her homework and her SUDS began decreasing through habituation to detailed descriptions of spiders.

The therapist began *in vivo* exposure exercises with a realistic plastic spider, which Cara was eventually able to place on her arm. She took a weekend trip to the zoo, during which she spent an hour watching several large tarantulas. Although she described them as "disgusting," she was able to remain in the insect exhibit while experiencing only mild anxiety. She also denied significant distress related to spiders in her home. At that point in treatment, Cara was assessed as no longer meeting criteria for the diagnosis of specific phobia, and treatment was terminated.

Clinical Vignette: Poor outcome with psychotherapy

Rick is a 42-year-old Caucasian male who works as a high school math teacher. He reported attending therapy at several points in the past, and described these experiences in mixed terms. He reported enjoying his work and having good social support, but also described himself as "a worrier by nature." Rick self-referred to a private psychotherapy practice for anxiety around receiving health care, having located the clinic through his insurance network and researched the psychologist online.

The psychologist conducted a thorough intake interview with Rick, focusing not just on his current symptoms but on current and historical life circumstances. During the intake, Rick disclosed that he has always felt afraid in medical settings because of the possibility of receiving an injection or incision. He stated that he had two minor foot procedures for ingrown toenails as a child that greatly increased his anxiety, and reported that 3 years earlier he was "traumatized" during a blood draw, when he fainted. Since then he has avoided health care despite ongoing gastrointestinal problems that require treatment. Rick reported that even thinking about a syringe or scalpel makes him feel panicked to the point that other people notice.

The psychologist made a diagnosis of specific phobia, blood-injection-injury type. After sensing his patient's discomfort with the extended conversation about his phobia, the psychologist assured Rick that the sessions could focus on material beyond that specific concern. Rick expressed relief that he would not have to talk about his phobia during every session, stating that even thinking about discussing it made him feel uneasy.

After establishing rapport with Rick, the psychologist introduced relaxation skills with the intention of reducing the patient's clear anxiety about discussing his phobia. Rick described the relaxation exercises themselves as enjoyable and helpful, but redirected the conversation when the psychologist attempted to return to the subject of his phobia. The psychologist recognized this pattern of avoidance and focused on helping Rick to cope with his distress.

After several more sessions, Rick agreed to try an imaginal exposure exercise. The psychologist asked Rick to visualize receiving a quick routine injection at a doctor's office. Halfway through the exercise, Rick became very anxious and felt as though he was about to pass out. He was unwilling to proceed and the session terminated early. At the next session, Rick expressed anger at the psychologist for "not fixing this problem like you said you would." When the psychologist prompted the patient to explain in his own words the rationale for doing exposure exercises, Rick could not do so. He requested that they focus on the relaxation exercises, which were "less painful." Several months later, the psychologist had not broached the subject of exposure therapy again, the patient's symptoms had not improved, and he was still avoiding necessary medical care.

COMBINED THERAPY

Several reviews have been written regarding the use of psychopharmacologic treatment of phobias in combination with behavioral or cognitive therapy. Sartory (1983) reviewed the evidence for combining benzodiazepines with behavioral treatment and concluded that this practice should be discouraged. Hofmann, Pollack, and Otto (2006) conclude that attempts to improve treatment outcomes for specific phobia by combining antidepressants or benzodiazepines with psychotherapy have been disappointing to date. In a comprehensive review of treatment studies for specific phobias from 1960 to 2005, Choy et al. (2007) state, "The general view is that medication has little benefit in specific phobia" (p. 280). However, they go on to state that only sparse data are available in the literature to support or negate the use of medication for specific phobia. In particular, Choy and associates (2007) found some indication suggesting that the use of a benzodiazepine in acute situations (e.g., flying phobia) may be beneficial in the short run. Davis, Ressler, Rothbaum, and Richardson (2006) evaluate the combination of SSRIs and benzodiazepines with psychological treatment of specific phobias as being of modest benefit at best. Norberg, Krystal, and Tolin (2008) report that the combination of antidepressants or anxiolytics with exposure therapy has not yielded long-term beneficial effects in excess of what is typically achieved by exposure/extinction training alone.

Randomized clinical trials

In a randomized, placebo-controlled, double-blind study of 111 adult phobic patients, Zitrin, Klein, and Woerner (1978) compared outcomes for three treatment groups: behavioral therapy plus imipramine, behavioral therapy plus placebo, and supportive psychotherapy plus imipramine. Participants were classified as mixed phobics, agoraphobics, and simple phobics. For the population of interest in this chapter, simple (or specific) phobics, the authors found significantly positive outcomes for all treatment groups, with no difference between behavioral therapy and supportive therapy, and no difference between imipramine and placebo. Therefore, there was no advantage to combining imipramine with behavioral therapy for specific phobia in this study.

In a similar and expanded study, Zitrin, Klein, Woerner, and Ross (1983) conducted a similar study of 218 adult phobic patients. Treatment groups included behavioral therapy plus imipramine, behavioral therapy and placebo, and supportive psychotherapy plus imipramine. For participants with simple or specific phobia there was no significant outcome difference between those treated with imipramine and those in the placebo condition.

Marks, Viswanathan, Lipsedge, and Gardner (1972) conducted a randomized, placebo-controlled, double-blind study of 18 phobic patients and their treatment response under three conditions. The phobias included spiders, dogs, cats, birds, balloons, blood, and heights. All three conditions involved two hours of flooding exposure to the feared stimulus during the "waning" effects of diazepam, during the "peak" effects of diazepam, or in the presence of placebo. The results revealed significant improvement across all three groups as a result of exposure. Improvement in anxiety was achieved most in the "waning" group, then in the "peak" group, and finally in the placebo group.

Whitehead et al. (1978) report on a small randomized, double-blind, placebo-controlled study that investigated treatment outcomes for 14 phobics of cats, roaches, snakes, and spiders. The study compared a behavioral treatment (flooding) plus diazepam (taken three times/day at 5 mg per dose) versus flooding plus placebo, also dosed three times daily. The authors concluded that diazepam did not improve the effectiveness of flooding when compared to flooding and placebo for phobic individuals.

Wilhelm and Roth (1997) investigated the response of 28 female flying phobics to the combination of a benzodiazepine (alprazolam, 1 mg) plus exposure therapy in a randomized, double-blind, placebo-controlled study. The participants were exposed to two flights. In the exposure plus benzodiazepine condition, for the first flight the participants reported acute anxiety improvement. A week later, upon the exposure to the second flight, the effects of the alprazolam were not maintained and anxiety increased for this group of participants. However, for the second flight the placebo condition group did report signs of fear extinction. As compared to the exposure plus placebo condition, the authors concluded that under acute stress conditions the addition of alprazolam may have increased physiological activation, perhaps as modified by cognitive expectations, and therefore interfered with the positive effects of exposure treatment for flying phobia.

A recent development in the combined (medication plus psychotherapy) treatment of specific phobias involves the use of D-cycloserine (DCS), a partial agonist at the glycine recognition site on the glutamatergic *N*-methyl-D-aspartate

(NMDA) receptor. Glutamate (GLU) is one of the brain's primary excitatory neurotransmitters and plays a role in the neurocircuitry involved in fear processing
(Hofmann, Meuret et al., 2006). There is evidence that the action of GLU at the
NMDA receptor has a significant role in learning and memory (e.g., Castellano,
Cestari, & Ciamei, 2001; Newcomer & Krystal, 2001; Bear, 1996). DCS may facilitate memory consolidation of extinction that occurs during cognitive and behavioral treatments for specific phobia (Hofmann, Meuret et al., 2006). DCS is being
investigated as an adjunct to enhance behavioral and cognitive treatments for
specific phobias (Norberg et al., 2008).

Ressler et al. (2004) conducted a study of 28 adults with acrophobia to compare exposure treatment results when combined with either DCS or placebo.
This randomized, double-blind study involved two sessions of exposure therapy using VR technology. DCS was dosed in either 50 mg or 500 mg formulations and administered before the onset of exposure therapy. The authors
found that when exposure therapy was combined with DCS, the results were
superior to those observed for the participants in the placebo condition.
Although reductions in anxiety were found for both groups, the DCS group
had significantly greater reductions in measures of anxiety. There was no significant difference in treatment outcome between those treated with 50 mg as
against 500 mg of DCS. This enhancement of treatment was maintained at 3
months post-treatment.

Two studies have not supported the use of DCS in combination with exposure therapy for patients with non-clinical levels of fear. Guastella, Dadds, Lovibond, Mitchell, and Richardson (2007a) randomized 100 spider-fearful
participants to exposure therapy plus DCS or exposure therapy plus placebo. As
in the Ressler et al. (2006) study, the dosing was either 50 mg or 500 mg of DCS
administered just prior to exposure treatment. Psychological treatment
involved psychoeducation, cognitive therapy, and an 11-step exposure session
that were all provided within a 2-hour time span or less. Neither study provided
any evidence that DCS enhanced reduction in fears, as compared to placebo,
when combined with exposure therapy. This failure to observe enhancing
effects was found at both the 50 mg and the 500 mg dosing of DCS. A critical
difference between this study and that of Ressler et al. (2004) is that in the
Guastella study the participants had non-clinical levels of spider fear.

In a second study, Guastella, Lovibond, Dadds, Mitchell, and Richardson
(2007b) used Pavlovian fear conditioning in 238 participants randomly assigned
to treatment with DCS (50 mg or 500 mg) or placebo after being subjected to a
differential shock conditioning paradigm. They then were engaged in extinction training, and anxiety reduction was evaluated by skin conductance and
self-report expectancy measures. The authors report that DCS had no effect on
these measures, either between dosing conditions (50 mg or 500 mg) or
between placebo and DCS conditions. They conclude that DCS may not

facilitate extinction of learned fear such as that found in specific phobias. As in the first Guastella et al. (2007a) study, the participants were non-clinical adults. Hofmann, Meuret et al. (2006) have suggested that the study design in the Guastella et al. (2007b) research may have resulted in a ceiling effect that made it difficult to show enhancement of treatment with DCS as compared to placebo.

Strengths and benefits of using a combined approach

The combination of antidepressants, anxiolytics, or beta-blockers with expo-sure/extinction therapy, while rational, has not yielded significantly positive effects as compared with behavioral/cognitive therapy alone for the treatment of specific phobia. There is recent evidence suggesting that DCS may be used to significantly enhance the effect of exposure/extinction therapy. While prom-ising, the use of DCS in conjunction with exposure/extinction therapy has not been evaluated comprehensively enough to recommend as a treatment at this time. Nevertheless, we may see the eventual use of DCS, in some form, to facilitate exposure/extinction therapy in the future. For the time being, the state of research evidence does not suggest that the use of medication in com-bination with exposure/extinction treatment is warranted in uncomplicated cases of specific phobia.

SUMMARY

This chapter has outlined how SPs develop and the history and current treat-ment with psychiatric medications and various psychotherapies. Most medica-tions have shown at best only modest benefit, with some evidence for the use of benzodiazepines in acute anxiety. Newer treatments such as D-cycloserine also show promise. The treatment of choice for SPs at this time is clearly some form of exposure-based therapy. At present there is not adequate evidence to recommend any particular combination of medication plus psychotherapy for the treatment of specific phobias.

Clinical Points to Remember

1. The onset of specific phobia typically occurs in childhood or early adolescence.
2. Having one phobia increases the likelihood that a person will have an additional phobia.
3. Evidence for pharmacological treatment of specific phobias has been less than stellar.

4. Evidence has shown that benzodiazepine use in specific phobia can hamper treatment.
5. Exposure therapy is highly useful in treating specific phobias; however, dropout rates are high, owing to the uncomfortable nature of the treatment.
6. Research on combined treatment has not yielded robust results.

REFERENCES

Abene, M. V., & Hamilton, J. D. (1998). Resolution of fear of flying with fluoxetine treatment. *Journal of Anxiety Disorders, 12*(6), 599–603.

American Psychiatric Association (APA). (1980). *Diagnostic and statistical manual of mental disorders* (3rd ed.). Washington, DC: APA.

American Psychiatric Association. (1987). *Diagnostic and statistical manual of mental disorders* (3rd ed., rev.). Washington, DC: APA.

American Psychiatric Association. (2000). *Diagnostic and statistical manual of mental disorders* (4th ed., text revision). Washington, DC: APA.

Antony, M. M., & Barlow, D. H. (2002). Specific phobias. In D. H. Barlow (Ed.), *Anxiety and its disorders* (2nd ed., pp. 380–417). New York: Guilford Press.

Bear, M. F. (1996). A synaptic basis for memory storage in the cerebral cortex. *Proceedings of the National Academy of Sciences of the United States of America, 93*(24), 13453–13459.

Becker, E. S., Rinck, M., Türke, V., Kause, P., Goodwin, R., Neumer, S., & Margraf, J. (2007). Epidemiology of specific phobia subtypes: Findings from the Dresden Mental Health Study. *European Psychiatry, 22*(2), 69–74.

Benjamin, J., Ben-Zion, I. Z., Karbofsky, E., & Dannon, P. (2000). Double-blind placebo-controlled pilot study of paroxetine for specific phobia. *Psychopharmacology, 149*(2), 194–196.

Bernadt, M. W., Silverstone, T., & Singleton, W. (1980). Behavioural and subjective effects of beta-adrenergic blockade in phobic subjects. *British Journal of Psychiatry, 137*, 452–457.

Bienvenu, O. J., & Eaton, W. W. (1998). The epidemiology of blood-injection-injury phobia. *Psychological Medicine, 28*(5), 1129–1136.

Booth, R., & Rachman, S. (1992). The reduction of claustrophobia–I. *Behaviour Research and Therapy, 30*(3), 207–221.

Botella, C., Bretón-López, J., Quero, S., Baños, R., & García-Palacios, A. (2010). Treating cockroach phobia with augmented reality. *Behavior Therapy, 41*(3), 401–413.

Castellano, C., Cestari, V., & Ciamei, A. (2001). NMDA receptors and learning and memory processes. *Current Drug Targets, 2*(3), 273–283.

Chambless, D. L., & Gillis, M. M. (1993). Cognitive therapy of anxiety disorders. *Journal of Consulting and Clinical Psychology, 61*(2), 248–260.

Choy, Y., Fyer, A. J., & Lipsitz, J. D. (2007). Treatment of specific phobia in adults. *Clinical Psychology Review, 27*(3), 266–286.

Craske, M. G., Antony, M. M., & Barlow, D. H. (2006). *Mastering your fears and phobias: Therapist guide* (2nd ed.). New York: Oxford University Press.

Curtis, G. C., Magee, W. J., Eaton, W. W., Wittchen, H.-U., & Kessler, R. C. (1998). Specific fears and phobias: Epidemiology and classification. *British Journal of Psychiatry, 173*, 212–217.

Davis, M., Ressler, K., Rothbaum, B. O., & Richardson, R. (2006). Effects of D-cycloserine on extinction: Translation from preclinical to clinical work. *Biological Psychiatry, 60*(4), 369–375.

Depla, M. F., ten Have, M. L., van Balkom, A. J., & de Graaf, R. (2008). Specific fears and phobias in the general population: Results from the Netherlands Mental Health Survey and Incidence Study (NEMESIS). *Social Psychiatry and Psychiatric Epidemiology, 43*(3), 200–208.

Emmelkamp, P. M. G., Bruynzeel, M., Drost, L., & van der Mast, C. A. P. G. (2001). Virtual reality treatment in acrophobia: A comparison with exposure in vivo. *CyberPsychology and Behavior, 4*(3), 335–339.

Emmelkamp, P. M. G., & Felten, M. (1985). The process of exposure *in vivo*: Cognitive and physiological changes during treatment of acrophobia. *Behaviour Research and Therapy, 23*(2), 219–223.

Emmelkamp, P. M. G., Krijn, M., Hulsbosch, A. M., de Vries, S., Schuemie, M. J., & van der Mast, C. A. P. G. (2002). Virtual reality treatment versus exposure in vivo: A comparative evaluation in acrophobia. *Behaviour Research and Therapy, 40*(5), 509–516.

Fredrikson, M., Annas, P., Fisher, H., & Wik, G. (1996). Gender and age differences in the prevalence of specific fears and phobias. *Behaviour Research and Therapy, 34*(1), 33–39.

Fyer, A. J. (1987). Simple phobia. *Modern Problems in Pharmacopsychiatry, 22*, 174–192.

Gamble, A. L., Harvey, A. G., & Rapee, R. M. (2010). Specific phobia. In D. J. Stein, E. Hollander, & B. O. Rothbaum (Eds.), *Textbook of anxiety disorders* (2nd ed., pp. 525–546). Arlington, VA: American Psychiatric Publishing.

Grös, D. F., & Antony, M. M. (2006). The assessment and treatment of specific phobias: A review. *Current Psychiatry Reports, 8*(4), 298–303.

Guastella, A. J., Dadds, M. R., Lovibond, P. F., Mitchell, P., & Richardson, R. (2007a). A randomized controlled trial of the effect of D-cycloserine on exposure therapy for spider fear. *Journal of Psychiatric Research, 41*(6), 466–471.

Guastella, A. J., Lovibond, P. F., Dadds, M. R., Mitchell, P., & Richardson, R. (2007b). A randomized controlled trial of the effect of D-cycloserine on extinction and fear conditioning in humans. *Behaviour Research and Therapy, 45*(4), 663–672.

Harvey, A., & Rapee, R. (2002). Specific phobia. In D. J. Stein & E. Hollander (Eds.), *Textbook of anxiety disorders*. Washington, DC: American Psychiatric Publishing.

Hayward, P., & Wardle, J. (1997). The use of medication in the treatment of phobias. In G. C. L. Davey (Ed.), *Phobias: A handbook of theory, research and treatment* (pp. 281–298). New York: John Wiley.

Hofmann, S. G., Meuret, A. E., Smits, J. A. J., Simon, N. M., Pollack, M. H., Eisenmenger, K. Otto, M. W. (2006). Augmentation of exposure therapy with D-cycloserine for social anxiety disorder. *Archives of General Psychiatry, 63*(3), 298–304.

Hofmann, S. G., Pollack, M. H., & Otto, M. W. (2006). Augmentation treatment of psychotherapy for anxiety disorders with D-cycloserine. *CNS Drug Reviews, 12*(3–4), 208–217.

LeBeau, R. T., Glen, D., Liao, B., Wittchen, H.-U., Beesdo-Baum, K., Ollendick, T., & Craske, M. G. (2010). Specific phobia: A review of DSM-IV specific phobia and preliminary recommendations for DSM-V. *Depression and Anxiety, 27*(2), 148–167.

Lipsitz, J. D., Barlow, D. H., Mannuzza, S., Hofmann, S. G., & Fyer, A. J. (2002). Clinical features of four DSM-IV-specific phobia subtypes. *Journal of Nervous and Mental Disease, 190*(7), 471–478.

Marks, I. M., Viswanathan, R., Lipsedge, M. S., & Gardner, R. (1972). Enhanced relief of phobias by flooding during waning diazepam effect. *British Journal of Psychiatry, 121*, 493–505.

Newcomer, J. W., & Krystal, J. H. (2001). NMDA receptor regulation of memory and behavior in humans. *Hippocampus, 11*(5), 529–542.

Norberg, M. M., Krystal, J. H., & Tolin, D. F. (2008). A meta-analysis of D-cycloserine and the facilitation of fear extinction and exposure therapy. *Biological Psychiatry, 63*(12), 1118–1126.

Öst, L.-G. (1989). One-session treatment for specific phobias. *Behaviour Research and Therapy, 27*(1), 1–7.

Öst, L.-G. (1997). Rapid treatment of specific phobias. In G. C. L. Davey (Ed.), *Phobias: A handbook of theory, research, and treatment* (pp. 227–246). New York: John Wiley.

Öst, L.-G., Alm, T., Brandberg, M., & Breitholtz, E. (2001). One vs five sessions of exposure and five sessions of cognitive therapy in the treatment of claustrophobia. *Behaviour Research and Therapy, 39*(1), 167–183.

Öst, L.-G., Salkovskis, P., & Hellström, K. (1991). One-session therapist-directed exposure vs. self-exposure in the treatment of spider phobia. *Behavior Therapy, 22*(3), 407–422.

Rachman, S. (1977). The conditioning theory of fear-acquisition: A critical examination. *Behaviour Research and Therapy, 15*(5), 375–387.

Ressler, K. J., Rothbaum, B. O., Tannenbaum, L., Anderson, P., Graap, K., Zimand, E., et al. (2004). Cognitive enhancers as adjuncts to psychotherapy: Use of D-cycloserine in phobic individuals to facilitate extinction of fear. *Archives of General Psychiatry, 61*(11), 1136–1144.

Rothbaum, B. O., Hodges, L., Kooper, R., Opdyke, D., Williford, J., & North, M. M. (1995). Effectiveness of virtual reality graded exposure in the treatment of acrophobia. *American Journal of Psychiatry, 152*(4), 626–628.

Rothbaum, B. O., Hodges, L., Smith, S., Lee, J. H., & Price, L. (2000). A controlled study of virtual reality exposure therapy for the fear of flying. *Journal of Consulting and Clinical Psychology, 28*(6), 1020–1026.

Sartory, G. (1983). Benzodiazepines and behavioural treatment of phobic anxiety. *Behavioural Psychotherapy, 11*, 204–217.

Task Force on Promotion and Dissemination of Psychological Procedures. (1995). Training in and dissemination of empirically validated psychological treatment: Report and recommendations. *Clinical Psychologist, 48*(1), 3–23.

Thom, A., Sartory, G., & Jöhren, P. (2000). Comparison between one-session psychological treatment and benzodiazepine in dental phobia. *Journal of Consulting and Clinical Psychology, 68*(3), 378–387.

Whitehead, W. E., Blackwell, B., & Robinson, A. (1978). Effects of diazepam on phobic avoidance behavior and phobic anxiety. *Biological Psychiatry, 13*(1), 59–64.

Wilhelm, F. H., & Roth, W. T. (1997). Clinical characteristics of flight phobia. *Journal of Anxiety Disorders, 11*(3), 241–261.

Wittchen, H.-U., Lecrubier, Y., Beesdo, K., & Nocon, A. (2003). Relationships among anxiety disorders: patterns and implications. In D. J. Nutt & J. C. Ballenger (Eds.), *Anxiety disorders* (pp. 25–37). Oxford: Blackwell.

Wolitzky-Taylor, K. B., Horowitz, J. D., Powers, M. B., & Telch, M. J. (2008). Psychological approaches in the treatment of specific phobias: A meta-analysis. *Clinical Psychology Review, 28*(6), 1021-1037.

Zitrin, C. M., Klein, D. F., & Woerner, M. G. (1978). Behavior therapy, supportive psychotherapy, imipramine, and phobias. *Archives of General Psychiatry, 35*(3), 307–316.

Zitrin, C. M., Klein, D. F., Woerner, M. G., & Ross, D. C. (1983). Treatment of phobias: I. Comparison of imipramine hydrochloride and placebo. *Archives of General Psychiatry, 40*(2), 125–138.

Zlomke, K., & Davis, T. E. III. (2008). One-session treatment of specific phobias: A detailed description and review of treatment efficacy. *Behavior Therapy, 39*(3), 207–223.

CHAPTER 12

Separation Anxiety Disorder

George M. Kapalka and Callandra Peters

INTRODUCTION

Separation anxiety disorder (SAD) was first introduced in the *DSM–III* (APA, 1980), along with overanxious disorder and avoidant disorder of childhood or adolescence, and is the only one of those three still included in the current version of the *DSM* system (*DSM–IV–TR*; APA, 2000). The core feature of SAD is excessive anxiety when separation from a parental figure takes place or is anticipated, and the fear and anxiety are evidenced by significant distress, avoidance of separation situations, and impairment in adaptive functioning. SAD is significantly different from the typical worries regarding separation from attachment figures in early childhood, and the diagnosis of SAD is usually made when developmental level of the child indicates that such fears are no longer commonplace among most children. Children with SAD are often preoccupied with the potential harm or negative events associated with the separation, such as illness, car accidents, or kidnapping. Children with SAD may experience persistent nightmares in which these events occur, and sleep disturbance is often associated with this disorder (APA, 2000). Children with SAD may refuse to sleep without the attachment figure nearby and may sleep outside the attachment figure's bedroom door. During the day, children with SAD typically follow the attachment figure around the home and may feel uncomfortable when left in a room alone.

As a result of the excessive fear of being away from the attachment figure, school refusal behaviors are very common in children with SAD (Doobay, 2008). Reluctance and refusal to attend school occur in conjunction with severe emotional distress that may be exhibited by somatic complaints, tantrums, refusal to get out of bed, tearfulness, difficulty concentrating, and irritability. Sleep disturbance is also common, as children with SAD tend to worry the night before in anticipation of separation from the attachment figure the following morning (when the child has to go to school).

The etiology of separation anxiety disorder is unknown; however, genetics is thought to play a role, as children of anxious adults are much more likely to present symptoms of various anxiety disorders, including SAD. In fact, comparing symptoms of anxious parents and their offspring, some have suggested that any differences are better thought of as dimensional rather than categorical (for example, frequency and intensity of symptoms, rather than presence or absence of any specific disorder) (Albano, Chorpita & Barlow, 2003). This tendency toward anxiety and resultant avoidant behaviors has been conceptualized as an inhibited temperamental style that is evident in up to 85% of children of adults with panic disorder with agoraphobia (Biederman, Rosenbaum, Bolduc, Faraone, & Hirshfeld, 1991), and twin studies have suggested that heritability accounts for about 29% and heritability–environment interaction accounts for another 33% of the occurrence of anxiety disorders (Stevenson, Batten, & Cherner, 1992). Hyperreactivity of the limbic system, especially the pituitary–hypothalamic–adrenal axis, is usually presumed to underlie the biological vulnerability, and life stressors, such as death or illness of a relative, changing schools, and moving commonly contribute to the development of SAD. Other family factors associated with SAD are family conflict, marital discord, frequent negative feedback from parents, and parental restriction (Barrett, 1998). Onset can occur during preschool age and up until before age 18, though onset in adolescence is uncommon. The course of the disorder usually involves exacerbation and remission phases, with relapses following significant life stressors. Furthermore, some have suggested that symptoms may persist throughout the lifespan, manifesting in social and affective limitations (Masi, Mucci, & Millipiedi, 2001).

Prevalence

According to the *DSM–IV–TR*, SAD has a prevalence of roughly 4% in children and adolescents (APA, 2000), and estimates from various studies range from 3.5% to 4.7% (Masi et al., 2001). A decrease in prevalence is generally seen from childhood to adolescence: a 6-month prevalence rate of 4.9% for children ages 6–8 and 1.3% for adolescents ages 12–14 has been reported (Breton et al., 1999, cf. Masi et al., 2001). Some studies have also found higher rates in females compared to males (Masi et al., 2001), but others report that the gender distribution is relatively equal in clinical samples (APA, 2000). Lower socioeconomic status (SES) and lower parental education level have also been found to be associated with a greater prevalence of SAD (Bird, Gould, Yager, Staghezza, & Canino, 1989). Interestingly, cultural variations have also been observed, with European children showing lower prevalence rates of anxiety disorders (Orvaschel, 1988), while SAD is the most frequently diagnosed childhood anxiety disorder in New Zealand (Anderson et al., 1987).

DSM Criteria

According to the *DSM–IV–TR*, the essential feature of Separation Anxiety Disorder (309.21) is excessive anxiety deemed inappropriate on the basis of developmental expectations (APA, 2000). The excessive anxiety is centered on separation from home or those persons to whom the individual is attached. To diagnose SAD, the persistence and excess of three or more of the following symptoms is needed: distress when separation occurs or is anticipated; worry about losing major attachment figures, such as parents; worry about an event that may lead to separation; unwillingness to go anywhere without the attachment figures, or school refusal behavior; fear of being alone; unwillingness or refusal to sleep without attachment figures nearby; ongoing nightmares involving separation; and repeated physical complaints when separation occurs or is anticipated (APA, 2000, p. 125).

The symptoms must persist for at least 4 weeks, and the onset must be before age 18. If the onset is before age 6, an "Early Onset" specifier should be used. The symptoms must also create clinically significant impairment in important areas of adaptive functioning (such as social or academic). SAD should not be diagnosed if the symptoms exclusively occur during the the the course of Pervasive Developmental Disorder, or Schizophrenia or another psychotic disorder, or if the symptoms are better accounted for by the diagnosis of Panic Disorder with Agoraphobia (APA, 2000).

General Clinical Considerations

Many clinical aspects should be considered. Because children with SAD commonly exhibit deficits in social skills and communication, some may mistake these signs as indications of a pervasive developmental disorder (such as Asperger's). Children with SAD often argue with adults and defy requests to engage in activities involving separation, and may tantrum when forced. Consequently, some may attribute these symptoms to a disruptive disorder (such as oppositional defiant disorder). Children with SAD may refuse to attend school, and school phobia may need to be ruled out. If these symptoms occur exclusively around issues of separation from the main attachment figure, SAD is the likely diagnosis. Other disorders that share some symptoms are social phobia, generalized anxiety disorder, and mood disorders (since agitation and/or sadness around the time of separation are common). Clinicians must carefully perform a differential diagnosis to assure that the symptoms are due to SAD rather than a broader anxiety or mood disorder. In addition, anxiety disorders are commonly comorbid with mood and disruptive disorders (especially tic disorders), further underscoring the need for a thorough diagnostic work-up and the need to develop a comprehensive treatment plan that will address all of the diagnoses and symptoms.

The course of SAD is not well understood. Some studies suggest that for many individuals SAD is the precursor for later onset of panic disorder with agoraphobia, but more recently this conclusion has been questioned and contradictory evidence has been published (Albano et al., 2003). What is clear, however, is that long-term consequences of untreated separation anxiety disorder may include substance abuse, further psychiatric difficulties, lack of social skills and support, and academic underachievement (Doobay, 2008). For example, college students with a history of separation anxiety disorder have been found to exhibit adjustment disorders, eating disorders, and depression (Ollendick, Lease, & Cooper, 1993, as cited in Doobay, 2008). Retrospectively, many adults with anxiety difficulties report symptoms of SAD during childhood (Barrett, 1998). This suggests that at least some symptoms of SAD, if not treated, may persist into adulthood, and it is important to diagnose and treat SAD symptoms early.

Parents may play a major role in development of SAD symptoms. As conceptualized by Chorpita (2001), a coercive process may take place by which parents reinforce the avoidance behaviors (avoidance of separation) by giving in to it, and further feed the symptoms by allowing the child to experience a sense of control over whether or not the separation will occur. This underscores the need to involve parents in the treatment of the youngster to reduce the effectiveness of avoidance behaviors and understand the dynamics driving the development of the symptoms, thus helping to prevent future relapse.

SOLITARY TREATMENT APPROACHES

Pharmacological Treatment

Deciding whether to treat a child with medication should be dependent on the efficacy of this treatment shown in controlled studies (Masi et al., 2001); however, studies on drug treatment in children are rare and findings have been inconsistent. Because separation anxiety disorder is rarely studied alone, evidence for efficacy data for pharmacological treatment is usually obtained from studies that include participants diagnosed with separation anxiety disorder and other anxiety disorders. Research supports the use of serotonin-specific reuptake inhibitors (SSRIs) in treatment of anxiety disorders in children and adolescents (Reinblatt & Walkup, 2005). These medications are being increasingly used, owing to reported tolerability and efficacy in this age group. Tricyclic antidepressants are used as the second line of pharmacological treatment because there is less supporting evidence of efficacy and more adverse effects (Reinblatt & Walkup, 2005). Few randomized clinical trials have examined this particular type of drug. Benzodiazepines are also reported as lacking research in treatment of anxiety disorders in children.

Randomized clinical trials

Birmaher et al. (2003) conducted a randomized clinical trial to assess the efficacy of fluoxetine in the treatment of childhood anxiety disorders, including generalized anxiety disorder, separation anxiety disorder, and social phobia. The participants ranged from age 7 to 17 ($M = 11.8$) and were randomly assigned to the fluoxetine group ($N = 37$) or the placebo group ($N = 37$). Fifty-four percent were female. Forty-seven percent of those in the sample were diagnosed with separation anxiety disorder, 54% with specific phobia, 63% with generalized anxiety disorder, 5% with selective mutism, 24% with simple phobia, and 1% with panic disorder. Following the 12-week trial period, 61% percent of participants in the fluoxetine group showed much or very much improvement, compared to 35% in the placebo group. At a 1-year follow-up, participants taking fluoxetine had maintained more significant improvement as compared to those taking the placebo (Clark et al., 2005).

Another controlled trial, conducted by the the Research Unit on Pediatric Psychopharmacology Anxiety Study Group (2001), included 128 children, ages 6–17 ($M = 9.7$), who had not responded to 3 weeks of psychological treatment and had a diagnosis of separation anxiety disorder, social phobia, or generalized anxiety disorder. The trial was 8 weeks in length, and participants were randomly placed into either the fluvoxamine treatment group or the placebo group. Seventy-eight percent of the fluvoxamine treatment group showed overall improvement, compared to only 29% in the placebo group. Eight percent of participants in the fluvoxamine group dropped out because of adverse effects, compared to 2% in the placebo group.

In another study on fluvoxamine, participants included 128 subjects, ages 12–17, who exhibited social phobia, separation anxiety disorder, or generalized anxiety disorder diagnoses. When compared to the placebo group, fluvoxamine significantly reduced anxiety symptoms and the drug was well tolerated. The most common adverse effect was abdominal pains.

Researchers conducted a double-blind trial to compare clomipramine and a placebo in the treatment of school refusal (Berney et al., 1981). Participants were randomly assigned to groups but stratified by gender. The trial was 12 weeks in length. After attrition, 27 participants remained in the clomipramine group and 19 in the placebo group. Eighty-seven percent exhibited marked to moderate severity of separation anxiety. Twenty-seven were female and 19 were male. Eighteen participants were younger than 12 years of age, and 28 participants were adolescents (12–18 years old). Results revealed that clomipramine had no significant impact on separation anxiety; however, when one looks at the data, some decrease in symptoms was reported.

Bernstein, Garfinkel, and Borchardt (1990) conducted a double-blind, placebo-controlled study to compare imipramine and alprazolam in the treatment of school refusal. Twenty-four children, between ages 7 and 17, participated in the trial. Thirteen were male and the mean age was roughly 14. Diagnoses included major depression or adjustment disorder with depressed mood ($N = 10$), separation anxiety disorder and overanxious disorder ($N = 4$), and a combination of both a depressive disorder and anxiety disorder ($N = 10$). Subjects were randomly assigned to one of three groups: imipramine, alprazolam, or placebo. Both medications were superior to the placebo in reduction of symptoms.

Klein, Koplewicz, and Kanner (1992) recruited children through a research clinic for anxiety disorders by both referrals and local media announcements. The participants were treated for a month with intensive behavioral treatment. Those children who did not improve entered a double-blind study to receive drug treatment. Twenty-one participants remained; 14 were male and the mean age was 9.5. All subjects were diagnosed with separation anxiety disorder. Eleven children were randomly assigned to the imipramine group and 10 were assigned to the placebo. The children received the treatment for 6 weeks. Roughly 50% in both groups showed overall improvement.

Open label

Following the completion of the researchers' previous study in 2001 (discussed on p. 264), participants were asked to join a 6-month open-label treatment (Research Unit on Pediatric Psychopharmacology Anxiety Study Group, 2002). Three groups were assessed: fluvoxamine responders who remained on fluvoxamine, fluvoxamine non-responders who changed to fluoxetine, and placebo non-responders who changed to fluvoxamine. During the 6 months, 94% of the participants who originally responded to fluvoxamine remained at low levels of anxiety; 71% of subjects who switched to fluoxetine showed significant improvement in anxiety; and among the placebo group that switched to fluvoxamine, 56% showed significant improvement in symptoms.

Strengths and weaknesses of pharmacological treatment as a sole approach

Pharmacological treatment is less time-consuming than psychological treatment, for both the child and the parents, and may be cheaper. Improvement may be more rapid; rather than there being the need to attend psychotherapy sessions for several months, beneficial effects of medications may be seen within only 6 weeks. Since many individuals in the United States have limited insurance coverage for psychotherapy, medical treatment may be more practical and easier to access. Although in the United States there is a well-documented shortage of pediatric psychiatrists, many pediatricians are comfortable prescribing anxiolytic medications.

Thus far, selective serotonin reuptake inhibitors have shown the most clearly evident efficacy in decreasing symptoms of anxiety in children (Reinblatt & Walkup, 2005), and usually the decrease in symptoms is significantly greater when compared to placebo groups. Adverse effects are usually limited, and SSRIs seem to be well tolerated. If SSRIs are not effective, other drugs may be useful, but research evidence for the efficacy of tricyclics and benzodiazepines in the treatment of anxiety disorders (especially separation anxiety disorder) is scarce. Unfortunately, it seems that some novel antidepressants (like venlafaxine) and buspirone, which have proven efficacy in treating anxiety disorders in adults, have not been researched in this population.

On the other hand, pharmacological treatment is less comprehensive than psychological treatment. Rather than addressing the environmental stressors and influences which likely contribute to the generation as well as maintenance of the symptoms of most mental health disorders in children and adolescents, medication seeks only to address the biological processes that may be underlying the symptoms. Thus, the child will not learn necessary coping skills, nor will the parents change any behaviors than may be influencing the child's conduct. Relapse of symptoms is also not addressed, making the long-term efficacy of medication-only treatment questionable. In addition, treatment with antidepressants, especially in the initial 2 weeks, has been associated with an increase in suicidality (primarily thoughts), and all antidepressants marketed in the United States carry a black box warning to alert both prescribers and patients to this potential risk. Although no actual suicides associated with onset of antidepressant therapy have been reported, and some feel that this risk has been exaggerated (Gibbons, Brown, Hur, Davis, & Mann, 2012), it is a factor that must be taken into consideration when deciding which treatment is best.

Because pharmacological treatment in children continues to lack empirical support for most diagnoses, including separation anxiety disorder, significant caution should be used when administering this type of treatment, and most mental health professionals suggest that medications are best used in conjunction with psychological treatment (Masi et al., 2001). This seems especially prudent in light of at least some risk of increase in suicidal tendencies in the first 2 weeks of treatment with an antidepressant, as clinicians delivering psychotherapeutic treatment are able to monitor patients' responses and any adverse effects (including suicidality).

Clinical Vignette: Good outcome with pharmacotherapy

John is a 9-year-old black male from a large urban community who lives with his mother. He is attending a local school but his mother must walk him to school every morning. In school he is described as active and somewhat bossy with his peers, and he usually gets average grades.

He does not have a relationship with his father, who never married the mother and was lost to contact after he found out that he had impregnated John's mother. John grew up with his mother and his two older half-sisters. John's grandmother lives nearby and has been extensively involved in his upbringing. For as long as the mother can remember, John has been exhibiting discomfort separating from her. In the morning he sometimes cries and shakes when she drops him off at school, but he calms down and usually seems free of anxiety while in school. However, he insists on being with his mother or grandmother at all times except for when he is in school. His mother must lie down with him at night when he goes to sleep, and he usually goes to sleep as long as she is there. He will separate from the mother when the grandmother comes over to watch him, but refuses to let anyone else watch him, including his two teenage half-sisters. He has verbalized to his family that he is afraid that something will happen to his mother when she is away from him, and his fear is exacerbated by the fact that the family lives in an urban environment in which occasional violence does occur, and sirens can regularly be heard from police, ambulances, or fire trucks passing down the street below. Whenever this happens and his mother is not home, John verbalizes fear that something has happened to his mother, and often starts to cry. When going to any activities or friends' houses for play dates, he must be accompanied by his mother or grandmother and they must wait for him, or he refuses to stay and becomes upset. When his mother goes shopping, if the grandmother cannot come over to watch him, he insists on going with her, and when the mother forced him to stay with his sisters a few times, he was reportedly crying and shaking for much of the time the mother was away.

John's family does not have good mental health coverage. His mother asked the school counselor to talk to John, and some counseling has been provided in school, but did not seem sufficient to reduce the anxiety. The mother consulted John's pediatrician, who initially referred John to a local public clinic, but when the family was told that John would wait about 3 months for the initial appointment, the pediatrician suggested that while the family awaited counseling at the public clinic, John could try a medication to see whether his symptoms improved. Although the mother was reluctant, she agreed because she wanted to try to help John become more comfortable without waiting 3 months for his treatment to commence.

After a thorough medical work-up, the pediatrician concluded that John was medically healthy and his anxiety symptoms were consistent with SAD. The pediatrician started by prescribing fluoxetine (10 mg) once daily in the mornings and asked the mother to check in with him about

2 weeks after John began taking the medication, unless he appeared to have significant adverse reactions. The mother was given literature about the medication, and the physician assistant working in the office further reviewed the treatment with her and answered any questions the mother had. John was also told that a medication was going to be given to him so that he might become a little more comfortable during times when he felt scared or upset, and John seemed receptive to the idea.

The mother returned to the office after about 3 weeks. John was reportedly tolerating the medication well. At first, his appetite decreased and some nausea was evident, but the mother had been warned about this beforehand and she waited to see whether this reaction continued; it dissipated after about 3 or 4 days, and since that time no adverse effects had been evident. The mother started to notice some improvement: for example, John became less reluctant to separate from her in the morning (he still exhibited fear, but fewer physical symptoms were evident), and seemed to separate more easily from her during nighttime; she now could tuck him in and leave, and he fell asleep more quickly. However, separation problems during the day continued, although with somewhat reduced intensity. The pediatrician decided to increase the dose to 20 mg/day, and advised the mother to return in a month.

During the next follow-up, which occurred about 6 weeks later, John and his mother reported to the pediatrician that he was feeling better and was now attending school regularly. Separation difficulties had all but disappeared. At times, he still asked Mom where she was going, but was able to stay at home with his siblings or a babysitter without difficulties or any visible discomfort.

Clinical Vignette: Poor outcome with pharmacotherapy

Linda is a 10-year-old Caucasian female from a small, suburban community who lives with her parents and two younger brothers. She is attending school regularly and maintains good grades, but she is described as shy and does not like to interact with her peers. At home, her mother describes Linda as "my shadow" and Linda is always by her side, and does not like to be anywhere in the house without her mother next to her. She is not involved in any activities outside of her home, and does not stay at home without her mother being there. When the mother goes out to the store or to run any other errand, Linda is always with her, and when attempts are made to leave her at home with her father or a babysitter, she starts crying and carrying on, which agitates her brothers, who then also start to cry, and so the parents usually back down. Linda's mother admits that as a child she was also very shy, and at this time she is still not comfortable in stores and other places with many people around, and so she does not mind Linda's company. However, Linda's mother would like some privacy from time to time—for example, at night (Linda refuses to sleep in her bed at night)—and Linda's father is becoming increasingly frustrated at the parents' lack of privacy, and so the father insisted that Linda's mother talk with Linda's pediatrician about this problem.

After interviews with the mother and Linda, the pediatrician diagnosed SAD and suggested counseling. Because the family had very limited health insurance, including minimal coverage of psychotherapeutic treatment, the mother sought treatment at a local public mental health center, but the wait list was about 3 months, and meanwhile Linda continued to exhibit problems, and the father was becoming increasingly frustrated. Thus, Linda's mother decided to return to the pediatrician. The doctor prescribed fluoxetine (10 mg) and asked to see Linda again in about 2 weeks. Linda, however, did not like to take the medication. She insisted there was nothing wrong with her, and when her parents insisted she take the medication, Linda complained that it did not make her "feel right" and that it bothered her stomach. Although her parents attempted to insist, it seemed they started to do so only on days when they anticipated that it was necessary for Linda to separate from her mom, and therefore they did not give Linda the medication every day. No improvement was observed, and when the family next saw the pediatrician a few months later, the mother admitted that she did not think the medication was working well for her and she was reluctant to have Linda on medications. The pediatrician reported that he was not comfortable trying any other medications with Linda and again referred the family for mental health treatment. The referral included a name of a local pediatric psychiatrist. The family did not return to see the pediatrician for about a year. During the next yearly visit, the mother reported that Linda was essentially unchanged, but they were learning to deal with it and were waiting for Linda to grow out of the problem. The mother also admitted that she and the father were about to separate. The pediatrician again attempted to connect the family with mental health treatment, but once again the family did not follow up.

Psychosocial Treatment

Because separation anxiety disorder is one of the most common disorders experienced by children and adolescents (Doobay, 2008), researchers have studied the efficacy of psychosocial interventions in the treatment of this disorder; however, most studies include participants with other anxiety disorders, such as generalized anxiety disorder and social anxiety disorder (Hirshfeld-Becker et al., 2010). The lack of research solely devoted to separation anxiety disorder is a concern that should be addressed in future studies. Many consider psychosocial treatment as the first-choice approach when treating children and adolescents with separation anxiety disorder, because of the demonstrated efficacy of these interventions (Masi et al., 2001).

Randomized clinical trials

Most research on psychosocial treatments has examined the cognitive-behavioral approach. Such treatment typically includes psychoeducation about anxiety and the fearful situation, cognitive restructuring of maladaptive thoughts, exposure methods, instruction on coping skills and management of somatic symptoms, and relapse prevention (Compton et al., 2010).

Kendall incorporated these components into the "Coping Cat Programme," which was developed in 1990 for children with anxiety disorders. The children attend 60-minute sessions for 12–16 weeks. New skills, such as identifying anxious feelings and cognitive distortions, learning new coping strategies and actions, and understanding behavioral exposure techniques, are taught within the first six to eight sessions, and the second eight sessions are utilized to apply these new skills *in vivo*. Homework tasks are assigned as a relapse prevention technique.

Two randomized clinical trials have provided empirical support for the use of this program (Kendall, 1994; Kendall et al., 1997). The first study included 47 children, ages 8–13, with separation anxiety disorder, generalized anxiety disorder, or social phobia (Kendall, 1994). Sixty-six percent of the children in the cognitive-behavioral treatment group no longer met the diagnostic criteria for their previous disorder at post-treatment. These children exhibited a significant decrease in symptoms compared to those in the wait-list condition. Results were similar at a 1-year follow-up. In the second study, researchers examined 94 children, ages 9–13, randomly placed in either the cognitive-behavioral therapy treatment or the wait-list control (Kendall et al., 1997). Over 50% of those in the CBT group did not meet the diagnostic criteria for their primary diagnosis post-treatment. Significant decreases in symptoms were also demonstrated by many of those who continued to experience anxiety symptoms after treatment. At a 1-year follow-up, results were similar, with many of the children showing greater improvement. This suggests that the program has a lasting impact and that teaching relapse prevention techniques is beneficial.

Family factors, such as marital conflict and parental anxiety and depression, have been associated with childhood anxiety (Barrett, 1998). Therefore, it is necessary for researchers to determine the efficacy of involving parents in treatment of separation anxiety disorder. Barrett (1998) evaluated the efficacy of a cognitive-behavioral group intervention for childhood anxiety disorders through a randomized clinical trial. Thirty-two males and 28 females, with ages ranging from 7 to 14, participated in the study. The two treatment conditions were child-only cognitive-behavioral treatment and cognitive-behavioral treatment with family management training. The control-group participants were placed on a wait list for treatment. Twenty-six of the participants had a diagnosis of separation anxiety disorder, 30 had a diagnosis of overanxious disorder, and 4 had a diagnosis of social phobia. Post-treatment, both treatment groups had a significant decrease in participants still diagnosable with anxiety disorders as compared to the wait-list group. At the 12-month follow-up, the treatment group with family management training showed significantly higher improvement than the child-only CBT group on six of the seven clinical scales, suggesting that involving family members may be better when considering relapse prevention.

Kendall et al. (2008) sought to evaluate the efficacy of treating children with anxiety disorders with individual cognitive-behavioral therapy, family cognitive-behavioral therapy, compared to family-based education, support, and attention (FESA). Their randomized controlled trial (RCT) included 161 participants, ages 7–14, of whom 44% were females. Eighty-eight participants were diagnosed with generalized anxiety disorder, 47 with separation anxiety disorder, and 63 with social phobia. Fifty-seven percent of participants in individual CBT, 55% in family CBT, and 37% in FESA had no anxiety diagnosis at post-treatment. Significant differences were noted when comparing each treatment group to FESA but not when comparing the treatment groups to each other. These results suggest that involving the family in CBT is comparable to individual CBT but not superior. Because parents are also involved as collaborators in individual CBT, the results may indicate that parental involvement may also be a necessary component in the child's individual treatment of the disorder.

Another randomized clinical trial that examined parent–child cognitive-behavioral therapy in younger children produced similar results. In 2010, Hirshfeld-Becker et al. studied 64 children ages 4–7. Fifty-three percent of the sample members were female. Thirty-four children received the CBT treatment, and 30 children were placed on the wait-list control condition. Forty-four percent of the sample had separation anxiety disorder, 67% had social anxiety disorder, 44% had generalized anxiety disorder, 36% had agoraphobia, and 48% had specific phobia. Fifty-nine percent of children in the CBT group no longer met diagnostic criteria post-treatment compared to 18% in the control condition. Specifically, participants who were diagnosed with social anxiety disorder, separation anxiety disorder, and specific phobia exhibited the most significant improvement compared to the wait-list condition.

Little research has compared individual and group treatment of separation anxiety disorder. Liber et al. (2008) sought to compare the two modalities. Participants ranged in age from eight to 12. Fifty-two of the participants were diagnosed with separation anxiety, 37 with generalized anxiety disorder, 22 with social phobia, and 16 with specific phobia. Forty-one percent of the participants in the cognitive-behavioral group no longer met diagnostic criteria post-treatment, compared to 48% in the individual cognitive-behavioral therapy condition. This difference was not statistically significant. The researchers concluded that children can benefit from either type of treatment; however, the results of this study were limited by the lack of a control group.

Other studies

Non-CBT approaches are sometimes used in the treatment of anxiety disorders in children (Muratori et al., 2005); however, very little research has been done on the efficacy of these approaches. For this reason, Muratori et al. conducted a study to examine the efficacy of psychodynamic psychotherapy in treating separation anxiety disorder. Fourteen participants were assigned to the treatment group and were compared to 10 participants in the control group. Post-treatment, researchers found that individuals in the treatment group were less impaired on global measures of functioning and exhibited fewer symptoms. It was suggested that clinicians may consider the use of psychodynamic psychotherapy in treatment of separation anxiety disorder in place of, or following, cognitive-behavioral therapy.

Strengths and weaknesses of psychosocial treatment as a sole approach

Results of many controlled studies support the efficacy of psychological interventions, especially cognitive-behavioral therapy, in treating separation anxiety disorder (Masi et al., 2001). Furthermore, compared to pharmacological treatment, psychological treatments pose less risk of adverse effects. Prescribing medication to children often poses a concern, especially because there are few controlled studies for this age group, and long-term effects of medications on the developing brain are not known. Thus, many recommend implementing psychological approaches before pharmacological treatment.

Psychological treatment often is more comprehensive than pharmacological treatment. Cognitive-behavioral treatment addresses anxiety reduction by teaching somatic management, cognitive restructuring, and problem solving

(Velting, Setzer, & Albano, 2004)—skills that will not only help decrease current symptoms but prepare individuals to handle future relapses as well. Family involvement is another benefit of psychological treatment (Hirshfeld-Becker et al., 2010).

Psychological treatment, however, also has weaknesses. This type of treatment can be expensive, and many families in the United States have very limited (or non-existent) insurance coverage for psychological care. Psychological treatment usually requires at least 3 months of weekly sessions, and symptom relief is not immediate. In addition, psychological treatment alone is not always successful. Often, researchers have reported that roughly 50% of the sample no longer met the diagnostic criteria post-treatment (e.g., Kendall, 1994; Kendall et al., 1997; 2008; Liber et al., 2008). Thus, although the treatment groups show significant improvement compared to placebo groups, psychological interventions alone are not helpful to some participants.

Clinical Vignette: Good outcome with psychotherapy

The following vignette is loosely based on Doobay (2008, pp. 268–270): Gabriella is a 7-year-old Latina girl from a small rural community who lives with her mother. She is doing well in school but was always described as shy. About 3 months ago, Gabriella started showing separation anxiety in situations when she could not be with her mother. She refused to sleep alone in her bed, reported nightmares about being abandoned by her mother, and became withdrawn and tearful when her mother left her with a babysitter. Over time, this behavior became more pronounced as Gabriella began reporting significant somatic symptoms on separation, and exhibited tantrums. Gabriella repeatedly told her mother that she believed that something terrible would happen to the mother on her way to work and that she would never see her again. Gabriella was also being hypervigilant about remaining close to her mother when they went to the grocery store, the mall, or a restaurant. Her mother began staying home with Gabriella because she thought Gabriella was ill, and Gabriella started to miss school. After a thorough medical exam, which showed no physical basis for her somatic complaints, Gabriella's doctor suggested that she see a mental health professional.

Gabriella and her mother started treatment, and Gabriella was diagnosed with SAD. The treatment was started by teaching Gabriella coping skills to help her return to school. Gabriella learned relaxation skills, including diaphragmatic breathing, and responded well. Both she and her mother received psychoeducation about the physiological effects of anxiety and the benefits of relaxation, and the need to practice between sessions. Next, Gabriella learned progressive muscle relaxation; the therapist tape-recorded the instructions and gave the tape to Gabriella for use at home. At this point her therapist started to talk with Gabriella about her fears (cognitions) about returning to school. Gabriella admitted to thinking that kids would ask her embarrassing questions about missing school and her teachers would be mad at her. The therapist modeled appropriate responses, and these were rehearsed by using role-playing techniques. Gabriella's mother learned contingency management and identified ways in which she reinforced Gabriella's separation avoidance. She also learned ways to reinforce Gabriella for her positive behavior (when Gabriella separates from her mother).

As treatment continued, Gabriella experienced graded exposure to situations involving separation. To start, she viewed a brief video of a girl with separation anxiety preparing for school, going to school, talking to teachers and classmates, and then returning home at the end of the day. This video modeling exercise was followed by Gabriella role-playing some of the scenes and reviewing the coping techniques that were used. Her mother was also included on some of those activities to promote more practice. Gabriella's mother also learned to set up a smooth routine for Gabriella when separation situations were forthcoming, reinforcing these through contingency management. The therapist also consulted with Gabriella's teachers to develop similar contingency management techniques in school. The teachers agreed to provide Gabriella with additional encouragement and social support. Gabriella's school counselor agreed to check in with Gabriella to see how she was doing, provide her with additional social support, and become the person Gabriella could seek if she needed to reduce her anxiety through relaxation.

As Gabriella returned to school and made progress, the therapist, Gabriella, and her mother explored the aspects of each separation that were positive and those that were negative. They used problem solving, social skills training, coping skills training, and modeling to find ways to improve the uncomfortable aspects of the day for Gabriella. They also explored Gabriella's cognitions to identify maladaptive thoughts that could be changed through cognitive restructuring. The therapist encouraged (and modeled) talking with Gabriella at home about her fears and concerns. This was part of the relapse prevention stage, in which Gabriella learned to generalize to other settings the skills she learned in counseling.

The psychotherapy continued in this manner for 12 sessions, during which Gabriella made progress, and gradually her separation anxiety diminished. The last three sessions focused specifically on relapse prevention and planning of activities in the future that might pose a risk of return of anxiety (for example, her mother's overnight trip to visit relatives while Gariella stayed with a family member). The last three sessions were delivered at a frequency of about 3–4 weeks between sessions. Upon termination, Gabriella attended school regularly, identified no symptoms of anxiety when she was away from her mother for any reason, and felt confident that she would be fine when her mother went away overnight.

Clinical Vignette: Poor outcome with psychotherapy

Nicky is an 8-year-old Caucasian male from a small suburban community who lives with his parents. He is maintaining average grades in school but his attendance is a problem and he is frequently absent from school. Since toddlerhood, Nicky has been exhibiting separation anxiety in situations when he is separated from his mother. He usually falls asleep in his room but most of the time he then comes into the parents' bed in the middle of the night. While he verbalizes motivation and lack of fear, he says he does not like to be away from his mother, and when asked why, he replies, "I don't know." When a separation is announced, he usually has no reaction, but when it is about to occur he starts to carry on, cry, and tantrum. When going to school, he insists on his mother driving him and he sometimes has difficulties separating from her when he arrives at school. When she is not able to drive him, Nicky refuses to leave the house. He is involved in a variety of activities, including sports and cub scouts, but he must be driven by his mother and refuses to go when someone else offers to take him. When his mother leaves the house to go to the store, he insists on going with her and tantrums when his parents attempt to make him stay home (for example, with the father while the mother goes out). A thorough medical exam revealed no physical problems, and because Nicky has been missing school, the school counselor referred him for mental health treatment.

Nicky and his parents entered treatment and Nicky was diagnosed with SAD. The therapist started by attempting to teach Nicky coping skills, at first to improve his school attendance. Nicky learned relaxation skills, including diaphragmatic breathing, and appeared to learn the techniques well, but did not seem to use them when separation was occurring, and his behaviors did not change. The therapist delivered psychoeducation about the physiological effects of anxiety and the benefits of relaxation, and the need to practice between sessions, but Nicky continued to tantrum when separations were about to occur, and his mother usually gave in and took him in order to stop the acting out. The therapist attempted to engage the mother in treatment in order to help her recognize that giving in likely exacerbates the behavior, but, while receptive in session to this feedback, she did not seem to change how she addressed these incidents. In addition, she indicated that Nicky's father tends to be explosive and she often gives in because she is afraid that he will start to scream and yell at Nicky, thus exacerbating the situation. The father was invited to attend, but after coming in for the initial appointment, he did not come again. When asked why, the mother always said that he could not come that day because he was working.

As treatment continued, it became evident that the mother wanted the therapist to "fix" Nicky primarily through individual treatment, and attempts to get her to change the way she was reacting to Nicky were unsuccessful. It became apparent that when separations were about to occur, she usually tried to talk to Nicky and get him to agree to the separation, and made an attempt to leave, but then, seeing how uncomfortable Nicky was, she usually gave in because she did not want him to feel so bad. There were a few occasions when she left despite his protests, but she could hear him carry on very loudly even after she was out the door, and she was afraid that the neighbors might call the authorities because Nicky made it sound as though he was getting hurt. Nicky's father was advised to help Nicky calm down, but it was apparent that the father was not really supportive of the relaxation techniques, and apparently tried them half-heartedly and gave up quickly when they were not effective. He then tried to get Nicky to calm down by yelling at him and telling him he was acting like a baby, which usually made Nicky feel worse.

It seemed that the therapy with the parents was at an impasse, and the therapist tried to work with Nicky alone to try to help him manage the anxiety. However, despite about 10 sessions of treatment being delivered, Nicky never admitted that he feels anxious when away from his mother and always changed the subject whenever any mention of fear or anxiety was brought up. Seeing no progress, the therapist referred the family for consideration of medications, but the parents refused to follow through on the recommendation and dropped out of treatment shortly thereafter.

COMBINED THERAPY

Often, pharmacological treatment with children or adolescents is not used unless psychosocial treatment has not been effective, and many suggest that pharmacological treatment should not be used in place of psychosocial treatment but rather as an adjunct (Masi et al., 2001). Unfortunately, few researchers have examined whether combination treatments offer superior benefits and greater efficacy as compared to solitary treatments. Consideration of combination therapy is particularly important because approximately 40–50% of children with anxiety disorders (including separation anxiety disorder) do not sufficiently respond to short-term treatment with either monotherapy.

Randomized clinical trials

The Child/Adolescent Anxiety Multimodal Study was designed to examine short-term efficacy (12 weeks) and long-term efficacy (36 weeks) of different treatments of separation anxiety disorder, generalized anxiety disorder, and social phobia (Compton et al., 2010). The four conditions included cognitive-behavioral therapy, sertraline, a combination of the two, and a placebo pill. Four hundred and eighty-eight children, ages 7–17, were included in the study and were randomly assigned to one of the four groups. The study was carried out over 6 years, and results revealed that all three treatment approaches significantly decreased symptoms in the participants, but the combination therapy was most beneficial. Of the combination therapy group, 80.7% participants responded to treatment, compared to 59.7% of cognitive-behavioral treatment alone and 54.9% in sertraline-alone groups. Only 23.7% of the placebo group members showed significant improvement. When comparing the monotherapy approaches, individuals in the CBT group experienced less insomnia, fatigue, and restlessness than those in the sertraline group.

Open label

Bernstein, Garfinkel, and Borchardt (1990) conducted an open-label drug study of imipramine and alprazolam on school refusal behaviors using 17 children (9 of them male) aged up to 17 ($M = 14$). Sixty-five percent of the sample met diagnostic criteria for both depressive disorder (major depression or adjustment disorder with depressed mood) and anxiety disorder (separation anxiety disorder or overanxious disorder). The children were assigned to multimodal treatment plans, including a school reentry program, psychotherapy, and medication. One group received alprazolam and the other group received imipramine. Nine participants in the alprazolam group completed the trial, and six (67%) showed moderate or marked improvement. Six participants in the imipramine group completed the trial, and four (also 67%) showed moderate to marked improvement.

Strengths and weaknesses of combination treatment

One major strength of combination treatment is that it is more comprehensive than either monotherapy. Unlike pharmacotherapy alone, this treatment may also include relapse prevention, psychoeducation, and learning of coping skills. This will likely improve long-term efficacy because it teaches the child and family how to decrease symptoms aside from the use of medication. It is also likely that children receiving combination treatment respond better than psychosocial treatment alone. The use of medication further helps to decrease symptoms and may speed up the improvement, making it easier for the child to continue to attend psychotherapy. The child may return to better adaptive functioning more quickly (reducing the most debilitating symptoms), and psychotherapeutic interventions may then allow the child and family to make further progress. In addition, because the child is being seen regularly the clinician can monitor any adverse effects, including increases in suicidality, and attend to those symptoms immediately.

On the other hand, combination treatment poses some similar concerns to those of pharmacotherapy monotherapy. Prescribing medications to children, even if only as an adjunct to psychological treatment, may still result in adverse effects and developmental impact of these compounds is unknown.

Clinical Vignette: Combined treatment

Paul is an 11-year-old Caucasian male from a large suburban community who lives with his mother, stepfather, and two older stepsiblings. He is attending a local school but he admits he does not like school; his grades are mostly fair. In the mornings he often complains of stomachaches and makes an attempt to stay home, but his mother insists he goes, and so he usually gives in. In school he is described as a loner and he does not make friends easily. His teacher noticed that other students sometimes pick on Paul and he then tends to get angry and has sometimes lashed out at them physically. In addition, he seems to be falling behind in schoolwork and his teachers have observed that he is a slow reader and does not seem to comprehend much of what he reads.

At home, Paul always stays close to his mother and does not like to stay home with anyone else when she goes out. When forced, he does so, but he precipitates many problems within the home and fights with his siblings or argues with his stepfather. The stepfather generally tries to avoid contact with Paul because Paul does not seem to like him and tells him regularly that he is not his father and so Paul does not have to listen to him. His two older brothers call Paul a "baby," which further agitates him.

His mother knows that Paul and the rest of the family do not get along well, and so she usually agrees to take him with her when she goes out. However, Paul does not seem to be developing many friendships and she recognizes that at his age, Paul should be much more independent, and so she asked the school counselor to speak with Paul about the situation.

The school counselor interviewed Paul and discovered that he may be struggling academically, and decided to refer him to the school's child study team for assessment. In talking with Paul, she also discovered that he verbalized a lot of worry about his mother when he is not with her. He said that since his father left the family when Paul was a baby, it was just the two of them and he got used to "being the man of the house" until the mother remarried about 2 years ago. Since then, he has been feeling left out and is afraid his mother may leave and not come back, because he knows that she is getting frustrated with his behaviors.

Recognizing the complexity of the case, the school counselor referred the family to a local child clinical psychologist. Upon completion of the intake, the psychologist tentatively diagnosed SAD but felt that notable family dynamics contributed to Paul's symptoms, and therefore the psychologist felt that initial treatment through family therapy seemed most appropriate.

As the treatment unfolded, it became evident that Paul and his step-father were not close and Paul felt that the stepfather was coming between him and his mother. The family worked through these issues and Paul and his stepfather started to become a little more comfortable with each other and started to spend more time together—for example, going fishing and attending baseball games of a local minor-league team. However, even though the relationship between Paul and his stepfather (and stepsiblings) was improving, Paul remained anxious about what happens to his mother when he is not with her. He admitted that this is something he always worried about, but when there were just the two of them they were almost always together, so this problem was not as obvious as it has been lately. Because the therapy was focusing on family issues and more important work remained in this area, and because the family was not able to afford (financially or timewise) separate psychological treatment to address Paul's anxiety, a referral was made to a local pediatric psychiatrist to consider the use of medications. However, the family reported that the psychiatrist had about a 2-month wait list for the first appointment, and therefore the family consulted Paul's pediatrician, who reached out to the psychologist for his thoughts.

Because the psychologist was also trained in psychopharmacology, he and the pediatrician were able to confer and decided to attempt a trial of fluoxetine (10 mg) for about a month. The pediatrician prescribed the medication, and the psychologist, who continued to see the family for regular sessions, monitored Paul's response and any adverse effects. Paul tolerated the medication well and no adverse effects were apparent. In family treatment the psychologist helped Paul express his concerns about his mom's safety, and, despite initial embarrassment, Paul was able to do so, which allowed the rest of the family to offer support and reassurance. The family, with the psychologist's guidance, also helped Paul handle the negative thoughts that were triggered whenever he was away from his mother. To further improve progress, the family agreed to purchase a cell phone for Paul and allow him to call his mother if he felt he needed to check in with her and see that she was OK. At first, Paul used the cell phone extensively when away from his mother, but after about 2 weeks the calls waned significantly. At the same time, Paul's anxiety appeared to dissipate.

When a month had elapsed, the psychologist and pediatrician consulted again and decided that the medication and the family therapy appear to be working well, and Paul was tolerating the medication very well. Thus, the medication was renewed (at the same dosage) and family therapy continued, with reduced frequency. Paul started to develop a group of friends and he was also becoming closer with his two stepbrothers, now going out with them regularly and meeting their friends. At the same time, the mother and stepfather also seemed to get closer and were spending more time with each other when their children were out. At this point the treatment terminated.

FUTURE DIRECTIONS

Overall, the literature on the treatment of children with separation anxiety disorder is scarce, and the majority of studies include individuals with other anxiety disorders, such as generalized anxiety and social phobia, and do not differentiate between disorders in the results. Thus, the specific response of children with separation anxiety usually is unknown. Future studies should focus more specifically on the treatment of individuals with separation anxiety disorder.

Another problem evident with the current literature is the inconsistent differentiation of SAD and school refusal. In some studies the two terms were used interchangeably, yet in others they had separate meanings. Future research should clearly define and distinguish between treatment of SAD and school refusal behavior in order to differentiate the two and clarify what works for which disorder.

Non-behavioral approaches, such as psychodynamic therapy, are sometimes used in the treatment of children with separation anxiety disorder (Muratori et al., 2005), and some clinicians continue to insist that psychodynamic therapy is an appropriate method of treating this disorder. However, randomized controlled trials on psychodynamic psychotherapy and other non-CBT therapies in treating SAD are lacking, and clinicians continue to use these treatments without valid and reliable evidence on the efficacy of these approaches. Research needs to clarify the validity of such a decision.

More research is also necessary to examine the efficacy of medications in treating SAD. Many professionals are hesitant to prescribe drugs for children and adolescents, not only because youngsters are still developing but also because findings of some available studies are inconsistent. While SSRIs show efficacy and acceptable tolerability, other medications continue to be used as second- and third-line treatments. For example, buspirone is considered to be a promising drug that may offer benefits in the pediatric population (Masi et al., 2001).

Clinical Points to Remember

1. SAD is most common in children but may persist into adolescence in some cases.
2. Although anxiety at the time of separation from a primary caretaker is the most prevalent symptom, tantrums, agitation, and acting out may mask anxiety in some individuals.
3. School refusal is common with SAD, and SAD may sometimes be mistakenly diagnosed as school phobia.
4. Antidepressants, especially serotonergic drugs (like SSRIs), seem to be the most effective pharmacological agents to treat the symptoms of SAD, although efficacy data specific to SAD are scarce.
5. Although antidepressants carry a black-box warning about increased suicidality, recent findings suggest that the drugs are safe and the risk of suicidality has been exaggerated.
6. As monotherapy, psychosocial treatments offer many benefits over pharmacotherapy, including the development of anxiety management skills and relapse prevention that will further enhance long-term maintenance of therapeutic gains. On the other hand, progress is likely to be gradual and may require weeks of treatment for onset of improvement.

7. Involvement of the youngster's caretakers is paramount in order for psychosocial treatments to be effective, as it will be difficult to extinguish the child's avoidance behaviors without the caretakers' cooperation.

8. Combination treatment may be the most effective and practical, allowing both modalities to contribute to the alleviation of the symptoms. However, research data are limited, and further work needs to examine the most effective combination of interventions to use when treating individuals with SAD.

REFERENCES

Albano, A. M., Chorpita, B. F., & Barlow, D. H. (2003). Childhood anxiety disorders. In E. J. Mash & R. A. Barkley (Eds.), *Child psychopathology* (2nd ed., pp. 279–329). New York: Guilford Press.

American Psychiatric Association (APA). (1980). *Diagnostic and statistical manual of mental disorders* (3rd ed.). Washington, DC: APA.

American Psychiatric Association. (2000). *Diagnostic and statistical manual of mental disorders* (4th ed., text revision). Washington, DC: APA.

Anderson, J. C., Williams, S., McGee, R., & Silva, P. A. (1987). DSM-III disorders in preadolescent children: Prevalence in a large sample from a general population. *Archives of General Psychiatry, 44*, 69–76.

Barrett, P. M. (1998). Evaluation of cognitive-behavioral group treatments for childhood anxiety disorders. *Journal of Clinical Child Psychology, 27*, 459–468.

Berney, T., Kolvin, I., Bhate, S. R., Garside, R. F., Jeans, J., Kay, B., & Scarth, L. (1981). School phobia: A therapeutic trial with clomipramine and short-term outcome. *British Journal of Psychiatry, 138*, 110–118.

Bernstein, G. A., Garfinkel, B. D., & Borchardt, C. M. (1990). Comparative studies of pharmacotherapy for school refusers. *Journal of the American Academy of Child and Adolescent Psychiatry, 29*, 773–781.

Biederman, J., Rosenbaum, J. F., Bolduc, E. A., Faraone, S. V., & Hirshfeld, D. R. (1991). A high risk study of children with panic disorder and agoraphobia with and without comorbid major depression. *Psychiatry Research, 37*, 333–348.

Bird, H. R., Gould, M. S., Yager, T., Staghezza, B., & Canino, G. (1989). Risk factors for maladjustment in Puerto Rican children. *Journal of the American Academy of Child and Adolescent Psychiatry, 28*, 847–850.

Birmaher, B., Axelson, D. A., Monk, K., Kalas, C., Clark, D. B., Ehmann, M., et al. (2003). Fluoxetine for the treatment of childhood anxiety disorders. *Journal of the American Academy of Child and Adolescent Psychiatry, 42*, 415–423.

Breton, J. J., Bergeron, L., Valla, J. P., Berthiaume, C., Gaudet, N., Lambert, J., et al. (1999). Quebec Child Mental Health Survey: Prevalence of DSM-III-R mental health disorders. *Journal of Child Psychology and Psychiatry, 40*, 375–384.

Chorpita, B. F. (2001). Control and the development of negative emotions. In M. W. Vasey & M. R. Dadds (Eds.), *Developmental psychopathology of anxiety* (pp. 112–142). New York: Oxford University Press.

Clark, D. B., Birmaher, B., Axelson, D., Monk, K., Kalas, C., Ehmann, M., et al. (2005). Fluoxetine for the treatment of childhood anxiety disorders: Open-label, long-term extension to a controlled trial. *Journal of the American Academy of Child and Adolescent Psychiatry, 44*, 1263–1270.

Compton, S. N., Walkup, J. T., Albano, A. M., Piacentini, J. C., Birmaher, B. Sherrill, J. T., et al. (2010). Child/Adolescent Anxiety Multimodal Study (CAMS): Rationale, design, and methods. *Child and Adolescent Psychiatry and Mental Health, 4*, 1–15.

Doobay, A. F. (2008). School refusal behavior associated with separation anxiety disorder: A cognitive-behavioral approach to treatment. *Psychology in the Schools, 45*, 261–272.

Gibbons, R. D., Brown, H., Hur, K., Davis, J. M., & Mann, J. J. (2012). Suicidal thoughts and behavior with antidepressant treatment: Reanalysis of the randomized placebo-controlled studies of fluoxetine and venlafaxine. *Archives of General Psychiatry, 69*, 580–587.

Hirshfeld-Becker, D., Masek, B., Henin, A., Blakely, L. R., Pollock-Wurman, R. A., et al. (2010). Cognitive behavioral therapy for 4- to 7-year-old children with anxiety disorders: A randomized clinical trial. *Journal of Consulting and Clinical Psychology, 4*, 498–510.

Kendall, P. C. (1990). *Coping Cat Workbook*. Ardmore, PA: Workbook Publishing.

Kendall, P. C. (1994). Treating anxiety disorders in children: Results of a randomized clinical trial. *Journal of Consulting and Clinical Psychology, 62*, 100–110.

Kendall, P. C., Flannery-Schroeder, E., Panicelli-Mindel, S. M., Southam-Gerow, M. A., Henin, A., & Warman, M. (1997). Therapy for youths with anxiety disorders: A second randomized clinical trial. *Journal of Consulting and Clinical Psychology, 65*, 366–380.

Kendall, P. C., Hudson, J. L., Gosch, E., Flannery-Schroeder, E. F., & Suveg, C. (2008). Cognitive-behavioral therapy for anxiety disordered youth: A randomized trial evaluating child and family modalities. *Journal of Consulting and Clinical Psychology, 76*, 282–297.

Klein, R. G., Koplewicz, H. S., & Kanner, A. (1992). Imipramine treatment of children with separation anxiety disorder. *Journal of the American Academy of Child and Adolescent Psychiatry, 31*, 21–28.

Liber, J. M., Van Widenfelt, B. M., Utens, E. M. W. J., Ferdinand, R. F., Van der Leeden, A. J., Van Gastel, W., & Treffers, P. D. A. (2008). No differences between group versus individual treatment of childhood anxiety disorders in a randomized clinical trial. *Journal of Child Psychology and Psychiatry, 49*, 886–893.

Masi, G., Mucci, M., & Millepiedi, S. (2001). Separation anxiety disorder in children and adolescents: Epidemiology, diagnosis, and management. *CNS Drugs, 15*, 93–104.

Muratori, F., Picchi, L., Apicella, F., Salvadori, F., Espasa, F. P., Ferretti, D., & Bruni, G. (2005). Psychodynamic psychotherapy for separation anxiety disorders in children. *Depression and Anxiety, 21*, 45–46.

Orvaschel, H. (1988). Structured and semistructured interviews for children. In C. J. Kestenbaum & D. T. Williams (Eds.), *Handbook of clinical assessment of children and adolescents* (Vol. 1, pp. 31–42). New York: New York University Press.

Reinblatt, S. P., & Walkup, J. T. (2005). Psychopharmacologic treatment of pediatric anxiety disorders. *Child and Adolescent Psychiatric Clinics of North America, 14*, 877–908.

Research Unit on Pediatric Psychopharmacology Anxiety Study Group. (2001). Fluvoxamine for the treatment of anxiety disorders in children and adolescents. *New England Journal of Medicine, 344,* 1279–1285.

Research Unit on Pediatric Psychopharmacology Anxiety Study Group. (2002). Treatment of pediatric anxiety disorders: An open-label extension of the research units on pediatric psychopharmacology anxiety study. *Journal of Child and Adolescent Psychopharmacology, 12,* 175–188.

Stevenson, J., Batten, N., & Cherner, M. (1992). Fear and fearfulness in children and adolescents: A genetic analysis of twin data. *Journal of Child Psychology and Psychiatry, 33,* 977–985.

Velting, O. N., Setzer, N. J., & Albano, A. M. (2004). Update on and advances in assessment and cognitive-behavior treatment of anxiety disorders in children and adolescents. *Professional Psychology: Research and Practice, 35,* 42–54.

Index

Page numbers in *italics* denote tables. Those in **bold** denote figures.

Printed in the United States
by Baker & Taylor Publisher Services